Anxiety and Depression Association of America

Patient Guide to Mood and Anxiety Disorders

Anxiety and Depression Association of America

Patient Guide to **Mood** and **Anxiety** Disorders

Edited by

Charles B. Nemeroff, M.D., Ph.D.
W. Edward Craighead, Ph.D., ABPP

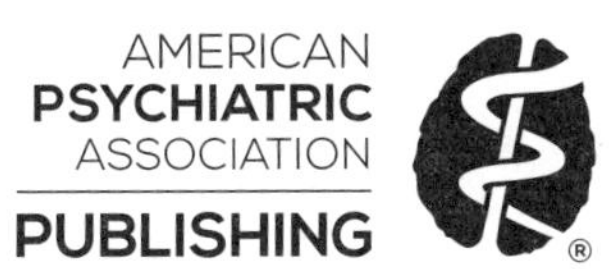

Note: The authors have worked to ensure that all information in this book is accurate at the time of publication and consistent with general psychiatric and medical standards, and that information concerning drug dosages, schedules, and routes of administration is accurate at the time of publication and consistent with standards set by the U.S. Food and Drug Administration and the general medical community. As medical research and practice continue to advance, however, therapeutic standards may change. Moreover, specific situations may require a specific therapeutic response not included in this book. For these reasons and because human and mechanical errors sometimes occur, we recommend that readers follow the advice of physicians directly involved in their care or the care of a member of their family.

First Edition

Manufactured in the United States of America on acid-free paper
28 27 26 25 24 5 4 3 2 1

Published by:
American Psychiatric Association Publishing
800 Maine Avenue SW, Suite 900
Washington, DC 20024-2812
www.appi.org

Library of Congress Cataloging-in-Publication Data
Names: Nemeroff, Charles B., editor. | Craighead, W. Edward, editor.
Title: Anxiety and Depression Association of America patient guide to mood and anxiety disorders / edited by Charles B. Nemeroff, M.D., Ph.D., W. Edward Craighead, Ph.D., ABPP
Other titles: Patient guide to mood and anxiety disorders
Description: First edition. | Washington, DC : American Psychiatric Association Publishing, [2024] | Includes bibliographical references and index.
Identifiers: LCCN 2023053409 (print) | LCCN 2023053410 (ebook) | ISBN 9781615375035 (paperback) | ISBN 9781615375042 (ebook)
Subjects: LCSH: Affective disorders--Popular works. | Anxiety disorders--Popular works.
Classification: LCC RC537 .A5925 2024 (print) | LCC RC537 (ebook) | DDC 616.85/22--dc23/eng/20231213
LC record available at https://lccn.loc.gov/2023053409
LC ebook record available at https://lccn.loc.gov/2023053410

Dedication:
To our patients and their families
who have taught us much.

Contents

Part I
The Disorders

Part II
Treatment of the Disorders

Part III
The Treatments: *Pharmacological*

Part IV
The Treatments: *Neuromodulation*

Part V
The Treatments: *Psychological*

Part VI
Special Populations and Special Topics

Contributors

Amy Adams, M.P.H.
M.D./Ph.D. student, Texas A&M University Health Sciences Center, Bryan, Texas

Arij Alarachi, B.Sc.
Department of Psychology, Neuroscience, and Behaviour, McMaster University and St. Joseph's Healthcare, Hamilton, Ontario, Canada

Jorge R.C. Almeida, M.D., Ph.D.
Associate Professor, Dell Medical School, University of Texas at Austin, Austin, Texas

Jonathan E. Alpert, M.D., Ph.D.
Professor, Department of Psychiatry and Behavioral Sciences, Dominick P. Purpura Department of Neuroscience, and Department of Pediatrics; Dorothy and Marty Silverman Chair in Psychiatry; and Chair, Department of Psychiatry and Behavioral Sciences, Montefiore Medical Center and Albert Einstein College of Medicine, Bronx, New York

Carol L. Alter, M.D.
Professor and Executive Associate Chair, Department of Psychiatry, Dell Medical School, University of Texas at Austin, Austin, Texas

Leslie K. Anderson, Ph.D.
Clinical Professor, Department of Psychiatry, and Director of Training, Eating Disorders Center for Treatment and Research, University of California, San Diego, San Diego, California

Joan R. Asarnow, Ph.D., ABPP
Professor of Psychiatry and Biobehavioral Sciences, University of California, Los Angeles, Los Angeles, California

David H. Barlow, Ph.D.
Professor of Psychology and Psychiatry Emeritus and Founder, Center for Anxiety and Related Disorders, Boston University, Boston, Massachusetts

Jessica Batten, PA-C, CAQ-Psych
Physician Assistant, Dell Medical School, University of Texas at Austin, Austin, Texas

Colleen Bloom, M.S.W.
Program Manager, Columbia University, New York, New York

Lisa Boyars, M.D.
Assistant Professor of Medicine, Department of Psychiatry and Behavioral Sciences, University of Texas at Austin, Austin, Texas

Kathleen T. Brady, M.D., Ph.D.
Director, South Carolina Clinical and Translational Research Institute, and Distinguished University Professor, Medical University of South Carolina, Charleston, South Carolina

Joshua C. Brown, M.D., Ph.D.
Department of Psychiatry, McLean Hospital, Harvard Medical School, Boston, Massachusetts

Linda L. Carpenter, M.D.
Professor, Department of Psychiatry and Human Behavior, Alpert Medical School, Brown University, Providence, Rhode Island

Katherine Chemakin, B.S.
Medical student, Albert Einstein College of Medicine, Bronx, New York

Eric Chen, M.D.
Resident Psychiatrist, Department of Psychiatry, Tufts Medical Center, Tufts University School of Medicine, Boston, Massachusetts

Fredrick Chin, Ph.D.
Postdoctoral Fellow, Indiana University School of Medicine, Indianapolis, Indiana

Amit Chopra, M.D.
Psychiatrist, Massachusetts General Hospital, Harvard Medical School, Boston, Massachusetts

Josh M. Cisler, Ph.D.
Associate Professor, Department of Psychiatry and Behavioral Sciences, University of Texas at Austin, Austin, Texas

Amy Claxton, Ph.D.
Senior Director for Clinical Development, Karuna Therapeutics, Boston, Massachusetts

Anita H. Clayton, M.D.
Wilford W. Spradlin Professor and Chair, Department of Psychiatry and Neurobehavioral Sciences, University of Virginia School of Medicine, Charlottesville, Virginia

Anahi Collado, Ph.D.
Assistant Research Professor, Renée Crown Wellness Institute, University of Colorado–Boulder, Boulder, Colorado

Susan K. Conroy, M.D., Ph.D.
Assistant Professor of Psychiatry, Indiana University School of Medicine, Indianapolis, Indiana

Charles R. Conway, M.D.
Professor, Department of Psychiatry, Washington University School of Medicine, St. Louis, Missouri

William Coryell, M.D.
Emeritus Professor of Psychiatry, University of Iowa, Iowa City, Iowa

W. Edward Craighead, Ph.D., ABPP
J. Rex Fuqua Professor and Endowed Chair and Vice Chair of the Child, Adolescent, and Young Adult Division, Department of Psychiatry and Behavioral Sciences, and Professor, Department of Psychology, Emory University, Atlanta, Georgia

Michelle G. Craske, Ph.D.
Distinguished Professor of Psychology and of Psychiatry and Biobehavioral Sciences and Director of the Anxiety and Depression Research Center, University of California, Los Angeles, California

Kimberly B. Day, M.A.
Graduate Student, Psychology Department, Washburn University, Topeka, Kansas

Elizabeth Deckler, M.D.
Jackson Behavioral Health Hospital, Miami, Florida

Jordan M. De Herrera, M.A.
Graduate Student, Psychology Department, Washburn University, Topeka, Kansas

Sona Dimidjian, Ph.D.
Director, Renée Crown Wellness Institute, and Professor, Department of Psychology and Neuroscience, University of Colorado–Boulder, Boulder, Colorado

Cody G. Dodd, Ph.D.
Assistant Professor, Department of Psychiatry and Behavioral Sciences, University of Texas Medical Branch, Galveston, Texas

Korrina A. Duffy, Ph.D.
Assistant Professor, Department of Psychiatry, University of Colorado Anschutz Medical Campus, Aurora, Colorado

C. Neill Epperson, M.D.
Robert Freedman Endowed Professor and Chair, Department of Psychiatry; Professor, Department of Family Medicine; and Executive Director, Helen and Arthur E. Johnson Depression Center, Department of Psychiatry, University of Colorado Anschutz Medical Campus, Aurora, Colorado

Alyssa L. Faro, Ph.D.
Instructor in Psychology, Department of Psychiatry, Harvard Medical School, Boston; Director of Clinical Services, OCD Institute for Children and Adolescents, McLean Hospital, Belmont, Massachusetts

Julie Farrington, M.D.
Assistant Professor, Department of Psychiatry and Behavioral Sciences, Dell Medical School, University of Texas at Austin, Austin, Texas

Jesse Finkelstein, Psy.D.
Postdoctoral Fellow, Columbia University, Irving Medical Center, New York, New York

Nicole R. Friedman, B.S., M.A.
Graduate Student, Department of Psychology and Center for Youth Development and Intervention, University of Alabama, Tuscaloosa, Alabama

Mark A. Frye, M.D.
Professor of Psychiatry, Mayo Clinic College of Medicine; Stephen & Shelly Jackson Family Professorship in Individualized Medicine, Department of Psychiatry and Psychology, Mayo Clinic, Rochester, Minnesota

Glen O. Gabbard, M.D.
Professor of Psychiatry, Baylor College of Medicine, Houston, Texas

Igor Galynker, M.D., Ph.D.
Clinical Professor of Psychiatry, Mount Sinai Suicide Prevention Research Laboratory, Icahn School of Medicine at Mount Sinai, New York, New York

Christopher Germer, Ph.D.
Lecturer on Psychiatry (part-time), Harvard Medical School, Cambridge, Massachusetts

Charles F. Gillespie, M.D., Ph.D.
Associate Professor, Department of Psychiatry and Behavioral Sciences, Emory University School of Medicine, Atlanta, Georgia

Deborah R. Glasofer, Ph.D.
Associate Professor of Clinical Medical Psychology (in Psychiatry), Columbia University Vagelos College of Physicians and Surgeons, New York, New York

Joseph F. Goldberg, M.D.
Clinical Professor of Psychiatry, Icahn School of Medicine at Mount Sinai, New York, New York

Inna Goncearenco, M.A.
Research Assistant, Mount Sinai Suicide Prevention Research Laboratory, New York, New York

Wayne K. Goodman, M.D.
D.C. and Irene Ellwood Chair in Psychiatry and Professor, Menninger Department of Psychiatry and Behavioral Sciences, Baylor College of Medicine, Houston, Texas

Britt M. Gott, M.S.
Clinical Lab Manager, Department of Psychiatry, Washington University School of Medicine, St. Louis, Missouri

Alexander Grieshaber, M.A.
Department of Psychology, Stony Brook University, Stony Brook, New York

Adrienne Grzenda, M.D., Ph.D.
Health Sciences Clinical Assistant Professor, Department of Psychiatry and Biobehavioral Sciences, David Geffen School of Medicine, University of California, Los Angeles, Los Angeles, California

Rebecca Hamblin, Ph.D.
Assistant Professor, Department of Psychiatry, University of Texas Medical Branch, Galveston, Texas

Philip D. Harvey, Ph.D.
Leonard M. Miller Professor of Psychiatry and Behavioral Sciences, Miller School of Medicine, University of Miami, Miami, Florida

Steven C. Hayes, Ph.D.
Foundation Professor of Psychology Emeritus, University of Nevada, Reno, Nevada

John M. Hettema, Ph.D.
Professor of Psychiatry, Department of Psychiatry and Behavioral Sciences, Texas A&M University Health Sciences Center, Bryan, Texas

Laurel Hicks, Ph.D.
Research Associate, Renée Crown Wellness Institute, University of Colorado–Boulder, Boulder, Colorado

Robert M. A. Hirschfeld, M.D., M.Sc.
Professor, Department of Psychiatry, Weill Cornell Medical College, New York, New York

Fatma Ozlem Hokelekli, M.D., Ph.D.
Resident Physician, General Psychiatry Residency Program, University of Texas Southwestern Medical Center, Dallas, Texas

Eric Hollander, M.D.
Professor, Department of Psychiatry and Behavioral Sciences; and Director, Autism and Obsessive Compulsive Spectrum Program, Psychiatry Research Institute of Montefiore Einstein, Albert Einstein College of Medicine, Bronx, New York

Steven D. Hollon, Ph.D.
Gertrude Conaway Vanderbilt Professor, Departments of Psychology and Psychiatry, Vanderbilt University, Nashville, Tennessee

Paul E. Holtzheimer, M.D., M.S.
Professor of Psychiatry and Professor of Surgery, Geisel School of Medicine, Dartmouth College, Hanover, New Hampshire

Jennifer L. Hughes, Ph.D., M.P.H.
Clinical Scholar, Big Lots Behavioral Health Services, Nationwide Children's Hospital; Associate Professor, Department of Psychiatry and Behavioral Health, College of Medicine and Division of Health Behavior and Health Promotion, College of Public Health, Ohio State University, Columbus, Ohio

Alissa Hutto, M.D.
Clinical Assistant Professor, Consultation Liaison Psychiatry, Department of Psychiatry, University of North Carolina, Chapel Hill, North Carolina

Neha Jain, M.D.
Associate Professor of Psychiatry, University of Connecticut School of Medicine, Farmington, Connecticut

Muhammad Youshay Jawad, M.B.B.S.
Resident Physician, Department of Psychiatry and Behavioral Health, Penn State Health Milton S. Hershey Medical Center, Hershey, Pennsylvania

Manish Kumar Jha, M.B.B.S.
Associate Professor of Psychiatry and O'Donnell Clinical Neuroscience Scholar, Center for Depression Research and Clinical Care, University of Texas Southwestern Medical Center, Dallas, Texas

Gregory H. Jones, M.D.
PGY-4 Resident, Center of Excellence in Mood Disorders, Faillace Department of Psychiatry, University of Texas, Houston, Texas

Lianna Karp, M.D.
Staff Psychiatrist, Massachusetts General Hospital, Boston, Massachusetts

Rebecca C. Kass, M.D.
Resident Physician IV, Department of Psychiatry and Behavioral Sciences, University of New Mexico School of Medicine, Albuquerque, New Mexico

Walter H. Kaye, M.D.
Professor, Department of Psychiatry, and Director, Eating Disorders Center for Treatment and Research, University of California, San Diego, San Diego, California

Reilly Kayser, M.D.
Assistant Professor of Clinical Psychiatry, Columbia University, New York, New York

Martin B. Keller, M.D.
Professor Emeritus, Department of Psychiatry and Human Behavior, Brown University, Providence, Rhode Island

Chris A. Kelly, Ph.D.
Postdoctoral Fellow, Icahn School of Medicine at Mount Sinai, New York, New York

Sean Kerrigan, M.D.
Assistant Professor, Department of Psychiatry and Behavioral Sciences, Dell Medical School, University of Texas at Austin, Austin, Texas

Jasmine Kim, M.D.
Resident Physician, Department of Psychiatry, Zucker School of Medicine at Hofstra/Northwell at Staten Island University Hospital, Staten Island, New York

Claire L. Kirk, Ph.D.
Assistant Professor, Department of Psychiatry and Behavioral Sciences, University of Texas Medical Branch, Galveston, Texas

Daniel N. Klein, Ph.D.
Distinguished Professor, Department of Psychology, Stony Brook University, Stony Brook, New York

Raymond Kotwicki, M.D., M.P.H.
President and Chief Medical Officer, Intensive Outpatient Services, Hightop Healthcare; Adjunct Professor, Department of Psychiatry and Behavioral Sciences, Emory University School of Medicine, Atlanta, Georgia

Andrew D. Krystal, M.D., M.S.
Professor, Department of Psychiatry, UCSF Weill Institute for Neurosciences, University of California, San Francisco, San Francisco, California

Grace Lethbridge, B.H.Sc.
Research Assistant, MacAnxiety Research Centre, McMaster University, Hamilton, Ontario, Canada

Israel Liberzon, M.D.
Department Head, Distinguished University Professor, and William and Dorothy Stearman Endowed Professor, Department of Psychiatry, Texas A&M University, College Station, Texas

Rodrigo Machado-Vieira, M.D., Ph.D.
Professor, Director of the UT Health Experimental Therapeutics and Molecular Pathophysiology Program, University of Texas, Houston, Texas

Cheri L. Marmarosh, Ph.D.
Associate Professor, George Washington University, Washington, D.C.

Luana Marques, Ph.D.
Director and Founder, Community Psychiatry PRIDE, Massachusetts General Hospital, Boston; Associate Professor, Department of Psychology, Harvard Medical School, Cambridge, Massachusetts

Sanjay J. Mathew, M.D.
Vice Chair for Research and Professor of Psychiatry and Behavioral Sciences, Menninger Department of Psychiatry and Behavioral Sciences, Baylor College of Medicine, Houston, Texas

Helen S. Mayberg, M.D.
Professor, Neurology, Neurosurgery, Psychiatry and Neuroscience, Mount Sinai Professor of Neurotherapeutics; Director, Center of Advanced Circuit Therapeutics, Icahn School of Medicine at Mount Sinai, New York, New York

Randi E. McCabe, Ph.D., C.Psych.
Professor, Department of Psychiatry and Behavioral Sciences, McMaster University; Director, Mood and Anxiety Services, and St. Joseph's Healthcare, Hamilton Anxiety Treatment and Research Clinic, Hamilton, Ontario, Canada

Roger S. McIntyre, M.D., FRCPC
Professor of Psychiatry and Pharmacology, University of Toronto, Toronto, Ontario, Canada

Sherri Melrose, Ph.D.
Adjunct Professor, Athabasca University, Athabasca, Alberta, Canada

Samantha Meltzer-Brody, M.D., M.P.H.
Assad Meymandi Distinguished Professor and Chair, Department of Psychiatry; Director, UNC Center for Women's Mood Disorders, University of North Carolina School of Medicine, Chapel Hill, North Carolina

Christina Metcalf, Ph.D.
Assistant Professor, Department of Psychiatry, University of Colorado Anschutz Medical Campus, Aurora, Colorado

Allison Metts, M.A.
Anxiety and Depression Research Center, University of California, Los Angeles, Los Angeles, California

Alicia E. Meuret, Ph.D.
Professor of Psychology and Director, Anxiety and Depression Research Center, Southern Methodist University, Dallas, Texas

David J. Miklowitz, Ph.D.
Distinguished Professor of Psychiatry and Biobehavioral Sciences, Semel Institute for Neuroscience and Human Behavior, David Geffen School of Medicine, University of California, Los Angeles, Los Angeles, California

Laura J. Miller, M.D.
Assistant Professor of Psychiatry and Behavioral Sciences, Department of Psychiatry and Behavioral Sciences, Emory University School of Medicine, Atlanta, Georgia

Cristina Montalvo, M.D., M.B.S.
Chief of Consultation-Liaison Psychiatry and Emergency Services, Tufts Medical Center; Assistant Professor, Department of Psychiatry, Tufts University School of Medicine, Boston, Massachusetts

Jennifer J. Mootz, Ph.D.
Assistant Professor of Clinical Medical Psychology (in Psychiatry), Columbia University; Department of Psychiatry, New York State Psychiatric Institute, New York, New York

James W. Murrough, M.D., Ph.D.
Professor of Psychiatry and Neuroscience, Icahn School of Medicine at Mount Sinai, New York, New York

Henry A. Nasrallah, M.D.
Professor of Psychiatry, Neurology, and Neuroscience, University of Cincinnati College of Medicine, Cincinnati, Ohio

Kristin Neff, Ph.D.
Associate Professor of Educational Psychology, University of Texas at Austin, Austin, Texas

Charles B. Nemeroff, M.D., Ph.D.
Matthew P. Nemeroff Professor and Chair, Department of Psychiatry and Behavioral Sciences and Mulva Clinic for the Neurosciences; Director, Institute of Early Life Adversity Research, Dell Medical School, University of Texas at Austin, Austin, Texas

Fabiano G. Nery, M.D., Ph.D.
Associate Professor of Psychiatry, University of Cincinnati College of Medicine, Cincinnati, Ohio

D. Jeffrey Newport, M.D., M.S., M.Div.
Associate Chair for Research and Professor, Department of Psychiatry and Behavioral Sciences; Professor, Department of Women's Health; and Director, Women's Reproductive Mental Health, The University of Texas at Austin, Austin, Texas

Richard J. Norton, M.A.
Department of Psychological Science, University of Vermont, Burlington, Vermont

Nicholas Ortiz, M.D.
Assistant Professor of Psychiatry, Dell Medical School, University of Texas at Austin, Austin, Texas

Sydney Parkinson, B.A.
Ph.D. Student in Clinical Psychology, Anxiety Treatment and Research Clinic, St. Joseph's Healthcare and McMaster University, Hamilton, Ontario, Canada

Beth Patterson, M.Sc.
Assistant Clinical Professor, Adjunct, Department of Psychiatry and Behavioural Neuroscience, MacAnxiety Research Centre, McMaster University, Hamilton, Ontario, Canada

Martin P. Paulus, M.D.
Scientific Director and President, Laureate Institute for Brain Research, Professor of Neuroscience, College of Health Sciences, Community Medicine, University of Tulsa, Tulsa, Oklahoma; Adjunct Professor, Department of Psychiatry, University of California, San Diego, San Diego, California

Giampaolo Perna, M.D., Ph.D.
Chief, Personalized Medicine Center for Anxiety and Panic Disorders, Humanitas San Pio X; Scientific Director, Psico Medical Care, Humanitas Medical Care; Professor of Psychiatry, Humanitas University, Milan, Italy

Grace S. Pham, D.O., Ph.D.
Resident in Psychiatry, Menninger Department of Psychiatry and Behavioral Sciences, Baylor College of Medicine, Houston, Texas

Katharine A. Phillips, M.D.
Professor of Psychiatry, DeWitt Wallace Senior Scholar, and Residency Research Director, Department of Psychiatry, Weill Cornell Medical College; Attending Psychiatrist, New York-Presbyterian Hospital, New York, New York

Robert M. Post, M.D.
Clinical Professor of Psychiatry, George Washington University School of Medicine, Washington, D.C.

Jessica Rao, M.P.H.
Executive Director, Center for Environmental Therapeutics, Worcester, Massachusetts

Sheila A.M. Rauch, Ph.D.
Mark and Barbara Klein Distinguished Professor in Psychiatry Professor of Psychology in Psychiatry, Department of Psychiatry and Behavioral Sciences, and Deputy Director, Emory Healthcare Veterans Program, Emory University School of Medicine; Director of Research and Program Evaluation, Mental Health Service Line, Atlanta VA Healthcare System, Atlanta, Georgia

Simon A. Rego, Psy.D., ABPP
Professor, Chief of Psychology, and Director of Psychology Training, Department of Psychiatry and Behavioral Sciences, Montefiore Medical Center and Albert Einstein College of Medicine, Bronx, New York

Patricia A. Resick, Ph.D., ABPP
Professor, Department of Psychiatry and Behavioral Sciences, Duke Health, Chapel Hill, North Carolina

Erin C. Richardson, M.S.N., R.N., APRN, PMHNP-BC
Psychiatric-Mental Health Nurse Practitioner, Women's Reproductive Mental Health of Texas, Mulva Clinic for the Neurosciences, University of Texas at Austin, Austin, Texas

Patricio Riva-Posse, M.D.
Associate Professor, Department of Psychiatry and Behavioral Sciences, Emory University School of Medicine, Atlanta, Georgia

Shireen L. Rizvi, Ph.D., ABPP
Professor of Clinical Psychology, Graduate School of Applied and Professional Psychology, Rutgers University, Piscataway, New Jersey

Donald J. Robinaugh, Ph.D.
Assistant Professor in the Department of Applied Psychology and the Department of Art + Design, Northeastern University, Boston, Massachusetts

Kelly J. Rohan, Ph.D.
Professor, Department of Psychological Science, University of Vermont, Burlington, Vermont

Laina E. Rosebrock, Ph.D.
Research Clinical Psychologist, University of Oxford, Oxford, United Kingdom

Jerrold Rosenbaum, M.D.
Stanley Cobb Professor of Psychiatry, Massachusetts General Hospital, Harvard Medical School, Boston, Massachusetts

Donald L. Rosenstein, M.D.
Professor, Departments of Psychiatry and Medicine; Director, Comprehensive Cancer Support Program; and Division Head, General Adult Psychiatry, University of North Carolina at Chapel Hill

Barbara O. Rothbaum, Ph.D., ABPP
Professor in Psychiatry, and Director, Emory Healthcare Veterans Program, Emory University, Atlanta, Georgia

Karen Rowa, Ph.D., C.Psych.
Psychologist and Professor, Anxiety Treatment and Research Clinic, St. Joseph's Healthcare and McMaster University, Hamilton, Ontario, Canada

David C. Rozek, Ph.D., ABPP
Associate Professor, Department of Psychology and Behavioral Sciences, School of Medicine, University of Texas Health Science Center at San Antonio, San Antonio, Texas

Michelle Rozenman, Ph.D.
Associate Professor, College of Arts, Humanities and Social Sciences, Department of Psychology, University of Denver, Denver, Colorado

Ihsan M. Salloum, M.D., M.P.H.
Professor and Founding Chair, Department of Neuroscience; and Director, Institute of Neuroscience, University of Texas Rio Grande Valley School of Medicine, Edinburg, Texas

Alan F. Schatzberg, M.D.
Kenneth T. Norris, Jr., Professor of Psychiatry and Behavioral Sciences, Department of Psychiatry and Behavioral Sciences, Stanford University School of Medicine, Stanford, California

Rebecca L. Schneider, Ph.D.
Assistant Professor, Department of Psychiatry and Behavioral Sciences, Emory University School of Medicine, Atlanta, Georgia

M. Katherine Shear, M.D.
Marion E. Kenworthy Professor of Psychiatry in Social Work, Columbia University, New York, New York

David V. Sheehan, M.D., M.B.A.
Distinguished University Health Professor Emeritus, Morsani College of Medicine, University of South Florida, Tampa, Florida

Naomi M. Simon, M.D.
Professor, Department of Psychiatry, NYU Grossman School of Medicine, New York, New York

H. Blair Simpson, M.D., Ph.D.
Professor of Psychiatry, Columbia University Irving Medical College, Columbia University; Director, Center for OCD and Related Disorders, New York State Psychiatric Institute, New York, New York

Balwinder Singh, M.D., M.S.
Assistant Professor, Department of Psychiatry and Psychology, Mayo Clinic, Rochester Minnesota

Natalia Skritskaya, Ph.D.
Adjunct Associate Research Scientist in the Faculty of Social Work, Columbia University, New York, New York

Jair C. Soares, M.D., Ph.D.
Professor, Pat R. Rutherford, Jr. Chair in Psychiatry, University of Texas, Houston, Texas

Isabella G. Spaulding, B.S.
San Diego State University/University of California, San Diego Joint Doctoral Program in Clinical Psychology, La Jolla, California

David C. Steffens, M.D., M.H.S.
Samuel "Sy" Birnbaum/Ida, Louis and Richard Blum Chair in Psychiatry and Professor, Department of Psychiatry, University of Connecticut School of Medicine, Farmington, Connecticut

Murray B. Stein, M.D., M.P.H.
Distinguished Professor, Department of Psychiatry and Herbert Wertheim School of Public Health and Human Longevity Science, University of California, San Diego, San Diego, California

Anne Louise Stewart, M.D.
Assistant Professor, Department of Psychiatry and Neurobehavioral Sciences, University of Virginia School of Medicine, Charlottesville, Virginia

Stephen M. Strakowski, M.D.
Professor of Psychiatry, Indiana University School of Medicine, Indianapolis, Indiana

Eric A. Storch, Ph.D.
Professor, Vice Chair, and McIngvale Presidential Endowed Chair, Menninger Department of Psychiatry and Behavioral Sciences, Baylor College of Medicine, Houston, Texas

Jong-Woo Suh, B.A., M.A.
Graduate Student, Department of Psychology, University of Alabama, Tuscaloosa, Alabama

Mark Sullivan, M.D.
Assistant Professor of Clinical Psychiatry, Weill Cornell Medical College, New York, New York

Paul Summergrad, M.D.
Formerly Psychiatrist-in-Chief, Tufts Medical Center, and Dr. Frances S. Arkin Professor and Chairman, Department of Psychiatry; currently Professor of Psychiatry and Medicine, Tufts University School of Medicine, Boston, Massachusetts

Amanda J. F. Tamman, M.Sc., Ph.D.
Assistant Professor, Department of Psychiatry and Behavioral Sciences, Baylor College of Medicine, Houston, Texas

Steven D. Targum, M.D.
Scientific Director, Signant Health, Boston, Massachusetts

Julia M. Terman, M.A.
Department of Psychological Science, University of Vermont, Burlington, Vermont

Michael Terman, Ph.D.
President, Center for Environmental Therapeutics, Worcester, Massachusetts; Professor of Clinical Psychology (in Psychiatry), Department of Psychiatry, Columbia University, New York

Tatiana Torti, Psy.D.
Scientific Director, ASIPSE School of Cognitive-Behavioral Therapy, Milan, Italy

Cynthia L. Turk, Ph.D.
Professor and Chair, Psychology Department, Washburn University, Topeka, Kansas

Michael Van Ameringen, M.D., FRCPC
Professor, Department of Psychiatry and Behavioural Neuroscience, MacAnxiety Research Centre, McMaster University, Hamilton, Ontario, Canada

Dina Vivian, Ph.D.
Clinical Professor, Department of Psychology, Stony Brook University, Stony Brook, New York

Karen Dineen Wagner, M.D., Ph.D.
Titus Harris Chair, Department of Psychiatry and Behavioral Sciences, University of Texas Medical Branch, Galveston, Texas

B. Timothy Walsh, M.D.
Ruane Professor of Psychiatry, Columbia University Vagelos College of Physicians and Surgeons, New York, New York

V. Robin Weersing, Ph.D.
Professor, Joint Doctoral Program in Clinical Psychology, San Diego State University/University of California, San Diego, La Jolla, California

Risa B. Weisberg, Ph.D.
Chief Clinical Officer, BehaVR Inc; Professor of Psychiatry, Chobanian and Avedisian School of Medicine, Boston University, Boston, Massachusetts

Myrna M. Weissman, Ph.D.
Diane Goldman Kemper Family Professor of Epidemiology and Psychiatry, Columbia University Vagelos College of Physicians and Surgeons; Codirector, Division of Translational Epidemiology and Mental Health Equity, New York State Psychiatric Institute, New York, New York

Susan W. White, Ph.D.
Professor and Doddridge Saxon Endowed Chair, Department of Psychology and Center for Youth Development and Intervention, University of Alabama, Tuscaloosa, Alabama

Anna E. Wise, Ph.D.
Assistant Professor of Psychology in Psychiatry, Department of Psychiatry and Behavioral Sciences, Emory University, Atlanta, Georgia

Kate Wolitzky-Taylor, Ph.D.
Associate Director, Anxiety and Depression Research Center, and Associate Professor, Department of Psychiatry and Biobehavioral Sciences, University of California, Los Angeles, Los Angeles, California

Lauren S. Woodard, B.A.
Clinical Research Coordinator, Center for Anxiety and Related Disorders, Boston University, Boston, Massachusetts

Disclosures

The following contributors to this book have indicated a financial interest in or other affiliation with a commercial supporter, a manufacturer of a commercial product, a provider of a commercial service, a nongovernmental organization, and/or a government agency, as listed below:

Jonathan E. Alpert, M.D., Ph.D. *Honoraria:* Belvoir Publications, MGH Psychiatry Academy; *Institutional Support:* Montefiore Medicine; *Research Support:* Janssen Pharmaceuticals, National Institutes of Mental Health, Patient Centered Outcomes Research Institute; *Royalties:* Cambridge University Press.

Joan R. Asarnow, Ph.D., ABPP *Editorial Committee:* Annual Review of Clinical Psychology; *Grant/Research Support:* American Foundation for Suicide Prevention, American Psychological Foundation, Association for Child and Adolescent Mental Health, National Institute of Mental Health, Patient Centered Outcome Research Institute, Society of Clinical Child and Adolescent Psychology (APA Division 53), Substance Abuse and Mental Health Services Administration; *Scientific Advisory Board:* Klingenstein Third Generation Foundation; *Scientific Council:* American Foundation for Suicide Prevention.

David H. Barlow, Ph.D. *Consultant/Honoraria:* Agency for Healthcare Research and Quality, Chinese University of Hong Kong, Foundation for Informed Medical Decision Making, Hebrew University of Jerusalem, Mayo Clinic, New Zealand Psychological Association, The Renfrew Center, Universidad Católica de Santa Maria (Arequipa, Peru), U.S. Department of Defense, various American and European universities, clinics, institutes; *Grants:* Colciencias (Government of Columbia Initiative for Science, Technology, and Health Innovation), National Institute of Alcohol and Alcohol Abuse, National Institute of Mental Health, The Templeton Foundation; *Royalties:* Cengage Learning, Guilford Publications, Oxford University Press, Pearson Publishing.

Linda L. Carpenter, M.D. *Clinical Trial:* Janssen Pharmaceuticals, Neurolief; *Consultant:* Magnus Medical, MAPS Public Benefit Corp., Motif Neurotech, Neuronetics, Sage Therapeutics; *Grant/Research Support:* Neuronetics.

Amit Chopra, M.D. *Publication/Writing Honoraria:* Slack; *Royalties:* Oxford University Press; *Speaker:* Psychopharmacology Institute.

Amy Claxton, Ph.D. *Employer:* Karuna Therapeutics.

Anita H. Clayton, M.D. *Advisory Board/Consultant Fee:* AbbVie, Brii Biosciences, Fabre-Kramer, Field Trip Health, Janssen Research & Development LLC,

Mind Cure Health, Ovoca Bio PLC, Praxis Precision Medicines, PureTech Health, S1 Biopharma, Sage Therapeutics, Takeda/Lundbeck, Vella Bioscience Inc., WCG MedAvante-ProPhase; *Grants:* Daré Bioscience, Janssen Pharmaceuticals, Praxis Precision Medicines, Relmada Therapeutics Inc., Sage Therapeutics; *Royalties/Copyright:* Ballantine Books/Random House, Changes in Sexual Functioning Questionnaire, Guilford Publications,; *Shares/Restricted Stock Units:* Euthymics, Mediflix LLC, S1 Biopharma.

Susan K. Conroy, M.D., Ph.D. *Site PI:* Janssen Pharmaceuticals.

Charles R. Conway, M.D. *Consultant/Research Support:* LivaNova PLC.

W. Edward Craighead, Ph.D., ABPP *Officer:* Hugarheill efh; *Publication/Writing Honoraria:* John Wiley & Sons; *Scientific Advisory Board:* AIM for Mental Health, Anxiety and Depression Association of America, George West M.H. Foundation.

Sona Dimidjian, Ph.D. *Founder/Co-founder:* Access Consulting LLC, Mindful Noggin Inc.; *Funding:* National Institutes of Health, philanthropic foundations; *Revenue:* Mindful Noggin Inc.; *Royalties:* Guilford Publications, Wolters Kluwer.

C. Neill Epperson, M.D. *Consultant:* Asarina Pharma, Sage Therapeutics; *Investigator:* Sage Therapeutics; *Research Support:* HealthRhythms; *Scientific Advisory Board:* Babyscripts.

Julie Farrington, M.D. *Expert Testimony:* Thornton Biechlin Reynolds & Guerra LC; *Grant/Research Support:* CPRIT grant; *Principal Investigator:* Boehringer Ingelheim, COMPASS Pathways, Jazz Pharmaceuticals, LivaNova PLC, Sage Therapeutics; *Study M.D.:* NIH R01–Grants Office ID 202201540001FP.

Jesse Finkelstein, Psy.D. *Consultant:* TheraHive; *Employer:* Columbia University Irving Medical Center.

Mark A. Frye M.D. *Grant/Research Support:* Assurex Health; *Officer/Director/Trustee:* Breakthrough Discoveries for Thriving With Bipolar Disorder; *Royalties:* Chymia LLC; *Speaker:* American Physician Institute, Carnot Laboratories.

Joseph F. Goldberg, M.D. *Consultant:* BioXcel, Jazz Pharmaceuticals, Lundbeck, Otsuka Pharmaceuticals, Sage Therapeutics, Sunovion, Supernus; *Royalties:* American Psychiatric Association Publishing, Cambridge University Press; *Speakers Bureau:* Abbvie, Alkermes, Axsome Therapeutics, Intracellular Therapies, Sunovion.

Wayne K. Goodman, M.D. *Consultant:* Biohaven; *Research Support:* NIH UH3NS100549; *Royalties:* Nview LLC, OCDscales LLC.

Adrienne Grzenda, M.D., Ph.D. *Consultant:* American Psychiatric Association; *Honoraria:* Carlat Publishing.

Philip D. Harvey, Ph.D. *Consulting/Travel Fees:* Alkermes, Aneurotech, Bio-Excel, Boehringer Ingelheim, BV, Karuna Pharmaceutical, Merck Pharma, Minerva Pharma, Sunovion; *Officer:* Chief Science Officer, i-Function Inc.; *Royalties:* WCG Verasci Inc.; Scientific Consultant: EMA Wellness Inc.

Eric Hollander, M.D. *Editorial Fees:* Elsevier Publishing; *Grants:* GW Pharmaceuticals, Roche, U.S. Department of Defense, U.S. Food and Drug Administration Orphan Products Division; *Royalties:* Body Dysmorphic Disorder Modification of the Y-BOCS (BDD-YBOCS).

Paul E. Holtzheimer, M.D., M.S. *Royalties:* Oxford University Press, Wolters Kluwer.

Manish Kumar Jha, M.B.B.S. *Consultant:* Boehringer Ingelheim, Eleusis Therapeutics US Inc, Janssen Scientific Affairs; *Data Safety and Monitoring Board:* Click, Eliem, Inversargo; *Grants/Research Support:* Neurocrine Bioscience, Navitor/Supernus and Janssen Research & Development; *Honoraria:* Clinical Care Options, Global Medical Education, Medscape/WebMD, North American Center for Continuing Medical Education, Psychiatry & Behavioral Health Learning Network.

Walter H. Kaye, M.D. *Consultant:* COMPASS Pathways, EDCare; *Grant/Research Support:* COMPASS Pathways.

Martin B. Keller, M.D. *Donation (to University of Miami):* The John J. McDonnell and Margaret T. O'Brien Foundation.

Andrew D. Krystal, M.D., M.S. *Consultant:* Axsome Therapeutics, Big Health, Eisai, Evecxia, Harmony Biosciences, Idorsia, Janssen Pharmaceuticals, Jazz Pharmaceuticals, Millenium Pharmaceuticals, Merck, Neurocrine Biosciences, Neurawell, Pernix, Otsuka Pharmaceuticals, Sage Therapeutics, Takeda; *Grant/Research Support:* Attune, Axsome Therapeutics, Harmony, Janssen Pharmaceuticals, National Institutes of Health, Neurocrine Biosciences, The Ray and Dagmar Dolby Family Fund, Reveal Biosensors; *Stock:* Big Health, Neurawell.

Sanjay J. Mathew, M.D. *Consultant:* Clexio Biosciences, COMPASS Pathways, Eleusis, Engrail Therapeutics Inc., Neumora, Neurocrine, Perception

Neurosciences, Praxis Precision Medicines, Sage Therapeutics, Seelos Therapeutics, Sunovion; *Research Support:* Boehringer Ingelheim, Neurocrine, Sage Therapeutics.

Helen S. Mayberg, M.D. *Consultant/IP Licensing:* Abbott Laboratories.

Roger S. McIntyre, M.D., FRCPC *Grant/Research Support:* CIHR/GACD/ National Natural Science Foundation of China; *Speaker/Consultation:* Abbvie, Alkermes, Atai Life Sciences, Axsome Therapeutics, Bausch Health, Biogen, Boehringer Ingelheim, Eisai, Intra-Cellular, Lundbeck, Janssen Pharmaceuticals, Kris, Mitsubishi Tanabe, Neumora Therapeutics, Neurocrine, NewBridge Pharmaceuticals, Novo Nordisk, Otsuka Pharmaceuticals, Pfizer, Purdue, Sage Therapeutics, Sanofi, Sunovion, Takeda; *Officer:* Chief Executive Officer of Braxia Scientific Corp.

Samantha Meltzer-Brody, M.D., M.P.H. *Consultant:* EmbarkNeuro; *Grant/ Research Support:* Sage Therapeutics; *Officer/Director/Trustee:* Modern Health; *Speaker:* grand rounds at academic institutions.

David J. Miklowitz, Ph.D. *Royalties:* Guilford Publications, John Wiley & Sons.

Jennifer J. Mootz, Ph.D. *Royalties:* Oxford University Press; *Speaker:* Interpersonal Psychotherapy Workshop.

James W. Murrough, M.D., Ph.D. *Consultant/Advisory Board:* Boehringer Ingelheim, Clexio Biosciences, COMPASS Pathways; *Patents*: neuropeptide Y as a treatment for mood and anxiety disorders (pending), use of KCNQ channel openers to treat depression and related conditions (pending).

Charles B. Nemeroff, M.D., Ph.D. *Consultant:* ANeuroTech, Autobahn Therapeutics, BioXCel Therapeutics, Clexio Biosciences Ltd, EcoR1, EmbarkNeuro, Engrail Therapeutics Inc., Galen, GoodCap Pharmaceuticals Inc., Heading Health LLC, Intracellular Therapies (ITI), MAPS Public Benefit Corp., Ninnion LLC, Pasithea Therapeutics Corp., Relmada Therapeutics, Sage Therapeutics, Senseye Inc., Signant, Silo Pharma, SynapseBio Inc., *Other:* Precisement Health, Lucy.

D. Jeffrey Newport, M.D., M.S., M.Div. *Grant/Research Support:* Navitor, Sage Therapeutics.

Martin P. Paulus, M.D. *Consultant:* Hoffmann La Roche, Spring Care; *Employer:* William K. Warren Foundation; *Grant/Research Support:* National Institute on Drug Abuse, National Institute of General Medical Sciences; *Publication/Writing Honoraria:* Wolters Kluwer.

Katharine A. Phillips, M.D. *Honoraria:* Informa Exhibitions, Merck Manual, OCD Scales, Simple and Practical Medical Education; *Royalties:* American Psychiatric Association Publishing, Guilford Publications, International Creative Management Inc., L'Oreal, Oxford University Press, Wolter's Kluwer; *Speaker:* Informa Exhibitions, Miami Cosmetic Surgery and Aesthetic Dermatology Conference, academic institutions and professional societies.

Sheila A. M. Rauch, Ph.D. *Grant/Research Support:* McCormick Foundation, National Institutes of Health, Tonix Pharmaceuticals, U.S. Department of Defense, Woodruff Foundation, Wounded Warrior Project; *Royalties:* American Psychological Association Press, Oxford University Press.

Patricia A. Resick, Ph.D., ABPP *Royalties:* Guilford Publications.

Erin C. Richardson, M.S.N., R.N., APRN, PMHNP-BC *Grant/Research Support:* Sage Therapeutics.

Patricio Riva-Posse, M.D. *Consultant:* Abbott Neuromodulation, Janssen Pharmaceuticals, LivaNova PLC, Motif Neurotech.

Shireen L. Rizvi, Ph.D., ABPP *Consultant:* Behavioral Tech LLC; *Royalties:* Guilford Publications,.

Kelly J. Rohan, Ph.D. *Funding:* National Institute of Mental Health; *Royalties:* Oxford University Press.

Jerrold Rosenbaum, M.D. *Consultant:* TaraMind; *Officer/Director/Trustee:* Cerebral Inc., Entheos Labs, Psy Therapeutics, Sensorium Therapeutics.

Barbara O. Rothbaum, Ph.D., ABPP *Advisory Board:* Aptinyx, Genentech, Jazz Pharmaceuticals, Neuronetics, Nobilis Therapeutics, Sophren; *Consultant:* Cerebral Therapeutics, Jazz Pharmaceuticals, Otsuka Pharmaceuticals, Senseye Inc., Virtually Better Inc.; *Equity:* Virtually Better Inc.; *Funding:* Bob Woodruff Foundation, Cohen Veteran Bioscience, The Hidden Heroes Fund (an initiative of the Elizabeth Dole Foundation), McCormick Foundation, National Science Foundation, U.S. Department of Defense Clinical Trial Grant No. W81XWH-10-1-1045, Wounded Warrior Project; *Royalties:* American Psychiatric Association Publishing, Emory University, Guilford Publications, Oxford University Press. The terms of these arrangements have been reviewed and approved by Emory University in accordance with its conflict of interest policies.

Michelle Rozenman, Ph.D. *Royalties:* Oxford University Press.

Alan F. Schatzberg, M.D. *Consultant:* ANeurotech, COMPASS Pathways, Douglas, NeuraWell, Sage Therapeutics; *Equity:* Alto Neurosciences, Corcept, Delphor, Magnus, Owl Insights, Seattle Genetics, Titan.

M. Katherine Shear, M.D. *Author Contract:* Guilford Publications,.

David V. Sheehan, M.D., M.B.A. *Advisor/Consultant:* Noema Pharmaceuticals, Sage Therapeutics, Seelos, Syneos; *Board Membership:* Sage Therapeutics; *Honoraria:* Eisai, Janssen Pharmaceuticals, MAPI/ICON Language Services, Seelos, Sunovion; *Stock:* Nview Health; *Royalties:* licensing of scales and structured diagnostic interviews including the MINI, the SDS, and the S-STS, and for books and publications, through multiple tiers.

Naomi M. Simon, M.D. *Grants/Research Support:* American Foundation for Suicide Prevention, Cohen Veterans Network, National Institutes of Health, Patient-Centered Outcomes Research Institute, U.S. Department of Defense; *Personal Fees:* BehaVR LLC, Bionomics Ltd, Cerevel, Engrail Therapeutics Inc., Genomind, Praxis Therapeutics, Vanda Pharmaceuticals; *Royalties/Fees:* American Psychiatric Association Publishing, Wiley, Wolters-Kluwer; *Stock (spouse):* G1 Therapeutics, Zentalis.

H. Blair Simpson, M.D., Ph.D. *Research Support:* Biohaven Pharmaceuticals; *Royalties:* Wolters Kluwer, Cambridge University Press; *Stipend:* American Medical Association.

Balwinder Singh, M.D., M.S. *Employer:* Mayo Clinic; *Grant/Research Support:* Mayo Clinic, National Network of Depression Centers.

Murray B. Stein, M.D., M.P.H. *Consultant:* Acadia Pharmaceuticals, Aptinyx, atai Life Sciences, BigHealth, Biogen, Bionomics, BioXcel Therapeutics, Boehringer Ingelheim, Clexio, Delix Therapeutics, Eisai, EmpowerPharm, Engrail Therapeutics Inc., Janssen Pharmaceuticals, Jazz Pharmaceuticals, NeuroTrauma Sciences, PureTech Health, Sage Therapeutics, Sumitomo Pharma, Roche/Genentech; *Editorial Fees:* Wiley, Elsevier, Wolters-Kluwer; *Research Support:* National Institutes of Health, U.S. Department of Defense, U.S. Department of Veterans Affairs; *Scientific Advisory Board:* Anxiety and Depression Association of America, Brain and Behavior Research Foundation; *Stock Options:* EpiVario, Oxeia Biopharmaceuticals.

Eric A. Storch, Ph.D. *Consultant:* Biohaven Pharmaceuticals, Brainsway; *Research Support:* International OCD Foundation, National Institutes of Health,

Ream Foundation; *Royalties:* American Psychological Association, Elsevier, Guilford Publications, Jessica Kingsley, Routledge, Springer, Oxford University Press, Wiley; *Stock:* NView.

Paul Summergrad, M.D. *Consultant:* COMPASS Pathways, Owl Health, Pear Therapeutics, Quartet Health; *Officer/Director/Trustee:* Health and Productivity Services; *Stock/Stock Options:* Eli Lilly, Health and Productivity Services, Karuna Pharmaceuticals, Owl Health, Pear Therapeutics, Quartet Health, Sensorium.

Steven D. Targum, M.D. *Employer:* Signant Health; *Grants/Consulting Fees:* AZ Therapies, BioXcel Therapeutics Inc., Denovo Biopharma, EMA Wellness LLC, Epiodyne, Frequency Therapeutics, Functional Neuromodulation, Johnson & Johnson PRD, Karuna Therapeutics, Merck, Methylation Sciences, Navitor Pharmaceuticals, Sunovion.

Michael Van Ameringen, M.D., FRCPC *Advisory Board:* Allergan, Almatica, Brainsway Lundbeck, Bausch Health, Otsuka Pharmaceuticals, Elvium, Empowerpharm, Jazz Pharmaceuticals, Tilray and Vistagen; *Clinical Trials:* Biohaven, Otsuka Pharmaceuticals; *Grants:* Canadian Institute of Health Research and Hamilton Academic Health Sciences Organization, Elvium; *Honoraria:* Wolters-Kluwer; *Speaker's Bureau:* Abbvie, Allergan, Elvium (Purdue), Lundbeck, Otsuka Pharmaceuticals, Pfizer, Sunovion, Takeda.

V. Robin Weersing, Ph.D. *Royalties:* Oxford University Press.

Risa B. Weisberg, Ph.D. *Officer:* Chief Executive Officer, BehaVR Inc.

Myrna M. Weissman, Ph.D. *Author Contract:* Guilford Publications.

The following contributors had no competing interests to declare:
Amy Adams, M.P.H.; Arij Alarachi, B.Sc.; Jorge R. C. Almeida, M.D., Ph.D.; Carol L. Alter, M.D.; Leslie K. Anderson, Ph.D.; Jessica Batten, PA-C, CAQ-Psych; Colleen Bloom, M.S.W.; Lisa Boyars, M.D.; Kathleen T. Brady, M.D., Ph.D.; Joshua C. Brown, M.D., Ph.D.; Katherine Chemakin, B.S.; Eric Chen, M.D.; Fredrick Chin, Ph.D.; Josh M. Cisler, Ph.D.; Anahi Collado, Ph.D.; William Coryell, M.D.; Michelle G. Craske, Ph.D.; Kimberly B. Day, M.A.; Elizabeth Deckler, M.D.; Jordan M. De Herrera, M.A.; Cody G. Dodd, Ph.D.; Korrina A. Duffy, Ph.D.; Alyssa L. Faro, Ph.D.; Nicole R. Friedman, B.S., M.A.; Glen O. Gabbard, M.D.; Igor Galynker, M.D., Ph.D.; Christopher Germer, Ph.D.; Charles F. Gillespie, M.D., Ph.D.; Deborah R. Glasofer, Ph.D.; Inna Goncearenco, M.A.; Britt M. Gott, M.S.; Alexander Grieshaber, M.A.; Rebecca Hamblin, Ph.D.; Steven C. Hayes, Ph.D.;

John M. Hettema, Ph.D.; Laurel Hicks, Ph.D.; Robert M.A. Hirschfeld, M.D., M.Sc.; Fatma Ozlem Hokelekli, M.D., Ph.D.; Steven D. Hollon, Ph.D.; Jennifer L. Hughes, Ph.D., M.P.H.; Alissa Hutto, M.D.; Neha Jain, M.D.; Muhammad Youshay Jawad, M.B.B.S.; Gregory H. Jones, M.D.; Lianna Karp, M.D.; Rebecca C. Kass, M.D.; Reilly Kayser, M.D.; Chris A. Kelly, Ph.D.; Sean Kerrigan, M.D.; Jasmine Kim, M.D.; Claire L. Kirk, Ph.D.; Daniel N. Klein, Ph.D.; Raymond Kotwicki, M.D., M.P.H.; Grace Lethbridge, B.H.Sc.; Israel Liberzon, M.D.; Rodrigo Machado-Vieira, M.D., Ph.D.; Cheri L. Marmarosh, Ph.D.; Luana Marques, Ph.D.; Randi E. McCabe, Ph.D., C.Psych.; Sherri Melrose, Ph.D.; Christina Metcalf, Ph.D.; Allison Metts, M.A.; Alicia E. Meuret, Ph.D.; Laura J. Miller, M.D.; Cristina Montalvo, M.D., M.B.S.; Henry A. Nasrallah, M.D.; Kristin Neff, Ph.D.; Fabiano G. Nery, M.D., Ph.D.; Richard J. Norton, M.A.; Nicholas Ortiz, M.D.; Sydney Parkinson, B.A.; Beth Patterson, M.Sc.; Giampaolo Perna, M.D., Ph.D.; Grace S. Pham, D.O., Ph.D.; Robert M. Post, M.D.; Jessica Rao, M.P.H.; Simon A. Rego, Psy.D., ABPP; Donald J. Robinaugh, Ph.D.; Laina E. Rosebrock, Ph.D.; Donald L. Rosenstein, M.D.; Karen Rowa, Ph.D., C.Psych.; David C. Rozek, Ph.D., ABPP; Ihsan M. Salloum, M.D., M.P.H.; Rebecca L. Schneider, Ph.D.; Natalia Skritskaya, Ph.D.; Jair C. Soares, M.D., Ph.D.; Isabella G. Spaulding, B.S.; David C. Steffens, M.D., M.H.S.; Anne Louise Stewart, M.D.; Stephen M. Strakowski, M.D.; Jong-Woo Suh, B.A., M.A.; Mark Sullivan, M.D.; Amanda J. F. Tamman, M.Sc., Ph.D.; Julia M. Terman, M.A.; Michael Terman, Ph.D.; Tatiana Torti, Psy.D.; Cynthia L. Turk, Ph.D.; Dina Vivian, Ph.D.; Karen Dineen Wagner, M.D., Ph.D.; B. Timothy Walsh, M.D.; Susan W. White, Ph.D.; Anna E. Wise, Ph.D.; Kate Wolitzky-Taylor, Ph.D.; Lauren S. Woodard, B.A.

Preface

Personal Use of This Book

This book primarily informs consumers of mental health services about the types of anxiety, depressive, and related disorders. If you have opened this book, you are probably seeking such information regarding the mental health of yourself or someone you care about. The first step in that process is to find a mental health professional who can provide the appropriate and effective clinical services that this book describes.

Once a provider has been identified, their process begins with assessing and diagnosing the problem for which the person is seeking treatment. At a practical level, correct diagnosis is essential regardless of whether the problem to be addressed is as simple as a basic broken bone or as complex as human behavior and the brain. The best mental health provider in the world, if they are treating the wrong problem, will not provide a viable solution. Although after reading this book it would be inappropriate for you to diagnose yourself or someone you seek to help, you will have a clearer idea of these types of clinical problems and how they might be treated. Then you can better select a competent professional to thoroughly and appropriately assess, diagnose, and treat the disorder with which you are presenting.

Barriers to Treatment

Even with the information in this book in hand, you may still find it difficult to find an appropriate mental health professional. Many significant barriers to treatment exist; first among these is the lack of available mental health providers near you, especially those with the proper training to treat your specific problem(s). Beyond the obvious solution of traveling to the nearest qualified professional, recent studies have shown that receiving evidence-based intervention via telehealth is essentially as effective as "in person" or "face-to-face" care. However, regardless of how you receive ongoing treatment, the initial assessment will likely always be conducted in person with your provider. If, in fact, the most appropriate treatment is medication, you will most likely need to see your prescribing professional in person on an intermittent basis. Sometimes in-person visits also are necessary to obtain laboratory tests to determine the levels of the medicine circulating in your body or to determine whether medical disorders may be contributing to your symptoms. In addition, in-person visits sometimes are necessary to comply with laws for prescribing of certain medications.

Financial costs are a second frequent barrier to treatment. Beyond the cost of traveling to your provider for assessment and treatment, mental health services are expensive for most individuals in society. This is particularly true for care provided by private clinics and clinicians. Fortunately, mental health professionals of all types now are more readily available in community mental health centers, government-supported specialty clinics, and philanthropic clinics, most of which take private insurance or government insurance such as Medicaid or Medicare, at least as partial payment. If you have difficulty locating a needed clinical service, internet searches can help, as can talking with your primary health provider, religious leaders, school counselors (typically, parents can ask for referrals for themselves as well as their children), or trusted friends who may have received treatment for a condition such as those in this book.

Clinical Assessment

Types of Assessment

Almost always, the treatment process begins with an assessment. Sometimes a particular problem might require specific testing, but most commonly the initial assessment is a *semistructured clinical interview*, which means the initial questions asked may be specific to the problems you present. However, over the course of the interview (typically one or two sessions), a range of symptoms or problems likely will be evaluated to ensure that the problem being experienced is the primary problem that needs to be addressed.

Frequently, a clinician may ask you to complete some self-report questionnaires about the symptoms you are experiencing at the time of your first visit or about additional problems uncovered during the interview. Such questionnaires usually contain 20–30 items asking about the behaviors, thoughts, or feelings you may have had during a specified time included in the instructions. For example, with questionnaires about depression, the instructions might ask how often or how much of the time during the past 2 weeks you felt sad, had trouble sleeping, experienced changes in your appetite, had difficulty concentrating or making decisions, and even had thoughts of death. Questionnaires used in the clinical situation have been shown to be stable and reliable indications of the degree of disorder severity; thus, they complement the interview questions and help the clinician understand your perception of the nature and severity of your disorder.

Less frequently, your provider may refer you for laboratory work, such as taking blood (typically from your arm) to determine whether something such as an underactive thyroid is related to your problem. Because many mental health issues may be related to unusual structures or dysregulated functions of certain areas in your brain, neuroimaging may be ordered to determine if some brain dysfunction may be related to your problem. The continuing advances in research and technology mean that, in addition to talking with you about your problem, your provider can use clinically relevant research findings to ensure the treatment they provide matches more specifically with your difficulties. This is referred to as *personalized treatment*, and, in addition to enhancing treatment in many areas of medicine (e.g., cancer, heart disease), it has begun to provide better treatment outcomes in mental health care. At this point in time, however, there may not be a laboratory test that would be useful for the particular problems you are experiencing.

Diagnosis

The mental health professional integrates the information they obtained during the assessment with their own clinical knowledge and experience to arrive at a diagnosis. The combination of assessment and diagnosis allows them to formulate a treatment plan for your specific problem. The diagnostic and classification system currently used in the United States is the *Diagnostic and Statistical Manual of Mental Disorders* (DSM) published by the American Psychiatric Association. The first such manual was published in 1952; a text revision of the DSM's fifth edition was published in 2022. The manual is organized by types of psychiatric and psychological disorders. Among the most frequently diagnosed disorders are anxiety and mood disorders (including major depressive disorder), which occur in approximately 20%–25% of the population at some point in their lives.

Although DSM can be used reliably and usefully by trained mental health professionals, it is important to understand that professional use of assessment procedures and DSM requires years of professional training. While you are reading this book you can get an idea of what might be bothering you; you may be able to identify whether you are experiencing a "diagnosable" level of a mental health disorder and even what the scientific research shows is likely to work best to treat your condition. Nevertheless, this information does not replace the necessity of seeking and receiving professional mental health services for assessment, diagnosis, and treatment. It is risky (if not dangerous) for someone with a disorder to try to use DSM to self-diagnosis their own or someone else's problems. The information in this book will point you in a helpful direction, but it is not intended to give you the detailed and necessary information, knowledge, and skills to make your own diagnosis. Its major purpose is to provide understandable information that will inform your selection of the best mental health professional for you and give you some idea about what types of treatment that professional might recommend to provide relief from your symptoms.

Picking a Mental Health Professional

A wide range of qualified and effective mental health professionals is available to conduct your assessment, diagnosis, and treatment. These include but are not limited to social workers, licensed professional counselors, psychiatrists (a type of physician), clinical psychologists (a type of psychologist), nurse practitioners, and others. It is important to select a licensed or certified professional to ensure you have a qualified provider who is guided by scientific and ethical guidelines. Despite the variety of professionals available, some disorders are best treated by psychiatrists because these disorders are likely to respond to medication or to other somatic treatments that psychiatrists can provide (e.g., schizophrenia and bipolar I [manic-depressive disorder of most severe type]). Even for these disorders, it generally is best if treatment includes an appropriate evidence-based psychotherapy or counseling as well in order to maximize benefit for the person receiving treatment. As you will see by reading this book, mental health treatments have improved in quality and effectiveness over the past few decades, and this has been especially true for treatment of anxiety and mood disorders. Unfortunately, mental health systems and training programs for professionals have not advanced rapidly enough to establish an adequate work force to meet the need for mental health services. However, effective evidence-based treatments for anxiety and mood disorders now exist, and these are becoming increasingly available on a wide-scale basis.

Conclusion

Progress has been made in matching the treatment to the diagnosed problem, although much more work is needed to improve the provision of these best treatments for each person on an individualized basis. Much progress has been made, and it is our hope that by reading this book you will become better informed so that you can find and receive the maximally beneficial treatment for whatever disorder you may be experiencing.

Introduction

Charles B. Nemeroff, M.D., Ph.D.
W. Edward Craighead, Ph.D., ABPP

Mental pain is less dramatic than physical pain, but it is more common and also more hard to bear. The frequent attempt to conceal mental pain increases the burden: it is easier to say "my tooth is aching" than it is to say "my heart is broken."

C.S. Lewis

There is no health without mental health.

Brock Chisholm, First Director–General
of the World Health Organization

This project was launched as the flagship of Dr. Nemeroff's term as president of the Anxiety and Depression Association of America (ADAA). With the full support of the ADAA Board of Directors, we entered into a collaboration with American Psychiatric Association Publishing to provide a user-friendly guide to patients and families seeking a better understanding of the often bewildering world of mental health diagnosis and treatment. We have been professional collaborators and close friends since 1986, so we have together seen the personal, familial, and societal devastation of mental health disorders and, more importantly, the tremendous value of achievable and successful treatment of the variety of problems presented in the chapters that follow. Thus, we undertook developing this book because it was our collaborative professional belief that a book of this nature would serve as a valuable and hope-inducing guide for individuals experiencing mental health problems and their loved ones. We then asked the authors of these brief chapters to write in a manner understandable to the lay public rather than the often jargon-filled prose of academic books and research journals.

The book is divided into six discrete sections. The first is a description of each of the mental health disorders, described in a manner to help patients and families truly understand how mental health professionals arrive at diagnoses. The second section is a brief summary of evidence-based treatment approaches for each disorder. The third is a chapter-by-chapter account of all the U.S. Food and Drug Administration (FDA)-approved medications for the treatment of psychiatric disorders. The fourth section summarizes neuromodulation treatments, including electroconvulsive therapy (ECT) and transcranial magnetic stimulation (TMS). The fifth section is a comprehensive review of all available evidence-based psychotherapies for various conditions, and the final section deals with relatively novel treatments still being investigated, including psychedelics and deep brain stimulation, as well as with special topics, such as inpatient hospitalization, partial hospitalization, and intensive outpatient treatment programs. Chapters on the assessment and treatment of females during pregnancy and the postpartum period and the treatment of children and elderly patients are also addressed. The goal of this book is to provide an easy-to-read guide for patients and families to aid in their decision-making so that they may obtain the optimal treatment in the best setting.

We are grateful to Kelly Puzdrak for her tireless editorial assistance, to the ADAA staff and Board of Directors for supporting the project, and to American Psychiatric Association Publishing for joining us on this journey.

Part I

The Disorders

1

Major Depression

Alan F. Schatzberg, M.D.

Definition

Depression is common and at times disabling for those who experience it. Historically, it was ranked second among disorders causing morbidity worldwide and is now in the number one position. Depression has been described for centuries—if not for millennia—but the classification of the depressive disorders, including major depressive disorder (MDD), and the criteria for diagnosing these disorders are relatively recent. A great deal of early work some 80 or 90 years ago was done in the United Kingdom by research psychiatrists who today are relatively unknown—Mapother, Lewis, and others. Their work was important in demarcating *endogenous* (not caused by external events or consisting of somatic type symptoms) from *nonendogenous* (reacting to events and less physical symptoms), but it was only after the development of usable, codified systems of classification based on specific symptom criteria as seen initially in the third edition of the *Diagnostic and Statistical Manual of Mental Disorders* (known as DSM) published in 1980 by the American Psychiatric Association or the complementary edition of the World Health Organization's *International Classification of Diseases* (ICD) that various psychiatric disorders (including MDD) could be reliably diagnosed. This chapter discusses the diagnosis, classification, hallmark features, and biology and genetics of MDD.

Depression as a disorder goes well beyond sadness, disappointment, or loss. All humans experience depressed mood at some point, but these are generally in response to external, generally negative, events: a student who receives a lower-than-expected grade; someone who is disappointed in relationships; or a child who loses a parent all experience a sense of sadness. However, these are usually transient and remit with positive events or after relatively brief periods of time. When the sadness is accompanied by other symptoms and persists for weeks, however, an episode of clinical depression is often emerging.

How Is Major Depressive Disorder Diagnosed?

The current edition of DSM (DSM-5-TR) includes several depression diagnoses: MDD, dysthymia (chronic mild depression), bipolar I or II depression, and depression associated with physical disorders. MDD is characterized by episodes of depression (i.e., major depressive episode) and is the most common form of a diagnosable depressive disorder. The 1-year prevalence of MDD in the United States is 7%, with a lifetime prevalence of some 17%. The disorder occurs at all ages and is more common in females than in males. In childhood, before puberty, the sexes are equal in prevalence of the disorder. To meet a diagnosis of MDD, patients must meet at least five of nine symptom criteria for at least 2 weeks. These symptoms must include either depressed mood most of the time or loss of interest or pleasure in daily activities, as well as symptoms such as psychomotor retardation (slowness in thinking), change in weight, insomnia or increased guilt, and loss of energy, with at least five criteria being met in total (Table 1–1).

By definition, MDD without a *bipolar* designation is a *unipolar* depression. In other words, a diagnosis of unipolar MDD indicates the patient does not have a history of hypomania or mania that would warrant a diagnosis of bipolar disorder. To meet criteria for a bipolar disorder, the patient must have had an episode of hypomania or mania at some time in the past. Mania and hypomania are the core hallmarks in bipolar I and bipolar II disorders, respectively, and require that patients meet three or four symptom criteria, including grandiosity or decreased need for sleep. A diagnosis of mania requires at least 1 week of symptoms and marked impairment in functioning, hospitalization, or psychotic features. Bipolar II disorder requires at least 4 consecutive days of symptoms and is milder in terms of impairment. Bipolar I and II major depressions are less common than unipolar depression, with current prevalence rates of approximately 1.5%.

The diagnosis of MDD has a number of descriptive qualifiers that either suggest specific subtypes or appear to actually designate a specific subtype. For example, severity of the episode is designated by indicating mild, moderate, or severe. In DSM-IV, published in 1994, the severity dimension was divided into "severe without psychotic features" and "severe with psychotic features." The change in DSM-5 in 2013 reflected accumulation of data that some patients with psychotic features are not necessarily those who demonstrate the most se-

Table 1–1. DSM-5 diagnostic criteria for major depressive episode

A. Five (or more) of the following symptoms have been present during the same 2-week period and represent a change from previous functioning; at least one of the symptoms is either 1) depressed mood or 2) loss of interest or pleasure.

   Note: Do not include symptoms that are clearly attributable to another medical condition.

   1. Depressed mood most of the day, nearly every day, as indicated by either subjective report (e.g., feels sad, empty, hopeless) or observation made by others (e.g., appears tearful). (**Note:** In children and adolescents, this can be irritable mood.)
   2. Markedly diminished interest or pleasure in all, or almost all, activities most of the day, nearly every day (as indicated by either subjective account or observation).
   3. Significant weight loss when not dieting or weight gain (e.g., a change of more than 5% of body weight in a month) or decrease or increase in appetite nearly every day. (**Note:** In children, consider failure to make expected weight gain.)
   4. Insomnia or hypersomnia nearly every day.
   5. Psychomotor agitation or retardation nearly every day (observable by others, not merely subjective feelings of restlessness or being slowed down).
   6. Fatigue or loss of energy nearly every day.
   7. Feelings of worthlessness or excessive or inappropriate guilt (which may be delusional) nearly every day (not merely self-reproach or guilt about being sick).
   8. Diminished ability to think or concentrate, or indecisiveness, nearly every day (either by subjective account or as observed by others).
   9. Recurrent thoughts of death (not just fear of dying); recurrent suicidal ideation without a specific plan; a specific suicide plan; or a suicide attempt.

B. The symptoms cause clinically significant distress or impairment in social, occupational, or other important areas of functioning.

C. The episode is not attributable to the physiological effects of a substance or to another medical condition.

Note: Criteria A–C represent a major depressive episode.

Note: Responses to a significant loss (e.g., bereavement, financial ruin, losses from a natural disaster, a serious medical illness or disability) may include the feelings of intense sadness, rumination about the loss, insomnia, poor appetite, and weight loss noted in Criterion A, which may resemble a depressive episode. Although such symptoms may be understandable or considered appropriate to the loss, the presence of a major depressive episode in addition to the normal response to a significant loss should also be carefully considered. This decision inevitably requires the exercise of clinical judgment based on the individual's history and the cultural norms for the expression of distress in the context of loss.

Table 1–1. DSM-5 diagnostic criteria for major depressive episode *(continued)*

D. The occurrence of the major depressive episode is not better explained by schizoaffective disorder, schizophrenia, schizophreniform disorder, delusional disorder, or other specified and unspecified schizophrenia spectrum and other psychotic disorders.

E. There has never been a manic episode or a hypomanic episode.

Note: This exclusion does not apply if all of the manic-like or hypomanic-like episodes are substance-induced or are attributable to the physiological effects of another medical condition.

Source. From American Psychiatric Association: *Diagnostic and Statistical Manual of Mental Disorders*, 5th Edition, Text Revision. Washington, DC, American Psychiatric Association, 2022.

vere of the core depressive symptoms. It was decided also to redesignate the psychotic features under a separate descriptor.

Common Co-Occurring Mental Health Disorders

MDD commonly occurs with medical disorders such as cardiovascular disease, diabetes, and cancer. The criteria for making a diagnosis of MDD do not change in the face of medical disorders, but care must be taken to delineate some symptoms as to whether they represent depression or the medical disease (e.g., lack of energy or hypersomnia), remembering that the core depressed mood or sadness or inability to experience any pleasure are required symptoms for making an MDD diagnosis. Co-occurrence of MDD in a physical disorder often connotes poorer outcome of the medical disorder. The common co-occurrence is thought to reflect shared inflammatory processes. Studies have demonstrated that MDD is often a risk factor for developing many medical disorders as well as occurring secondary to the medical disorder.

In addition to these subtypes, a number of dimensions are used to further describe a patient's MDD. These modifiers include MDD with anxious distress, mixed features, melancholic features, atypical features, mood-congruent psychotic features, mood-incongruent psychotic features, catatonia, peripartum onset, or seasonal pattern. Physicians are encouraged to use these specifiers, although their adoption has been inconsistent.

Anxious distress requires two of four symptoms: feeling of being keyed up or tense, feeling restless, worry that causes concentration problems, fearing negative events, and feeling a loss of control. It is of particular importance because anxious distress is associated with a poorer response to monotherapy with antidepressants and several combination approaches. In the large-scale Sequenced Treatment Alternatives to Relieve Depression (STAR*D) and the International Study to Predict Optimised Treatment–in Depression (ISPOT-d) studies, MDD in patients who demonstrated anxiety symptoms—but did not necessarily meet full criteria for a comorbid anxiety disorder—responded significantly more poorly to antidepressants and to combinations explored in the STAR*D than did MDD in non-anxious patients. Data from some smaller size studies have shown that adding a benzodiazepine or an atypical antipsychotic (e.g., quetiapine) to a selective serotonin reuptake inhibitor (SSRI) medication produces greater antidepressant effects. Recently, the γ-aminobutyric acid (GABA)-ergic neurosteroids appear effective in patients with the disorder.

The specifier *with melancholic features* is now the moniker for melancholic MDD, and the designation is based largely on a near-complete loss of ability to enjoy pleasure. This is common in hospitalized patients with more severe illness and those with psychotic features. The dimension requires first either loss of pleasure in virtually all activities or a lack of ability to react to pleasurable stimuli and then requires three or more of the typical somatic (or vegetative) depressive features, such as early morning sleep disturbance, diurnal variation (feeling worse in the morning), marked psychomotor retardation, and so on.

Another specifier is *atypical depression*. This designation requires mood reactivity as well as two of the following differentiating symptoms: weight gain, hypersomnia, leaden paralysis, mood reactivity, rejection sensitivity, and others. It has long been thought that these patients preferentially responded to monoamine oxidase inhibitor (MAOI) medications rather than to tricyclic antidepressants (TCAs) or SSRIs, but this latter assertion has not been borne out in clinical trials because depression in patients with this subtype has responded to SSRIs.

Patients who have MDD with psychotic features represent about 18% of current patients with MDD, which translates to a 1-month prevalence of 0.3%–0.4%. Psychotic features often include delusions of guilt, nihilism, paranoia, or somatic illness. These patients often require the addition of an antipsychotic medication to their antidepressant regimen. The *with psychotic features* designation is further subdivided into mood-congruent and mood-incongruent features. *Mood-congruent* represents delusions related to the core themes of depression, such as guilt, nihilism, and death. *Mood-incongruent* refers more toward a less clear-cut depressive misperception, such as frank paranoia that may not reflect deserved punishment or retribution or certain hallucinations. The hallmark biological feature of MDD with psychotic features is increased levels of cortisol, the stress hormone produced in the adrenal gland that acts on the brain.

Catatonia is a nominal descriptor that is largely related to psychotic depression and is uncommonly used in contrast with the psychotic features specifier.

Catatonia is seen in other disorders as well, such as schizophrenia, and appears to respond to benzodiazepines, such as intravenous lorazepam.

There are two dimensions that reflect a temporal dimension to patients with MDD—*with peripartum onset* and *seasonal pattern*. The former refers to onset of MDD during pregnancy or shortly after delivery. Estimates are that 3%–6% of females experience onset during that time frame. GABA-ergic neurosteroids have now been specifically approved for treatment of this disorder (see Chapter 4, "Postpartum Depression and Related Disorders," and Chapter 18, "Treatment of Postpartum Depression and Related Disorders"). *With seasonal pattern* refers to major depressive episodes that occur during certain calendar seasons. These typically are depressions with onset in the fall and winter months, associated with the shortening of daylight hours. The disorder frequently has been treated with the use of light boxes.

There has been considerable interest in exploring other clinical constructs to delineate underlying biological mechanisms as well as to develop new treatments. These are related to the National Institute of Mental Health (NIMH)–sponsored Research Domain Criteria (RDoC) effort to develop agreed-upon, biologically determined clinical pictures for study. One in particular—anhedonic depression—has become the focus of a recent foundation-sponsored international collaboration to elucidate its biology. Anhedonic depression does touch up against MDD with melancholic features; as a symptom, anhedonic depression is seen in patients with depression that is more severe and more treatment refractory. Anhedonia appears to have a functional magnetic resonance imaging (fMRI) signature that can be seen in several disorders in addition to MDD (e.g., borderline personality disorder) and can be used to assess possible treatments. One recent study demonstrated that fMRI signatures as well as patients' anhedonic symptoms were improved by treatment with a kappa antagonist, a nonaddicting opioid agent not yet approved for clinical use.

Finally, data from the ISPOT-d study showed that approximately 28% of participants demonstrated poor cognition, and their depression responded more poorly to monotherapy with SSRIs and serotonin-norepinephrine reuptake inhibitors (SNRIs) than did that in patients without cognitive impairment. Specific antidepressants appear to have procognitive effects, and this area is becoming a focus of new drug development. Cognitive deficits in patients can be diagnosed by performing standard neuropsychological tests.

Are Genetics Involved?

The genetics of MDD are complex or heterogeneous, which indicates that they are likely to involve a large number of genes or underlying biologies. Searches for specific genetic variations in MDD have now yielded a number of genetic variations among large populations of patients with the disorder. These variants can be combined to calculate a polygenic risk score to connote the degree of risk that a person will develop MDD.

A recent meta-analysis revealed that across 10 polygenic methods used, the polygenic risk score explains—at most—3.5% of the variability of MDD. These data suggest that other factors play key roles in connoting risk, such as stress and early childhood abuse or neglect, and point to the involvement of the stress diathesis in the biology of MDD.

Conclusion

MDD is a common disorder with a definable construct of symptoms and other clinical characteristics. Recent years have witnessed renewed interest in potential MDD subtypes with differentiating features (e.g., anhedonia), underlying biologies, and brain imaging markers and potentially genetic markers.

Recommended Reading

Ni G, Zeng J, Revez JA, et al: A comparison of ten polygenic score methods for psychiatric disorders applied across multiple cohorts. Biol Psychiatry 90(9):611–620, 2021 34304866

Otte C, Gold SM, Penninx BW, et al: Major depressive disorder. Nat Rev Dis Primers 2:16065, 2016 27629598

2

Bipolar Disorder

Jessica Batten, PA-C, CAQ-Psych
Jorge R. C. Almeida, M.D., Ph.D.
Stephen M. Strakowski, M.D.

Definition

Bipolar disorder is a brain disease that causes extreme changes in mood, energy, and activity levels. In 1957, Dr. Karl Leonhard coined the term *bipolar* to describe individuals who experienced mania and depression (i.e., two poles) as distinct from those who experienced only depression (i.e., one pole, or *unipolar* depression). Currently, the term *bipolar disorder* includes two diagnoses: bipolar I disorder and bipolar II disorder. These conditions affect around 3% of the population, with equal impact across sex, geography, and ethnic/racial groups.

Bipolar I disorder is defined by the occurrence of mania. *Mania* is an extreme euphoric, expansive, or irritable mood that is accompanied by a marked increase in activation, as well as three or four of the additional symptoms listed in Table 2–1. The symptoms must represent a change in typical behavior, must significantly impair function, and must persist for at least 7 days or require hospitalization. Episodes of depression are not needed for a diagnosis of bipolar I disorder; however, a single manic episode predicts a lifetime course of recurrent manic and depressive episodes in 80% of individuals.

Table 2–1. DSM-5 diagnostic criteria for bipolar disorder

Bipolar I disorder

A. Criteria have been met for at least one manic episode (Criteria A–D under "Manic Episode").

B. The occurrence of the manic and major depressive episode(s) is not better explained by schizoaffective disorder, schizophrenia, schizophreniform disorder, delusional disorder, or other specified or unspecified schizophrenia spectrum and other psychotic disorder.

Manic episode

A. A distinct period of abnormally and persistently elevated, expansive, or irritable mood and abnormally and persistently increased goal-directed activity or energy, lasting at least 1 week and present most of the day, nearly every day (or any duration if hospitalization is necessary).

B. During the period of mood disturbance and increased energy or activity, three (or more) of the following symptoms (four if the mood is only irritable) are present to a significant degree and represent a noticeable change from usual behavior:

   1. Inflated self-esteem or grandiosity.
   2. Decreased need for sleep (e.g., feels rested after only 3 hours of sleep).
   3. More talkative than usual or pressure to keep talking.
   4. Flight of ideas or subjective experience that thoughts are racing.
   5. Distractibility (i.e., attention too easily drawn to unimportant or irrelevant external stimuli), as reported or observed.
   6. Increase in goal-directed activity (either socially, at work or school, or sexually) or psychomotor agitation (i.e., purposeless non-goal-directed activity).
   7. Excessive involvement in activities that have a high potential for painful consequences (e.g., engaging in unrestrained buying sprees, sexual indiscretions, or foolish business investments).

C. The mood disturbance is sufficiently severe to cause marked impairment in social or occupational functioning or to necessitate hospitalization to prevent harm to self or others, or there are psychotic features.

D. The episode is not attributable to the physiological effects of a substance (e.g., a drug of abuse, a medication, other treatment) or to another medical condition.

Bipolar II disorder

A. Criteria have been met for at least one hypomanic episode (Criteria A–F under "Hypomanic Episode") and at least one major depressive episode.

B. There has never been a manic episode.

Table 2–1. DSM-5 diagnostic criteria for bipolar disorder *(continued)*

C. The occurrence of the hypomanic episode(s) and major depressive episode(s) is not better explained by schizoaffective disorder, schizophrenia, schizophreniform disorder, delusional disorder, or other specified or unspecified schizophrenia spectrum and other psychotic disorder.

D. The symptoms of depression or the unpredictability caused by frequent alteration between periods of depression and hypomania cause clinically significant distress or impairment in social, occupation, or other important areas of functioning.

Hypomanic episode

A. A distinct period of abnormally and persistently elevated, expansive, or irritable mood and abnormally and persistently increased goal-directed activity or energy, lasting at least 4 consecutive days and present most of the day, nearly every day.

B. During the period of mood disturbance and increased energy and activity, three (or more) of the symptoms (four if the mood is only irritable) from the prior list for mania have persisted, represent a noticeable change from usual behavior, and have been present to a significant degree.

C. The episode is associated with unequivocal change in functioning that is uncharacteristic of the individual when not symptomatic.

D. The disturbance in mood and the change in functioning are observable by others.

E. The episode is not severe enough to cause marked impairment in social or occupational functioning or to necessitate hospitalization. If there are psychotic features, the episode is, by definition, manic.

F. The episode is not attributable to the physiological effects of a substance (e.g., a drug of abuse, a medication, other treatment).

Source. From American Psychiatric Association: *Diagnostic and Statistical Manual of Mental Disorders*, 5th Edition, Text Revision. Washington, DC, American Psychiatric Association, 2022.

In contrast, bipolar II disorder is defined by hypomania plus a major depressive episode. Hypomanic symptoms are the same as manic symptoms, but although they do represent a change in typical behavior, they are not severe enough to produce significant functional impairment, and they may last a minimum of only 4 days. The criteria for major depression in bipolar disorder are the same as for (unipolar) major depressive disorder.

Some individuals develop *rapid cycling*, defined as four or more distinct affective episodes within a single year. Furthermore, roughly one-half of episodes present as "mixed states," during which depressive and manic symptoms occur simultaneously.

How Is Bipolar Disorder Diagnosed?

Several conditions share symptoms with bipolar disorder, and should be considered before making a diagnosis. Typically, a thorough medical and psychiatric evaluation is required. Common psychiatric illnesses that may be confused with bipolar disorder include major depressive disorder, dysthymia, cyclothymia, schizophrenia, schizoaffective disorder, borderline personality disorder, substance use disorder, and attention-deficit/hyperactivity disorder (ADHD). Head trauma, neurological abnormalities, metabolic diseases, and infection also must be considered, although these are uncommon causes of mania in general.

Risk Factors

Bipolar disorder risk depends primarily on genetic factors (80%–85%) but also on environmental factors (15%–20%). Although the genes and neurofunctional changes predictive of bipolar disorder have yet to be identified, abnormalities in the ventral cortical prefrontal networks, including white matter connectivity, may underlie and predate the illness. Other hypotheses propose that mitochondrial dysfunction, neurotransmitter dysfunction, circadian rhythm dysfunction, and impaired cellular calcium modulation contribute to bipolar disorder risk. Environmental stressors that can precipitate illness in genetically susceptible individuals include trauma, substance abuse, and sleep deprivation.

The presence of certain mood symptoms increases the likelihood of an eventual bipolar diagnosis. For example, depression with early age at onset, psychosis, catatonia, and other atypical symptoms (e.g., hypersomnia instead of insomnia, weight gain instead of weight loss) increase the risk of an emerging bipolar disorder.

Common Co-Occurring Mental Health Disorders

A number of psychiatric conditions occur in patients with bipolar disorder at rates much higher than in the general population. Anxiety disorders, including posttraumatic stress disorder (PTSD), are three to four times more common in bipolar disorder. Co-occurring ADHD affects one-third of adults with bipolar disorder. Significantly higher rates of alcohol, cigarette, illicit drug, and prescription medication misuse have also been observed.

Sadly, individuals with bipolar disorder tend to die from various medical illnesses at younger ages than their unaffected counterparts. Suicide is a major component of this increased risk; up to 15% of individuals with bipolar disorder die from suicide. The second major cause of premature death in bipolar disorder is cardiovascular disease. Individuals with bipolar disorder are two to three times more likely to die prematurely from heart disease than the general population. One major contributor to this statistic is elevated rates of *metabolic syndrome,* a constellation of symptoms—specifically elevated cholesterol, blood pressure, blood sugar, and waist circumference—that increases the risk of heart disease, stroke, and diabetes mellitus type II. Metabolic syndrome is present in up to 50% of individuals with bipolar disorder, a twofold increase over the general population. Correspondingly, diabetes mellitus type II is up to three times more common in patients with bipolar disorder than the general population. Studies suggest that even after controlling for certain risk factors (e.g., psychotropic medications, substance abuse), individuals with bipolar disorder continue to have an increased risk of diabetes mellitus type II and cardiovascular disease. This suggests a possible underlying dysregulation of metabolic, hormonal, or inflammatory processes as part of this condition.

How Bipolar Disorder Starts and Progresses

Bipolar disorder commonly begins in late adolescence and then exhibits progressive shortening of euthymic periods with increasingly frequent mood episodes. Although several treatments decrease the frequency and duration of mood episodes, bipolar disorder is typically a lifelong illness for which there is no known cure. A long-term, large study of bipolar patients supported by the National Institute of Mental Health (NIMH) showed that individuals with bipolar disorder spent 32% of the time with depressive symptoms, compared with 9% of the time with manic symptoms and 6% of the time with mixed symptoms. Overall, bipolar disorder is the sixth leading cause of disability worldwide.

Are Genetics Involved?

A number of genes potentially underlying the expression of bipolar disorder have been identified, including D-amino acid oxidase activator (*DAOA*), brain-derived neurotrophic factor (*BDNF*), disrupted in schizophrenia 1 (*DISC1*), the serotonin transporter (*5HTT*), catechol-*O*-methyl transferase (*COMT*), monoamine oxidase A (*MAOA*), tryptophan hydroxylase (*TPH1*, *TPH2*), ankyrin 3 (*ANK3*), and calcium voltage-gated channel subunit alpha1 C (*CACNA1C*). Accumulating evidence suggests these genetic variations likely interact in combinations, rather than all of these "risk" genes occurring in all people. It is hoped that an increased understanding of the genetic contributions may guide future treatments.

Conclusion

Bipolar disorder is a common psychiatric condition that is associated with unusual shifts in mood, energy, and activity levels. Research to better understand its etiology and its relationships to other physical and mental health conditions is ongoing.

Recommended Reading

Miklowitz D: The Bipolar Disorder Survival Guide: What You and Your Family Need to Know, 3rd Edition. New York, Guilford Press, 2019

Strakowski SM: Bipolar Disorder. New York, Oxford University Press, 2014

3

Dysthymia and Cyclothymia

Muhammad Youshay Jawad, M.B.B.S.
Roger S. McIntyre, M.D., FRCPC

Dysthymia

Case Vignette

Andrea, a 20-year-old college student, came to the clinic after being encouraged by her friends. She begins with a complaint of feeling generally "not happy" for a long time now. She says she gradually moved into an "emotional pitfall" and has been there for some years. She feels "perpetually sad" for no apparent reason and rarely does anything excite her "in a real sense." On further questioning about her psychosocial environment, she says she experiences no chronic stress other than with her usual college quizzes and assignments. When asked about how her sadness manifests, she shares that she does not feel "loved anymore"—not worthy of love, not as intelligent as other girls—and cannot enjoy college as other people around her do. Although she can maintain her grades, her interpersonal relations are declining due to her "persistent low mood." There was not a single day on which the transition from happy to sad began; it was a gradual transformation that has affected her life significantly over the past few years.

Definition

In this patient case, Andrea is experiencing persistent depressive disorder (also known as *dysthymia*). Dysthymia entails low mood along with changes in appetite, sleep, energy, self-esteem, concentration, and hope toward life. The symptoms must persist for at least 2 years (or at least for 1 year in adolescents) to meet the criteria set forth by the *Diagnostic and Statistical Manual of Mental Disorders*, 5th Edition (DSM-5) as shown in Table 3–1.

How Does Dysthymia Start and Progress?

It has been estimated that the prevalence of dysthymia ranges from 1% to 6% among the world's population. The clinical course of dysthymia is significantly longer than that of other acute forms of depression (i.e., major depressive disorder) and can often last several years. Due to the milder and longer presentation of symptoms, individuals with dysthymia are commonly late to present for professional help, which significantly affects their quality of life, overall well-being, and treatment prognosis. Patients with dysthymia are often said to have "sad personalities" by their peers, which adds to their interpersonal strains. These patients often describe their lives as "hollow" or "incomplete" and are often unable to see their lives beyond their "colorless" perspective. Although they may experience periods of normal mood, these usually last only a few days or a few weeks (with a maximum of 2 months). Their chronic low mood makes patients with dysthymia especially susceptible to acute severe depressive episodes, and they often also meet the criteria for major depressive disorder (a combination also known as "double depression") during this period of life.

It has also been found that chronic forms of depression (including dysthymia) follow a greater familial pattern than other acute forms of depression. However, multiple studies have postulated that family environment might be a greater causal factor than family history alone. Predictors of dysthymia include childhood adversity or maltreatment and earlier age at onset of depression (before age 21 years). Furthermore, dysthymia is associated with a greater probability of anxiety and personality disorders. Patients who have had dysthymia for a long time have been known to develop personality traits (e.g., inability to put emotions into words, bodily pains, fatigue, ruminative thoughts, interpersonal attachment problems) that lead to greater impairment and compromised quality of life.

On a neurobiological scale, patients with dysthymia often show dysfunctions across serotonergic, neuroendocrine, and immune systems. Similarly, functional neuroimaging studies in these patients have found stark differences among the various parts of the brain involved in mood, sleep, and cognitive regulation when the results are compared with those of healthy patients. It is important for individuals to seek professional help for this condition because the untreated dysthymic phase increases the risk of suicide, substance use disorder, and failure to remit to normal mood.

Table 3–1. DSM-5 diagnostic criteria for persistent depressive disorder

A. Depressed mood most of the day, more days than not, for at least 2 years

B. At least two of the following six symptoms:
   1. Poor appetite or overeating
   2. Insomnia or hypersomnia
   3. Low energy or fatigue
   4. Low self-esteem
   5. Poor concentration or difficulty making decisions
   6. Hopelessness

C. Never without the symptoms in criteria A and B for more than 2 months at a time

D. Criteria for a major depressive disorder can be continuously present for 2 years

E. No history of mania or hypomania

F. Not better explained by a non-mood psychotic disorder

G. Not due to physiological effects of a substance or another medical condition

H. Symptoms cause pronounced distress or impairment

Source. From American Psychiatric Association: *Diagnostic and Statistical Manual of Mental Disorders*, 5th Edition, Text Revision. Washington, DC, American Psychiatric Association, 2022.

Cyclothymia

Case Vignette

Bradley is a 40-year-old investment banker who has come to the clinic today at the suggestion of his wife. He describes his mood as "constantly changing." Over the past 10 years, he has very frequently experienced "good and bad weeks." During the good weeks, he can work hard, have the energy to come up with new ideas, and go above and beyond his work to uplift his profit goals. During his bad weeks, however, he does not feel like working, has low energy, and feels sad about his "current worth" in the company. His wife has also suggested that he is "more irritable" during some weeks than the others. These cyclical changes have caused him to "work inconsistently," which has now come to higher management's attention. Also, the periodic irritability is putting strain on his marriage.

Definition

The patient in this case is facing *cyclothymia*. Cyclothymia is considered an attenuated form of bipolar II disorder in which the mood changes are comparatively milder and do not meet the DSM criteria for bipolar disorder. However, the cyclical changes are more severe than the normal flow of mood. People with cyclothymia usually have bursts of physical and mental energy helping them to adapt to their work (this is somewhat similar to hypomania but never meets the exact DSM criteria for it). Concurrently, the bad weeks are very similar to persistent depressive disorder and are described as feelings of hopelessness, fatigue, and lack of mental energy. The bursts of energy can also manifest as irritability that can be sensed by people around. These repeated mood changes should be present for at least 2 years in adults and 1 year in adolescents to meet the DSM-5 criteria for cyclothymic disorder (Table 3–2). It must be noted that during this whole period, symptoms are not ever severe enough to meet the criteria for either major depressive disorder or bipolar disorder.

Patients with cyclothymia are often called "impulsive" or "temperamental." Some clinicians consider cyclothymia to be a co-occurring condition with certain personality disorders such as borderline or histrionic. Other consider it to be a part of the bipolar disorder spectrum. Whatever the case, mood dysregulation and reactivity toward the environment are considered the main culprits.

Are Genetics Involved?

Cyclothymia is highly influenced by genetics, with a concordance rate of 57% observed in monozygotic twins. However, the prevalence remains low, with an estimate of approximately 1% of the world's population. Psychological factors in general and early life events in particular influence the pathogenesis of cyclothymic disorder to a great extent. It has been speculated that early-life emotional abuse or neglect can lead to dysfunctional emotional regulation due to the abnormal development of key brain emotional regulatory regions. Emotional dysregulation is thought to be the primary framework behind reactive mood in cyclothymic patients (i.e., feeling euphoric in presence of positive factors and feeling dejected in face of subjective negative factors). The differential diagnosis for someone showing abrupt mood changes includes borderline personality disorder, bipolar disorder, depression with mixed features, and illicit substance use. These diagnoses must be ruled out satisfactorily to meet the criteria for cyclothymia.

Rapid mood changes in cyclothymia can be a predictor of full-blown bipolar disorder episodes down the line. Patients with cyclothymia face difficulties in showing consistency in their personal, professional, and social lives, which is often seen as a major personality drawback. Moreover, reactivity and hypersensitivity to interpersonal emotions can lead to problems with their partners in particular. Cyclothymia also increases the risk for suicide, impulse control disorder, and substance use disorder. Professional help is often needed for patients with cyclothymia to live a normal life with minimal disruption.

Table 3–2. DSM-5 diagnostic criteria for cyclothymic disorder

The patient must meet all six criteria:

A. For at least a 2-year period, there have been episodes of hypomanic and depressive experiences that do not meet the full DSM-5 diagnostic criteria for hypomania or major depressive disorder.

B. The above criteria had been present at least half the time during a 2-year period, with not more than 2 months of symptom remission.

C. There is no history of diagnoses for manic, hypomanic, or a depressive episode.

D. The symptoms in Criterion A cannot be accounted for by a psychotic disorder, such as schizophrenia, schizoaffective disorder, schizophreniform disorder, or delusional disorder.

E. The symptoms cannot be accounted for by substance use or a medical condition.

F. The symptoms cause distress or significant impairment in social or occupational functioning.

Source. Reprinted from American Psychiatric Association: *Diagnostic and Statistical Manual of Mental Disorders*, 5th Edition, Text Revision. Washington, DC, American Psychiatric Association, 2022. Copyright © 2022 American Psychiatric Association. Used with permission.

Conclusion

It is common for people to think of mood changes as inherent parts of personalities rather than acute problems needing proper diagnosis and management. Mental health disorders may vary from mild to severe symptoms. Although people often seek medical help for more severe symptoms, they tend to overlook the milder ones. It is important to identify these milder symptoms on a personal level and to seek mental help in order to stop illness progression and have a better prognosis. Individuals with symptoms that are chronic and milder forms of major depressive disorder (i.e., dysthymia) and bipolar disorder (i.e., cyclothymia) should see a doctor to further analyze and treat their condition and to prevent the development of severe pathologies.

Recommended Reading

GoodTherapy: Persistent Depressive Disorder (Dysthymia). Olympia, WA, GoodTherapy, 2015. Available at: https://www.goodtherapy.org/blog/psychpedia/dysthymia.

Vitche M: Cyclothymia: the rare bipolar disorder type we don't talk about. The Mighty, September 13, 2023. Available at: https://themighty.com/topic/bipolar-disorder/cyclothymia-bipolar-disorder-mild-type.

4

Postpartum Depression and Related Disorders

Lisa Boyars, M.D.
D. Jeffrey Newport, M.D., M.S., M.Div.

Definition

Pregnancy and the postpartum period is a vulnerable time for developing maternal mental illnesses, collectively called *perinatal mood and anxiety disorders* (PMADs). According to the classification scheme of the *Diagnostic and Statistical Manual of Mental Disorders* (DSM), PMADs are not distinct syndromes but instead are perinatal occurrences (or exacerbations) of other generally recognized mental illnesses including depression, bipolar disorder, and anxiety disorders. Left untreated, these disorders can cause devastating consequences for the new or expectant parent, the baby, and the family.

Historical accounts of postpartum mental illness date back thousands of years. This was finally codified in DSM-IV in 1994 with the introduction of the *with postpartum onset* specifier for major depression and other disorders. However, growing awareness that pregnancy also lies within the window of risk for illness led this diagnostic specifier to be updated in 2013 in DSM-5 to *with peripartum onset,* which DSM-5 defines as "occurring during pregnancy as well as in the 4 weeks following delivery." However, a consensus has emerged that the

DSM-5 definition is still too restrictive and that the window of risk for PMADs extends from pregnancy to 6 months after delivery.

Case Vignette

Dr. Smith notes that her pregnant patient, Teresa, is no longer gaining weight as expected as she enters the third trimester. When Dr. Smith raises her concern, Teresa explains that she has had little appetite, being under a lot of stress at work and taking on additional duties to prepare the substitute who will provide coverage during her maternity leave. Despite her husband's assistance, Teresa still feels she is falling behind and letting everyone down. Over the past 2 months, she has felt very down, has had difficulty staying focused at work and at home, wakes up several more times a night than normal, and feels exhausted all the time, even on the weekends when she is able to sleep late. After the birth of her son Miles 2 years ago, she recalls being very depressed and having difficulty bonding with him. She assumed it was normal to feel this way and found this gradually resolved over the year after giving birth.

Perinatal Depression

Undoubtedly, perinatal depression is the most well-known PMAD and may arise as a perinatal depressive episode of major depression or bipolar disorder. Its symptoms are identical to those of major depressive disorder (see Chapter 1, "Major Depression"); nevertheless, diagnosing perinatal depression does present challenges. For example, the so-called neurovegetative symptoms of depression (e.g., sleep disturbance, low energy, appetite or weight changes) are also commonly experienced during a normal pregnancy; thus, careful consideration must be given as to whether such physical symptoms are related to depression or to pregnancy itself. In addition, "baby blues," a brief but normal postpartum mood disturbance, must be distinguished from perinatal depression. Symptoms of baby blues include sadness, irritability, and tearfulness and may be experienced by up to 80% of postpartum females. Baby blues begins within a few days of delivery but, unlike perinatal depression, resolves in a few days.

Postpartum Psychosis

Like perinatal depression, postpartum psychosis (PPP) is not a formal DSM-5 diagnosis. Instead, it appears in DSM-5 as the peripartum onset of a psychotic episode of bipolar disorder, major depression, or brief psychotic disorder. PPP, which is fortunately rare but most often experienced by those with bipolar disorder, develops rapidly, often a few days to a few weeks after birth. It may start with mood changes, including depression, mania, or a mixture of the two, before progressing to psychotic symptoms such as delusions and hallucinations. Other common symptoms of PPP include confusion, paranoia, irritability, and agitation. It is considered a medical emergency because patients are at risk of harming themselves (suicide) or their infant (infanticide).

Perinatal Anxiety and Related Disorders

DSM-5 does not include peripartum diagnostic specifiers for anxiety and other disorders; however, these conditions have received heightened attention in recent years because they may worsen during pregnancy and the postpartum period and thereby compromise patient and child well-being, akin to perinatal depression.

Anxiety during pregnancy and childbirth is often considered a normal phenomenon; therefore, generalized anxiety disorder (GAD) may be underdiagnosed. Perinatally, the hallmark symptom of GAD—excessive worry—is often about the health and safety of the pregnancy or baby. This anxiety may be accompanied by restlessness, fatigue, irritability, difficult concentrating, and sleep disturbance. Childbearing females with perinatal obsessive-compulsive disorder (OCD) may develop intrusive thoughts of harm befalling their baby, including fears that they themselves may harm their own child. However, unlike PPP, such thoughts are unwanted, intrusive, and very disturbing to individuals with perinatal OCD. To counteract this, some patients with perinatal OCD may obsessively check on their baby or delegate infant care to others in order to allay their fears.

Posttraumatic stress disorder (PTSD) may emerge in patients who experience traumatic events during pregnancy or labor such as miscarriage, stillbirth, or severe newborn complications. In addition, those with preexisting PTSD related to a personal history of childhood trauma may experience an exacerbation of PTSD symptoms following the birth of their child. Symptoms of PTSD include intrusive memories, flashbacks, or nightmares of the event, coupled with efforts to avoid reminders of the trauma as well as symptoms of excessive arousal (e.g., exaggerated startle, insomnia). Those who experience a pregnancy loss may not develop PTSD; however, they will invariably experience grief. Grief is a natural response to loss as seen with miscarriage, loss during labor, or early infancy death. Symptoms of grief include longing for the deceased, strong emotional pain, and difficulty engaging with others socially. Although grief can be an expected part of healing, for some the symptoms can turn into prolonged grief disorder, a condition introduced in the 2022 DSM-5 text revision (DSM-5-TR) and discussed in Chapter 14, "Prolonged Grief Disorder," and Chapter 28, "Treatment of Prolonged Grief Disorder."

Risk Factors

The strongest risk factor for developing perinatal depression is a personal history of depression. Only 1% of pregnant patients without a past history of depression will experience perinatal depression; however, 25% of those with any prior history of depression and 50% of those with a prior history of perinatal depression will experience a return of depression during or following their current pregnancy. Individuals who discontinue their antidepressant treatment while pregnant are at especially high risk. Patients with premenstrual syndrome; relationship stressors; a stressful life event, including unplanned or unwanted conception, pregnancy, or newborn complications; or lack of social support or those experiencing abuse or violence (sexual, emotional, or physical) also are at highest risk. Risk factors for other PMADs are similar (Table 4–1).

In addition to these clinical and psychosocial risk factors, there appears to be a subgroup of females for whom abrupt shifts in reproductive hormones, such as those occurring following delivery, can trigger depression, anxiety, and other psychiatric symptoms. This biological vulnerability to PMADs may interact with other risk factors, increasing the risk of illness.

How Is It Treated?

Clinical decision-making for PMADs begins with recognizing that the dangers posed by perinatal mental illness, for both parent and child, are considerable. PMADs have been associated with increased risk of preterm delivery, low birth weight, gestational hypertension, newborn complications, and poorer developmental outcomes for children. In addition, depressed pregnant patients are less likely to attend routine prenatal appointments, have poorer nutrition, and have greater use of prescription opiates, hypnotics, alcohol, tobacco, and other substances. These risks are then weighed against the potential risks of available treatments. The optimal choice minimizes the risk attributable to both the illness and its treatment; consequently, it is important when selecting a treatment to choose one with both a favorable safety profile and a likelihood of being effective.

Conclusion

The perinatal period represents a time of psychological vulnerability. In addition to perinatal depression, other PMADs include diagnoses such as PPP, perinatal anxiety, or PTSD. A personal history of PMADs or preexisting mental

Table 4–1. Risk factors for perinatal mood and anxiety disorders

Postpartum psychosis	Personal or family history of bipolar disorder
	Sleep disruption
	Mood stabilizer discontinuation
	Pregnancy or newborn complications
Perinatal anxiety (generalized anxiety disorder, panic disorder)	Personal or family history of anxiety disorder
	Discontinued anxiety medication
	Lower socioeconomic status
	Less education
	Younger age
	Previous or family history of mental illness
	Pregnancy or newborn complications
	Hyperemesis gravidarum
Perinatal obsessive-compulsive disorder (OCD)	Personal or family history of OCD
	Personal history of depression
	Discontinued OCD medication
	First-time mothers
	Previous or current depression
	Pregnancy or newborn complications
	Hyperemesis gravidarum
Perinatal posttraumatic stress disorder (PTSD)	Traumatic pregnancy outcome
	History of childhood maltreatment or trauma

health illness is often a risk factor for developing a PMAD. When considering treatment options, it is important to weigh the risk of possible pharmacological treatment and also the risks of untreated PMADs.

Recommended Reading

Hyman J, Newport DJ: Management of bipolar disorder during pregnancy and lactation, in The Bipolar Book: History, Neurobiology, and Treatment. Edited by Yildiz A, Ruiz P, Nemeroff CB. New York, Oxford Academic, 2015

Newport DJ, Lanza di Scalea T, Richardson E, et al: Psychopharmacology during pregnancy and lactation, in The American Psychiatric Publishing Textbook of Psychopharmacology, 6th Edition. Edited by Schatzberg AF, Nemeroff CB. Washington, DC, American Psychiatric Association Publishing, 2024, pp 537–598

5

Seasonal Affective Disorder

Julia M. Terman, M.A.
Richard J. Norton, M.A.
Kelly J. Rohan, Ph.D.

Definition

Many people get the "winter blues"—mild to moderate wintertime changes in mood, appetite, sleep length, or energy. This phenomeon is common, especially at northern latitudes where winters are particularly dark. In northern U.S. states (e.g., Washington, Minnesota, Maine, and North Dakota) and Southern Canada, about one in five people experience the winter blues. Unlike the winter blues, however, winter seasonal affective disorder (SAD) is a recognized mental health condition because it includes more severe and distressing symptoms that impair everyday functioning. Winter SAD is a form of clinical depression that regularly occurs in the fall or winter. People can also experience "summer SAD," clinical depression in the summer, but we focus on winter SAD because it is much more common and more widely researched.

How Is Seasonal Affective Disorder Diagnosed?

The symptoms of SAD are the same as those of clinical depression (major depressive disorder) and fall into four general categories: physical, emotional, cognitive, and behavioral. *Physical symptoms* are symptoms people can feel in their bodies, including low energy, significant change in appetite, and feeling physically weighed down or sped up. People with winter SAD most commonly experience an *increase* in appetite, specifically cravings for carbohydrate-rich foods such as starches (e.g., pasta, bread, potatoes) or sugars (e.g., chocolate, candy). *Emotional symptoms* are the feelings that accompany depression, such as sadness and loss of interest. *Cognitive symptoms* involve thought processes, such as negative thoughts about one's self-worth, trouble making decisions, and thinking about death or suicide. *Behavioral symptoms* affect people's actions, such as being less active, socially isolating, sleeping more or fewer hours per day, and eating a lot more or less than usual. People with winter SAD most commonly report *increases* in eating and sleep length (including naps).

In SAD, symptoms of depression tend to develop gradually over a period of days or weeks during seasonal transitions. For example, many people with winter SAD report that their symptoms trickle in as they notice signals of seasonal changes (e.g., fall foliage, end of daylight saving time, winter solstice). During spring and summer, most people with winter SAD return to their "normal" selves without these symptoms, but those with bipolar-type mood disorder may experience elevated mood states (hypomania or mania). If not treated, the annual seasonal pattern of depression can leave people with SAD constantly dreading changes of season.

To qualify for a diagnosis of SAD, patients must meet the diagnostic criteria for major depressive disorder (i.e., they experience several depression symptoms most of the day nearly every day for 2 weeks or longer) during the same season for at least the past 2 years in a row. Across one's lifetime, the seasonal pattern of depression must stand out, with depression occurring during the affected season(s) much more frequently than during other seasons. The person must experience their symptoms as bothersome and as negatively impacting life. Annual depression symptoms that are better explained by "anniversary reactions" (i.e., negative emotions and symptoms around the date marking a negative life event), the "holiday blues" (i.e., feelings of loneliness associated with the holidays), or cyclical stressors that happen to occur seasonally (e.g., regular unemployment in a certain season) are *not* considered SAD. In SAD, the assumed triggers of depression include the shorter day length for winter SAD and the intense heat and humidity for summer SAD. We caution against self-diagnosing SAD and recommend seeking a qualified mental health provider to determine whether there is a seasonal pattern to your symptoms. SAD typically begins in early adulthood, but cases have been reported in children and adolescents. New cases can emerge in people who relocate to a new climate, especially with a substantial change in latitude. Like the sex difference in clinical depression, SAD affects more females than males.

Risk Factors

The causes of SAD remain unknown, but several lines of thinking (hypotheses) have developed. Genetic factors play some role, because people who have a close relative with SAD (or with another type of clinical depression) are more likely to have SAD themselves. No single "SAD gene" has been identified, and multiple different genes each likely contribute risk. A popular theory about winter SAD relates to the biological clock (i.e., a tangle of neurons located in the brain's hypothalamus), which is responsible for regulating daily (or *circadian*) biological rhythms. According to the phase-shift hypothesis, winter SAD is associated with either a slow- or fast-running biological clock in the winter, such that the person's circadian rhythms are out of sync with the light/dark cycle or with their sleep/wake cycle. For example, in response to later dawns, the pineal gland may begin to release the hormone of darkness, melatonin, very late at night, which contributes to difficulty falling asleep, and may stop releasing melatonin very late in the morning, which contributes to difficulty waking up. This example represents a mismatch between the person's "biological night" (when melatonin is released) and the times they need to be asleep and awake to function properly—in this case, a slow-running biological clock (a *circadian phase delay*). Another hypothesis suggests that people with winter SAD are like photoperiodic mammals, those that track seasonal changes in the day-night cycle to determine when to hibernate, breed, and forage for food. This theory proposes that people with SAD have a unique biological signal of season (evidenced by a longer duration of melatonin release at night in the winter than in summer) contributing to their symptoms. Another theory proposes that people with winter SAD have retinas that are subsensitive to light, meaning their retinas do not compensate for lower light availability in the winter, contributing to their symptoms.

How Is It Treated?

Three treatments are effective for treating SAD: antidepressant medication, light therapy, and cognitive-behavioral therapy for SAD (CBT-SAD).

Antidepressant Medication

As with other types of clinical depression, antidepressant medications, such as the selective serotonin reuptake inhibitors (SSRIs), can help reduce SAD symptoms. Only one antidepressant medication, bupropion hydrochloride XL (extended release), has received U.S. Food and Drug Administration (FDA) approval for the prevention of winter SAD when it is taken before symptoms typically start.

Light Therapy

Clinical trials from around the world support the use of light therapy—timed daily exposure to bright artificial light—as an effective treatment for winter SAD. Light therapy is a cottage industry, and many products on the market claim to improve SAD. Light therapy devices most widely tested and supported in clinical trials for SAD emit 10,000 lux of full-spectrum or cool-white fluorescent light behind an ultraviolet screen to filter out harmful ultraviolet rays and have a surface area large enough such that the full dose of light reaches the user's retinas even if they slightly move their head. Note that 10,000 lux is much brighter than regular household lighting but is not nearly as bright as can be obtained outside on a clear summer day. Clinical guidelines for light therapy recommend consistent (daily) use during the affected seasons to achieve benefit. There is no "one-size-fits-all" light therapy prescription for the duration (number of minutes per day) and timing (specific time[s] of day) one needs in order to benefit from the treatment. Thirty minutes first thing in the morning upon waking is a common starting light therapy dose in clinical trials for winter SAD, with later adjustment based on individual response and side effects.

Mental health provider oversight is essential to tailor the prescription to the person and maximize benefit while minimizing side effects. Providers can also inform the selection of an effective light therapy device and the correct positioning and distance required. Side effects of light therapy tend to be mild and diminish with increased tolerance; these include headaches, eye strain, feeling wired, and changes in sleep such as difficulty falling asleep or waking up earlier than desired. Serious side effects to light therapy include mania/hypomania (especially in people with bipolar disorder) and increased thoughts of suicide. Ideally, light therapy practitioners will have expertise in *chronotherapeutics*, the field concerned with administering treatments to affect the body's circadian rhythms.

Limitations of light therapy include that it must be resumed every year during the affected months and that the regimen may require people to wake up earlier than they prefer to complete sessions before other daily responsibilities. Portable light therapy glasses have the potential to overcome the burden associated with stationary light therapy use, but their effectiveness for SAD is uncertain because they are currently in early testing phases.

Cognitive-Behavioral Therapy

CBT is a psychotherapy (talk therapy) that has been used to treat clinical depression for more than 50 years. It focuses on changing patterns of thoughts and behaviors that contribute to depression. CBT-SAD is a form of CBT specifically adapted to winter SAD and is the only psychotherapy intervention to date with research studies to support its effectiveness for SAD. In CBT-SAD, individuals learn to recognize their SAD symptoms early on, identify and schedule enjoyable wintertime activities, and think more flexibly and positively about things in general and the winter season specifically. One benefit of CBT-SAD is learning coping strategies that may be used to prevent future SAD episodes. Clinical trials suggest that people treated with CBT-SAD are less likely to experience future episodes of winter depression after treatment compared with those initially treated with light therapy.

Conclusion

SAD overlaps substantially with nonseasonal depression in many symptoms, risk factors, and effective treatment options. SAD is unique for its predictable seasonal pattern, which provides an opportunity for early detection, treatment, and prevention during seasonal transitions. Mental health providers can help determine the optimal treatment or combination of treatments for a particular individual with SAD.

Recommended Reading

Partonen T, Pandi-Perumal SR: Seasonal Affective Disorder: Practice and Research, 2nd Edition. New York, Oxford University Press, 2009

Rosenthal NE: Defeating SAD (Seasonal Affective Disorder): A Guide to Health and Happiness Through All Seasons. New York, G&D Media, 2023

6

Posttraumatic Stress Disorder

Amanda J. F. Tamman, M.Sc., Ph.D.
Israel Liberzon, M.D.
Josh M. Cisler, Ph.D.

Definition

Case Vignette

Brooke is a 16-year-old female who was sexually assaulted by a male peer at a party 6 months ago. Ever since the event, her teachers and parents notice that she starts to "blank out," seeming preoccupied and needing things to be repeated. She also appears very tired during the day, reporting to her parents that she has been having bad dreams. Brooke, who was previously social with a small but trusted circle of friends, started to withdraw and has become cautious and distrustful of others. She is quieter, sits alone during lunchtime, and has stopped attending an afterschool art club. Brooke's parents notice that she has become very fearful about going out at night, for instance, refusing to go out for dinner with her friends or parents, particularly on cooler nights that resemble the night of the assault. Whereas Brooke was previously excited about applying for out-of-state colleges, she has stopped planning for college and her future and expresses a lack of confidence in her ability to keep herself safe if she leaves home.

> Teachers have noticed that Brooke appears more edgy than before, becoming jumpy at the slightest noise and looking around the room and behind her persistently. Although she was previously cooperative with teachers and performed well in school, her grades have declined, and teachers have noted she is increasingly irritable and is engaging in self-destructive behaviors, such as smoking during recess, that are out of character for her.

Posttraumatic stress disorder (PTSD) develops in some people in response to traumatic events. PTSD has a lifetime prevalence of about 8%. In news and popular culture, PTSD is often described in veterans who have experienced combat trauma. However, it can also develop in response to other types of traumas, including rape, assault, child abuse, natural disasters, and witnessing domestic violence. We call these severe types of traumas "Criterion A" traumas, in which people are exposed to threat of death, serious injury, or sexual violence or witness such injury to others (Table 6–1).

Four clusters of symptoms are experienced by people with PTSD. The first cluster is *intrusion symptoms,* in which people have repetitive, painful thoughts or memories of the trauma that come into their minds without them wanting to remember the event. These memories often cause people to feel emotionally upset and experience uncomfortable physical symptoms. Sometimes, people can even experience the trauma as if it is happening *right now* in what is known as a "flashback."

The second cluster is *avoidance symptoms.* Because these memories are so painful, people often want to avoid thoughts and reminders of the trauma. They may go out of their way to distract themselves or to prevent these memories from coming into their mind by avoiding things that often trigger the trauma.

The third cluster is *negative alterations in cognitions and mood.* These are negative thoughts and feelings that come about or get worse after the trauma. Because trauma can change how one feels about oneself and the world they live in, trauma can shift the lens through which we view the world. For instance, individuals may start blaming themselves for what happened or begin seeing the world or others as always extremely dangerous and untrustworthy. People often describe low mood, losing interest in activities, and feeling very distant and cut off from people. This is an understandable response to trauma, because trauma can make it difficult to trust others, and people exposed to trauma can have the isolating perception that no one else will understand this experience.

The fourth symptom cluster is *alterations in arousal and reactivity.* People with PTSD can find that they are on edge, constantly watching for the next sign of danger (called *hypervigilance*), and becoming more easily scared, jumpy, and startled than they had been previously. This hypervigilance can be extremely distracting and can undermine their ability to concentrate on other things that are important to them. It can also be difficult to sleep properly.

Table 6–1. DSM-5 diagnostic criteria for posttraumatic stress disorder

Cluster	Criterion
A. Exposure	Exposure to actual or threatened death, serious injury, or sexual violence in one (or more) of the following ways: 1. Directly experiencing the traumatic event(s). 2. Witnessing, in person, the event(s) as it occurred to others. 3. Learning that the traumatic event(s) occurred to a close family member or close friend. In cases of actual or threatened death of a family member or friend, the event(s) must have been violent or accidental. 4. Experiencing repeated or extreme exposure to aversive details of the traumatic event(s) (e.g., first responders collecting human remains; police officers repeatedly exposed to details of child abuse).
B. Intrusion symptoms	Presence of one (or more) of the following intrusion symptoms associated with the traumatic event(s), beginning after the traumatic event(s) occurred: 1. Recurrent, involuntary, and intrusive distressing memories of the traumatic event(s). 2. Recurrent distressing dreams in which the content and/or affect of the dream are related to the traumatic event(s). 3. Dissociative reactions (e.g., flashbacks) in which the individual feels or acts as if the traumatic event(s) were recurring. (Such reactions may occur on a continuum, with the most extreme expression being a complete loss of awareness of present surroundings.) 4. Intense or prolonged psychological distress at exposure to internal or external cues that symbolize or resemble an aspect of the traumatic event(s). 5. Marked physiological reactions to internal or external cues that symbolize or resemble an aspect of the traumatic event(s).

Table 6–1. DSM-5 diagnostic criteria for posttraumatic stress disorder *(continued)*

Cluster	Criterion
C. Avoidance symptoms	Persistent avoidance of stimuli associated with the traumatic event(s), beginning after the traumatic event(s) occurred, as evidenced by one or both of the following: 1. Avoidance of or efforts to avoid distressing memories, thoughts, or feelings about or closely associated with the traumatic event(s). 2. Avoidance of or efforts to avoid external reminders (people, places, conversations, activities, objects, situations) that arouse distressing memories, thoughts, or feelings about or closely associated with the traumatic event(s).
D. Negative alterations in cognition and mood	Negative alterations in cognitions and mood associated with the traumatic event(s), beginning or worsening after the traumatic event(s) occurred, as evidenced by two (or more) of the following: 1. Inability to remember an important aspect of the traumatic event(s) (typically due to dissociative amnesia and not to other factors such as head injury, alcohol, or drugs). 2. Persistent and exaggerated negative beliefs or expectations about oneself, others, or the world (e.g., "I am bad," "No one can be trusted," "The world is completely dangerous," "My whole nervous system is permanently ruined"). 3. Persistent, distorted cognitions about the cause or consequences of the traumatic event(s) that lead the individual to blame themself or others. 4. Persistent negative emotional state (e.g., fear, horror, anger, guilt, or shame). 5. Markedly diminished interest or participation in significant activities. 6. Feelings of detachment or estrangement from others. 7. Persistent inability to experience positive emotions (e.g., inability to experience happiness, satisfaction, or loving feelings).

Table 6–1. DSM-5 diagnostic criteria for posttraumatic stress disorder *(continued)*

Cluster	Criterion
E. Alterations in arousal and reactivity	Marked alterations in arousal and reactivity associated with the traumatic event(s), beginning, or worsening after the traumatic event(s) occurred, as evidenced by two (or more) of the following: 1. Irritable behavior and angry outbursts (with little or no provocation), typically expressed as verbal or physical aggression toward people or objects. 2. Reckless or self-destructive behavior. 3. Hypervigilance. 4. Exaggerated startle response. 5. Problems with concentration. 6. Sleep disturbance (e.g., difficulty falling or staying asleep or restless sleep).
F. Duration	Criteria B, C, D, and E occurring for more than 1 month
G. Distress/Impairment	The disturbance causes clinically significant distress or impairment in social, occupational, or other important areas of functioning.
H. Attribution	The disturbance is not attributable to the physiological effects of a substance (e.g., medication, alcohol) or another medical condition.
Specify whether: **with dissociative symptoms**	Criteria are met for PTSD in addition to persistent or recurring symptoms of either of the following: **Depersonalization:** Persistent or recurrent experiences of feeling detached from, and as if one were an outside observer of, one's mental processes or body (e.g., feeling as though one were in a dream; feeling a sense of unreality of self or body or of time moving slowly). **Derealization:** Persistent or recurrent experiences of unreality of surroundings (e.g., the world around the individual is experienced as unreal, dreamlike, distant, or distorted).
Specify whether: **delayed expression**	If full diagnostic criteria are not met until 6 months after the event.

Source. Adapted from American Psychiatric Association: *Diagnostic and Statistical Manual of Mental Disorders*, 5th Edition, Text Revision. Washington, DC, American Psychiatric Association, 2022.

Most people who experience trauma develop these symptoms in the days and weeks after the event but naturally recover because these symptoms are our bodies' way of trying to keep us safe after being exposed to danger. However, these symptoms can persist into environments that are, for the most part, safe, thus limiting one's ability to function properly. For this reason, PTSD is defined as these symptoms lasting for *more than a month*. When these symptoms persist, they can cause a lot of problems, disrupt our work and relationships, and prevent us from living the type of life we want to live.

Risk Factors

The key risk factors for developing PTSD tend to fall into three categories: pre-trauma characteristics of the individual, characteristics of the trauma, and post-trauma characteristics of the environment. Some people are more at risk for developing PTSD following a traumatic event. Factors that increase one's risk of developing PTSD include having a history of mood or anxiety disorders. For example, someone who has struggled with depression in the past may be more likely to develop PTSD when faced with a traumatic event. People with female sex assigned at birth are more likely to develop PTSD than those with male sex assigned at birth, even if they are exposed to similar trauma. People who have previously gone through traumatic events are also at greater risk of developing PTSD following a new trauma. Indeed, the risk for PTSD increases with each traumatic event exposure. For example, the likelihood of developing PTSD following a fifth traumatic event is much higher than the likelihood of developing PTSD following the first traumatic event. Similarly, traumas that occur during childhood, including sexual abuse, emotional abuse and neglect, and physical abuse and neglect, are a notable risk factor for PTSD. Individuals who experienced these forms of early-life trauma tend to experience more traumas across their lifetime and are more likely to develop symptoms associated with complex PTSD (discussed in the next section), resulting in more comorbidity and resistance to treatment.

Some types of traumatic events also lead to different risk for developing PTSD. Interpersonal traumas, such as being physically or sexually assaulted, tend to carry a higher risk for developing PTSD than non-interpersonal traumas, such as car accidents and natural disasters. Traumatic events that lead to a physical injury or in which the individual perceived a life threat also tend to carry greater risk for PTSD. Experiencing dissociation during the traumatic event, such as a sense of unreality or disconnectedness from one's experience, also tends to lead to greater risk for PTSD.

Finally, factors in the environment during the time of the traumatic event or shortly after can influence the likelihood of developing PTSD. Having greater social support during or shortly following the traumatic event is associated with less likelihood of developing PTSD. Receiving evidence-based treatments, such as prolonged exposure, within the first few weeks following the trauma can reduce the likelihood of developing PTSD. However, receiving some treatments can increase the likelihood of developing the disorder. For example, taking benzodiazepines or undergoing critical incident stress debriefing shortly after experiencing a trauma might not be beneficial and may even be harmful for some people. Thus, individuals should make sure they receive evidence-based care from a qualified professional after exposure to a traumatic event.

Common Co-Occurring Mental Health Disorders

Individuals with PTSD often meet criteria for other mental health disorders as well. The most common mental health disorders that co-occur with PTSD include major depressive disorder, anxiety disorders, and substance use disorders. For example, someone with PTSD might also develop fear of having panic attacks and begin to avoid situations that might trigger those attacks in addition to experiencing the symptoms of PTSD mentioned earlier. Although less common, PTSD can also co-occur with other mental health disorders such as schizophrenia and bipolar disorder.

There are many reasons why PTSD commonly co-occurs with other mental health disorders. One reason is simply that there is symptom overlap between PTSD and other mental health disorders. For example, loss of interest in activities, sleep problems, irritability, and problems concentrating are symptoms of both major depressive disorder and PTSD. A second reason is that an individual may develop symptoms of another mental health disorder as a means of coping with or trying to manage symptoms of PTSD. For example, individuals may use substances such as alcohol or cannabis to reduce the persistent hyperarousal associated with PTSD, which in turn leads to excessive drinking or cannabis use and ultimately the development of a substance use disorder. A third reason for comorbidity is the shared neurobiological pathways between PTSD and other mental health disorders. For instance, trauma exposure and PTSD are associated with changes in neurocircuitry pathways that overlap with other anxiety disorders; as such, the development of PTSD through these neurocircuitry pathways then makes developing these related anxiety disorders more likely.

A fourth factor contributing to comorbidity in PTSD is the concept of complex PTSD (CPTSD). *Complex PTSD* refers to a distinct "type" of PTSD marked by specific developmental, interpersonal, and co-occurring symptom patterns that result in a more complicated symptom profile and resistance to treatment. Individuals with CPTSD tend to have experienced trauma early in life that was both chronic and included multiple forms of interpersonal trauma (e.g., emotional abuse, sexual abuse, and physical abuse). In addition to the symptoms of PTSD noted earlier, these patients also tend to have significant interpersonal difficulties (e.g., difficulties with trust, intimacy, and excessive negative beliefs about other people) and problems regulating their emotions. Individuals with CPTSD often also meet criteria for personality disorders, such as borderline personality disorder. Consistent with the idea of this diagnosis as a distinct type of PTSD with its own unique treatment needs, individuals with CPTSD often benefit from modified forms of treatment that focus on skill building in emotion regulation and interpersonal skills prior to beginning more standard forms of treatment.

Recommended Reading

National Institute of Mental Health: Post-traumatic stress disorder, in Mental Health Information: Health Topics. Bethesda, MD, National Institute of Mental Health, 2023. Available at: https://www.nimh.nih.gov/health/topics/post-traumatic-stress-disorder-ptsd.

U.S. Department of Veterans Affairs: PTSD: National Center for PTSD, in What Is PTSD: PTSD Basics. Washington, DC, U.S. Department of Veterans Affairs, 2023. Available at: https://www.ptsd.va.gov/understand/what/ptsd_basics.asp.

7

Social Anxiety Disorder

Allison Metts, M.A.
Kate Wolitzky-Taylor, Ph.D.

Definition

Social anxiety disorder, also known as *social phobia*, is one of the most common anxiety disorders, with around 12% of people experiencing this disorder at some point during their lifetimes. The main feature of social anxiety disorder is consistently feeling afraid in social situations or avoiding social situations due to fear or anxiety. At the core of social anxiety disorder, people are afraid of receiving negative judgment and evaluation from others, feeling embarrassed or humiliated, or offending others. Physical symptoms might occur when faced with social situations for some people, including blushing, trembling, or sweating. Table 7–1 displays criteria that need to be met for a social anxiety disorder diagnosis.

Common social situations that individuals with social anxiety disorder avoid or endure with distress include meeting unfamiliar people, initiating conversations, performing in front of others, and being observed by others (e.g., being observed while eating, writing). If the feared situation is limited to public speaking or performing, a "performance only" subtype is specified. This subtype would be given if the performance fear impairs the individual's professional life, school life, or other role that requires public speaking. Public speaking fear is thought to be the most common type of fear, affecting around 15%–30% of people. If individuals are afraid of or avoid multiple types of social situations, they would be considered to have *generalized social phobia*, which means social anxiety occurs in various types of social situations.

Avoidance, or intense fear, of social situations can negatively impact quality of life and important areas in the lives of individuals with social anxiety disorder. Consider the case that follows.

Case Vignette

Fiona is a 19-year-old female in her freshman year in college. Fiona spends most of her time alone and has struggled to make new friends in college. She fears that she may be rejected if she reaches out to classmates to initiate friendships. Despite having excellent grades in high school, Fiona's grades in college have been low. Fiona's anxiety prevents her from asking questions in her seminars, attending office hours, or joining study groups. Fiona also avoids classes on presentation days.

From Fiona's case, it is clear that social anxiety disorder can interfere in the social and school domains of her life.

How Is Social Anxiety Disorder Diagnosed?

Most cases of social anxiety disorder develop in childhood or adolescence and are diagnosed in adolescence and early adulthood. To diagnose social anxiety disorder, individuals must meet specific criteria (see Table 7–1). It is important to distinguish social anxiety disorder from other anxiety disorders, which can be done by assessing the thoughts and beliefs that accompany the individual's anxiety (e.g., a concern about embarrassment or fear of negative evaluation being the reason why a person is afraid of, or avoiding, the situation). In order to distinguish social anxiety, other disorders or causes must be ruled out, including other anxiety disorders, other psychiatric diagnoses, more normative emotional experiences, or medical conditions that may explain the presenting symptoms.

Common psychiatric diagnoses that are considered in the process of diagnosing social anxiety disorder include agoraphobia, panic disorder, generalized anxiety disorder, separation anxiety disorder, specific phobias, body dysmorphic disorder, delusional disorder, major depressive disorder, or personality disorder. In children, other psychiatric conditions considered in the diagnostic process include selective mutism, autism spectrum disorder, and oppositional defiant disorder. One common and normal emotional experience that is considered when diagnosing social anxiety disorder is shyness. Medical conditions may be considered as well, including obesity and Parkinson's disease. Because comorbidity is so common in social anxiety disorder, diagnosing the disorder is more often about assigning more than one diagnosis and prioritizing among these diagnoses to ensure adequate clinical care.

Table 7–1. DSM-5 diagnostic criteria for social anxiety disorder

A. Fear of social situation(s) in which the individual is exposed to possible scrutiny from others.

B. Fear of negative evaluation in response to behaviors or anxiety symptoms.

C. The social situation almost always provokes fear or anxiety.

D. Social situations are avoided or endured with intense fear or anxiety.

E. The fear or anxiety is out of proportion to the actual threat posed by the social situation and to sociocultural context.

F. The fear, anxiety, or avoidance is persistent (lasts at least 6 months).

G. The fear, anxiety, or avoidance causes clinically significant distress or impairment in important areas of functioning (e.g., social, occupational).

H. The fear, anxiety, or avoidance is not attributable to physiological effects of a substance or another medical condition.

I. The fear, anxiety, or avoidance is not better explained by symptoms of another mental disorder.

J. The fear, anxiety, or avoidance is clearly unrelated or excessive if another medical condition is present.

Source. From American Psychiatric Association: *Diagnostic and Statistical Manual of Mental Disorders*, 5th Edition, Text Revision. Washington, DC, American Psychiatric Association, 2022.

An important diagnostic question a clinician might ask is: "what are you afraid will happen?" This can help to distinguish social anxiety from other anxiety disorders. If the fear in the social situation (e.g., a crowded party) is exclusively about having a panic attack and the consequences of that panic attack, then a diagnosis of panic disorder might be more appropriate (if other criteria are also met). However, if the person is afraid people at the party will think they are stupid or boring, that would indicate a diagnosis of social anxiety disorder would be more likely (even if that fear resulted in a panic attack, which could occur in any anxiety disorder). It is also possible that individuals may be so afraid of negative evaluation at the party that they become afraid they will have a panic attack and then *also* fear that the panic attack will lead to negative consequences. In this case, this individual may have social anxiety disorder *and* panic disorder.

Risk Factors

Temperamental risk factors (i.e., relating to a person's nature) for social anxiety disorder that make an individual susceptible to this disorder include an underlying fear of evaluation or the tendency to react with nervousness in new situations (known as *behavioral inhibition*). Behavioral inhibition is a genetic risk factor for social anxiety disorder. A trait called *rejection sensitivity*, or the propensity to experience distress in response to a negative evaluation or social rejection, is also associated with developing social anxiety disorder.

Environmental factors that increase one's risk of developing social anxiety disorder include stressful life events and maltreatment during childhood. In addition, some research suggests that peer victimization (i.e., being the victim of bullying) during childhood and adolescence can put someone at risk for developing social anxiety disorder.

Interactions between genetic and environmental factors also elevate the risk for social anxiety disorder. For example, children who inherit the trait of behavioral inhibition may also be more likely to be influenced by their environments, such as learning from and imitating anxious behaviors from their parents. However, research on gene and environment interactions has produced mixed results. Social anxiety disorder is heritable, although the performance-only subtype is less so. This heritability is thought to be due to the interaction between factors specific to social anxiety, such as fear of scrutiny, and more general factors, such as a tendency toward negative emotions.

Common Co-Occurring Mental Health Disorders

Approximately 70%–80% of individuals with social anxiety disorder also meet criteria for other disorders. Comorbidity in individuals with social anxiety disorder is often associated with more severe impairment. It is more common in individuals who have a wide range of social fears as opposed to those with the performance-only subtype. Social anxiety disorder often precedes the onset of other anxiety disorders, with the exception of specific phobia and separation anxiety disorder. Social anxiety disorder also co-occurs with major depressive disorder, often because of social isolation. Because substance use may be employed to self-medicate in instances of experiencing social fears, substance use disorders are commonly co-occurring disorders. Social anxiety disorder can also co-occur with body dysmorphic disorder, bipolar disorder, and avoidant personality disorder. Social anxiety disorder in children can often co-occur with autism spectrum disorder and selective mutism.

How Social Anxiety Disorder Starts and Progresses

Social anxiety disorder is nearly twice as common among females than among males. Sex differences also exist regarding common fears and co-occurring disorders. Specifically, females are more likely to experience social fears and to have co-occurring depression, bipolar disorder, or other anxiety disorders. Males are more likely to experience fears related to dating and using the restroom in front of others as well as have comorbid oppositional defiant disorder, conduct disorder, or substance use disorders.

In terms of age differences, social anxiety disorder comorbidities often depend on age. Specifically, social anxiety disorder often co-occurs with autism spectrum disorder in children, whereas a broader array of comorbid diagnoses, including depression, are more likely to co-occur with social anxiety disorder in adolescents or adults.

Are Genetics Involved?

Approximately one-third of social anxiety disorder is attributable to genetics. First-degree relatives of individuals with the disorder are two to six times more likely to experience it themselves. Thus, parents who are aware of social anxiety within their families may want to be particularly sensitive to the social anxiety tendencies in their children and a potential need for treatment. Genetic influence generally occurs at the trait level, such as behavioral inhibition, but it may be related to factors that are specific to social anxiety disorder, such as a fear of evaluation from others.

Conclusion

In sum, social anxiety disorder is one of the most common anxiety disorders and is typically diagnosed in adolescence or young adulthood. The hallmark feature of social anxiety disorder is feeling fearful in social situations or avoiding social situations due to anxiety. There are a variety of risk factors for this disorder, including those that are temperamental, environmental, and genetic in nature. Social anxiety disorder will often co-occur with other mental disorders, which may vary depending on sex and age.

Recommended Reading

Heimberg R: Social anxiety disorder, in Clinical Handbook of Psychological Disorders: A Step-by-Step Treatment Manual, 5th Edition. Edited by Barlow DH. New York, Guilford Press, 2014

Stein MB, Stein DJ: Social anxiety disorder. Lancet 371(9618):1115–1125, 2008 18374843

8

Obsessive-Compulsive Disorder

Reilly Kayser, M.D.
H. Blair Simpson, M.D., Ph.D.

Definition

Obsessive-compulsive disorder (OCD) is a mental illness that affects around 2% of people, making it more common than schizophrenia. As the name suggests, people with OCD experience two types of symptoms: obsessions and compulsions. *Obsessions* are intrusive, unwanted thoughts, images, or impulses that are difficult to control and cause anxiety, disgust, or discomfort. *Compulsions* are repetitive actions or mental rituals that a person does, often in response to their obsessions. Although most people have unwanted thoughts or repeat certain behaviors from time to time, in OCD, these symptoms are distressing, can take hours each day, and interfere with their ability to do the things they care about. A full list of the criteria for OCD according to the *Diagnostic and Statistical Manual for Mental Disorders*, 5th Edition (DSM-5) is shown in Table 8–1. These are the criteria a clinician uses to make a diagnosis of OCD.

When many people think about OCD, they imagine someone who worries about illness or germs and spends hours cleaning their home or washing their hands. Although it is true that many people with OCD have fears about contam-

Table 8–1. DSM-5 diagnostic criteria for obsessive-compulsive disorder

Criterion	Symptom criteria
A	Presence of obsessions, compulsions, or both **Obsessions** are defined by 1. Recurrent and persistent thoughts, urges, or images that are experienced, at some time during the disturbance, as intrusive and unwanted and that in most individuals cause marked anxiety or distress. 2. The individual attempts to ignore or suppress such thoughts, urges, or images or to neutralize them with some other thought or action (i.e., by performing a compulsion). **Compulsions** are defined by 1. Repetitive behaviors (e.g., hand washing, ordering, checking) or mental acts (e.g., praying, counting, repeating words silently) that the individual feels driven to perform in response to an obsession or according to rules that must be applied rigidly. 2. The behaviors or mental acts are aimed at preventing or reducing anxiety or distress or preventing some dreaded event or situation; however, these behaviors or mental acts are not connected in a realistic way with what they are designed to neutralize or prevent or are clearly excessive.
B	The obsessions or compulsions are time consuming (e.g., take more than 1 hour per day) or cause clinically significant distress or impairment in social, occupational, or other important areas of functioning.
C	The obsessive-compulsive symptoms are not attributable to the physiological effects of a substance (e.g., a drug of abuse, a medication) or another medical condition.
D	The disturbance is not better explained by the symptoms of another mental disorder.

Source. Adapted from American Psychiatric Association: *Diagnostic and Statistical Manual of Mental Disorders*, 5th Edition, Text Revision. Washington, DC, American Psychiatric Association, 2022.

ination and engage in cleaning or washing rituals, these represent just one of several different themes of OCD symptoms that can occur. For example, other common obsessions and associated compulsions include fears about unintentionally harming a loved one; a need to know or remember certain information, which may lead to re-reading, rewriting, or retracing one's steps; or a disturbing sense that something is not "just right." Common compulsions in people with

Table 8–2. Common obsessive-compulsive disorder symptom types

Dimension	Example of obsession	Example of compulsion
Contamination/ Washing	"I will get sick because I touched that contaminated surface."	Excessive bathing, showering, hand washing
Violent/Harm	"I may have poisoned my children because I was not careful enough while cooking dinner."	Mentally reviewing the recipe followed, asking the children repeatedly if they feel okay
Symmetry/ Ordering	"Something about my desk just feels 'off.' I can't stop thinking about it!"	Repeatedly realigning objects on the desk until it feels "just right."
Unacceptable/ Taboo	Intrusive sexual thoughts about children that are unwanted and distressing.	Mentally listing all of the reasons why the person is "good," avoiding gatherings where children may be present
Other	"What if I am actually gay/ straight (even though I am otherwise clear about my orientation)?"	Scanning body for signs of arousal when someone of the same/ opposite sex is present
	"What if my partner is not actually 'the one'?"	Repeatedly asking partner if relationship is right, excessive internet research about relationship problems

OCD include repeatedly checking that they did not or will not hurt anyone (e.g., retracing their route on the highway or inspecting power outlets to make sure they will not cause a fire), re-reading the same passage again and again (e.g., on homework or tax paperwork), or ordering and arranging objects (e.g., making sure their books are perfectly aligned with the edge of the shelf). Table 8–2 provides more information about different types of OCD symptoms.

How Is Obsessive-Compulsive Disorder Diagnosed?

The obsessions and compulsions just described are some of the most common OCD symptoms, but there are many others. If you are unsure about whether you or a loved one may have OCD, we recommend working with an experienced mental health professional who can help determine whether OCD is the correct diagnosis. An excellent resource to find a clinician with OCD experience is the International OCD Foundation (https://iocdf.org), which hosts an online directory of professionals that is searchable by zip code.

Once you have made an appointment with a mental health professional, the first meeting usually involves working with the clinician to diagnose the problems you are facing. At this appointment, the clinician may ask questions about your history, different obsessions and compulsions, and other symptoms you may have had. They will also explore how these symptoms affect your everyday life. The first assessment also involves ruling out other conditions that share common symptoms with OCD, sometimes known as *obsessive-compulsive (OC) spectrum disorders*. This category includes conditions such as body dysmorphic disorder, hoarding disorder, and body-focused repetitive behaviors (e.g., trichotillomania). Each of these conditions has similar characteristics to OCD; for example, difficulty throwing away objects can be seen in patients with OCD and those with hoarding disorder. However, OC spectrum disorders also have important differences from OCD: although the main focus of hoarding disorder is the difficulty discarding or parting with possessions, in OCD this may be just one of several different themes.

Your clinician will also ask you questions to rule out other conditions that are easily confused with OCD. These include obsessive-compulsive personality disorder (OCPD), autism spectrum disorder, tic disorders, and schizophrenia, all of which mimic OCD in some ways but have key differences that set them apart. For example, people with both OCD and OCPD may want things to be perfect or "just right"; for those with OCD, this symptom tends to be upsetting, whereas people with OCPD may not see this as a problem. Similarly, having unwanted religious thoughts (e.g., "If I forget to pray at least five times a day, God will send me to hell") can be part of both OCD and schizophrenia. However, someone with OCD will often have a sense that such thoughts are irrational, even if they may doubt this from time to time. In contrast, schizophrenia frequently involves delusions, in which the individual is completely convinced that their thoughts are true.

Finally, your clinician will also check for symptoms of other conditions that may be present at the same time (known as *comorbid* conditions). Depressive disorders such as major depressive disorder and anxiety disorders such as generalized anxiety disorder or illness anxiety disorder are particularly common among individuals who have OCD. Other conditions such as autism spectrum disorders, eating disorders, and bipolar disorder are not quite as common, but they are still observed more often in people with OCD than in the general population.

Risk Factors

In the United States, around 2% of adults will experience OCD in their lifetime. OCD appears to affect the sexes equally and has similar rates among people of different racial and ethnic backgrounds. Although the disorder is most often first recognized in a person's teens or twenties, OCD symptoms may begin as early as preschool or develop later in adulthood. Historically, there has been a long gap between when a person's OCD symptoms first emerge and when the person first starts treatment. Yet the earlier someone is diagnosed and receives treatment, the better their chances of overcoming OCD. Because of this, we suggest that seeking a diagnostic assessment as soon as possible if you are concerned that you or a loved one may have OCD.

Are Genetics Involved?

Although we do not know exactly what causes OCD, we believe there are both genetic and environmental risk factors. Researchers have learned that OCD can run in families but is not always passed down from one generation to the next. Genetics studies have identified some genes that may increase risk for OCD and discovered that genes may be a more important factor when OCD starts during early childhood. At the same time, a person's environment also plays a role. Environmental risk factors for OCD include social isolation, exposure to physical violence or abuse, and other stressful experiences. Certain medical issues, including head injuries, recurrent infections, or being born prematurely may also increase the risk. Finally, rapid onset of OCD symptoms has been reported in children after an untreated streptococcal infection, a condition known as *pediatric autoimmune neuropsychiatric disorder associated with streptococcal infections* or PANDAS. It is important to speak with your pediatrician if you have concerns about symptoms such as these.

Conclusion

OCD can be disabling if it is not diagnosed and treated. Fortunately, we are increasingly learning about the range of symptoms that people with OCD experience and finding new and more effective ways to identify them in real-world settings. Although plenty of work remains, today more people are able to receive a diagnosis and treatment for OCD than ever before. If you or someone you care about may have symptoms of OCD, we encourage you to see a mental health professional as soon as possible, because early intervention matters.

Recommended Reading

Abramowitz JS: The Family Guide to Getting Over OCD: Reclaim Your Life and Help Your Loved One. New York, Guilford Press, 2021

Center for Practice Innovations: IMPACT OCD: Individual and Family Resources. New York, Columbia University, 2023. Available at: https://practiceinnovations.org/initiatives/impact-ocd/resources/impact-ocd-toolkit/individuals-and-families.

9

Panic Disorder

Giampaolo Perna, M.D., Ph.D.
Tatiana Torti, Psy.D.

Definition

Panic disorder (PD) is one of the most common "physical" psychiatric disorders. It manifests physical symptoms to such an extent that most patients with PD are referred to emergency departments or to cardiologists, pulmonologists, otolaryngologists, and neurologists. They usually undergo several medical and organic tests before consulting a mental health specialist. The key characteristic of PD is the recurrent unexpected panic attacks that are common in the first phases. The duration of a panic attack can vary from 15 to 30 minutes, but in some cases it can last for a few hours. However, a more important characteristic of a panic attack is the acute nature of distress from the onset of mental and physical sensations to the time when the peak is experienced (e.g., terror, sensations of dying or losing control). The time can range from a few seconds to a few minutes.

The frequency and severity of panic attacks may vary, and some people might experience sporadic panic attacks with minimal effect on their quality of life. Another key aspect of an unexpected panic attack is the absence of an instant trigger preceding the attack. A panic attack is often attributed to a stressful event that occurred a few hours or days before the actual onset of panic attacks; however, an immediate trigger or specific stressful event preceding the attack is often absent. These attacks, not to be confused with nightmares, might also occur during sleep and result in awakening the person with a sense of terror and physical danger. Notably, fear is not a necessary component of a panic attack because a person might experience a strong sensation of discomfort or distress without a clear sensation of fear, suggesting that a panic attack cannot be equated to a strong fear.

How Is Panic Disorder Diagnosed?

Panic attacks are characterized by somatic and mental sensations of distress (Table 9–1). Somatic sensations are more predominant and appear before mental sensations. However, the intense fear of dying experienced during panic attacks is not caused by the somatic sensations but is manifested during the attack. In other words, the sensation of dying is triggered by the panic attack and is not simply a consequence, which explains the persistence of this sensation even after surviving several harmless attacks. In most cases, the fear of dying persists despite having several experiential proofs of the attacks not being fatal. A major cause of worry in patients having panic attacks is the fear of having an underlying life-threatening illness, particularly a cardiac disease, and thus they tend to avoid physical exertion and sports. This maladaptive behavior leads to the patients' maintained susceptibility to panic attacks.

Although recurrent unexpected panic attacks are the key feature of PD, its clinical pathology seems to be complex. We can categorize the different clinical manifestations of panic vulnerability into four levels:

1. Unexpected panic attacks as described in the *Diagnostic and Statistical Manual of Mental Disorders*, 5th Edition (DSM-5)
2. Unexpected panic attacks with one or more symptoms associated with an intense sense of distress
3. "Missed" unexpected panic attacks in patients experiencing a clear sensation of an imminent panic attack but without the occurrence of the typical manifestation
4. A more subtle "shadow" panic attack in a patient experiencing just a sensation of being unfit due to somatic sensations that are not concordant with the patient's physical condition.

Risk Factors

As with many mental disorders, panic arises from a combination of genetic and environmental factors, in which the former are unchangeable and the latter are modifiable. Having a relative with PD, experiencing childhood trauma, or losing a parent in the first year of life are possible risk factors for PD. Being fearful

Table 9–1. DSM-5 diagnostic criteria for panic disorder

A. Recurrent unexpected panic attacks. A panic attack is an abrupt surge of intense fear or intense discomfort that reaches a peak within minutes, during which time four (or more) of the following symptoms occur:

   Note: The abrupt surge can occur from a calm state or an anxious state.

   1. Palpitations, pounding heart, or accelerated heart rate
   2. Sweating
   3. Trembling or shaking
   4. Sensations of shortness of breath or smothering
   5. Feelings of choking
   6. Chest pain or discomfort
   7. Nausea or abdominal distress
   8. Feeling dizzy, unsteady, light-headed, or faint
   9. Chills or heat sensations
   10. Paresthesias (numbness or tingling sensations)
   11. Derealization (feelings of unreality) or depersonalization (being detached from oneself)
   12. Fear of losing control or "going crazy"
   13. Fear of dying

   Note: Culture-specific symptoms (e.g., tinnitus, neck soreness, headache, uncontrollable screaming or crying) may be seen. Such symptoms should not count as one of the four required symptoms.

B. At least one of the attacks has been followed by 1 month (or more) of one or both of the following:

   1. Persistent concern or worry about additional panic attacks or their consequences (e.g., losing control, having a heart attack, "going crazy")
   2. A significant maladaptive change in behavior related to the attacks (e.g., behaviors designed to avoid having panic attacks, such as avoidance of exercise or unfamiliar situations)

C. The disturbance is not attributable to the physiological effects of a substance (e.g., a drug of abuse, a medication) or another medical condition (e.g., hyperthyroidism, cardiopulmonary disorders).

D. The disturbance is not better explained by another mental disorder (e.g., the panic attacks do not occur only in response to feared social situations, as in social anxiety disorder; in response to circumscribed phobic objects or situations, as in specific phobia; in response to obsessions, as in obsessive-compulsive disorder; in response to reminders of traumatic events, as in posttraumatic stress disorder; or in response to separation from attachment figures, as in separation anxiety disorder).

Source. From American Psychiatric Association: *Diagnostic and Statistical Manual of Mental Disorders*, 5th Edition, Text Revision. Washington, DC, American Psychiatric Association, 2022.

of the possible consequences of physical sensations (i.e., anxiety sensitivity) and being behaviorally avoidant and inhibited might also predispose a person to PD. Among the most modifiable risk factors, quitting smoking, increasing aerobic physical activity, and controlling stress and stressors are important.

Common Co-Occurring Mental Health Disorders

PD is often present with other concomitant psychiatric syndromes that should be correctly interpreted. The co-occurrence of a depressive episode needs to be evaluated while keeping the person's context in mind. The several negative consequences of PD might easily induce a secondary depressive syndrome, which is more of a coherent and normal mood reaction (demoralization) than an expression of a mood disorder. The co-occurrence of alcohol or benzodiazepine abuse can be a desperate attempt to self-medicate rather than a specific vulnerability to substance abuse or dependence. Agoraphobia and severe anticipatory anxiety are often adaptive emotional and behavioral reactions to panic attacks. It is not uncommon for the presence of comorbidity with bipolar disorder or obsessive-compulsive disorder (OCD) to make the clinical picture more complex.

The National Institute of Mental Health estimates that almost 10 million individuals in the U.S. population are affected by PD; most patients are in their early adulthood years (20–25 years of age). The incidence rate of panic attacks among females is twice as high as among males, and females experience a larger impact on quality of life and relapse more frequently than males. The clinical course of untreated PD is chronic, with varying intensity of symptoms; however, anticipatory anxiety and phobic avoidance tend to persist for longer. PD is rare in childhood, but "fearful spells" are often retrospectively reported and might be considered antecedents of PD. The prevalence of PD is lower in elderly individuals. Finally, it is important to remember that a person's attribution of unexpectedness might depend on the cultural context (i.e., Latin Americans experience *ataque de nervios* as a consequence of interpersonal arguments; Vietnamese individuals relate panic to wind).

How Panic Disorder Starts and Progresses

The course of PD typically follows the so-called march of panic. After experiencing their first panic attack with sensations that are often strongly rooted in the body, patients might focus their attention on the medical-physical sensations and thus be referred to medical doctors specializing in other diseases. When the undiagnosed panic attacks become more frequent, the patient might develop health and anticipatory anxiety, also known as the "fear of fear." This anticipatory anxiety can induce acute episodes of panic when the patient is exposed to situations in which seeking help or escaping might be challenging. The possibility of being embarrassed by a panic attack can also trigger acute anxiety in some cases. The secondary anxiety and fear might induce the development of avoidant behavior known as *agoraphobia,* in which patients "keep themselves in a cage" by limiting their own autonomy and freedom as a preventive strategy to avoid the risk of panic attacks. At this stage, patients often become dependent on other people, who become their phobic companions, to regain a part of their movement freedom.

The final stage of PD is the development of secondary depression or substance abuse (e.g., alcohol, benzodiazepines), along with the possible presence of suicidal thoughts and behaviors. Depression is usually a reaction to all the limitations and sufferings caused by panic attacks and dependence on alcohol. Benzodiazepine abuse is a strategy for overcoming anxiety and panic by facilitating social activities. Overall, PD is characterized by a high level of occupational, social, and economic costs due to the frequent absences from work and repeated requests for emergency department visits.

In clinical practice, patients might be in any of these stages and might shift from one stage to another regardless of sequence. Therefore, it is crucial that clinicians collect a detailed history of the patient's disorder from a longitudinal perspective and not simply look at the distress described "here and now."

Another key clinical aspect of PD is the mandatory need to rule out medical and pharmacological causes of acute phenomena that can resemble panic attacks. Endocrine disturbances (e.g., hyperthyroidism, hyperparathyroidism, pheochromocytoma), vestibular dysfunctions, seizure disorders, cardiopulmonary conditions (e.g., asthma, chronic obstructive pulmonary disease, arrhythmias, mitral valve prolapse, supraventricular tachycardia), and hypoglycemic episodes related to diabetes might resemble panic attacks. The onset of panic attacks after 45 years of age suggests an underlying medical ailment or substance abuse. To rule out these factors, clinicians must consider some peculiar clinical features of the acute episodes described instead of solely conducting multiple blood and diagnostic tests. A regular attack that occurs temporally distant from meals might be caused by hypoglycemic episodes in someone who is diabetic. A significant increase in blood pressure during panic attacks might indicate the presence of a pheochromocytoma, and heat intolerance and weight loss might be related to hyperthyroidism. In addition, sex hormones can also induce acute anxiety episodes. The (ab)use of stimulants such as caffeine, some antiasthmatic medications, cocaine, amphetamines, cannabis, and other substances may induce panic-like attacks. Therefore, an acute episode of somatic discomfort and fear experienced by a patient should be discussed with a medical practitioner in order to avoid diagnostic mistakes.

Conclusion

PD is a common but very easy to diagnose anxiety disorder. However, to avoid misdiagnosis that may mislead the choice of the appropriate treatment, the longitudinal course of the disorder should be carefully assessed, and the possible medical causes leading to panic-like attacks must be ruled out.

Recommended Reading

LeDoux J: Anxious: Using the Brain to Understand and Treat Fear and Anxiety. New York, Viking Press, 2016

Perna G: A La Vida: Comprende y Supera la Ansiedad. Barcelona, Plataforma Editorial, 2013

10

Generalized Anxiety Disorder

John M. Hettema, M.D., Ph.D.
Amy Adams, M.P.H.

Definition

Generalized anxiety disorder (GAD) involves persistent feelings of worry, anxiety, nervousness, or tension that interfere with daily activities. Individuals with GAD worry more than necessary about multiple areas of their lives (e.g., home, health, family, work). This chronic worry and anxiety can be tiresome, distracting, and distressful. It frequently leads to additional symptoms such as agitation, fatigue, difficulty concentrating, irritability, muscle tension, and sleep disturbances. These symptoms can cause significant problems in one's life.

How Is Generalized Anxiety Disorder Diagnosed?

Two documents guide the diagnosis of GAD: the *Diagnostic and Statistical Manual of Mental Disorders,* 5th Edition (DSM-5) and the *International Classification of Diseases,* 11th Edition (ICD-11). Both define GAD based on similar key symptoms. Table 10–1 lists the DSM-5 diagnostic criteria for GAD along with a simplified interpretation.

Table 10–1. DSM diagnostic criteria for generalized anxiety disorder

DSM-5 text	Condensed version
A. Excessive anxiety and worry (apprehensive expectation), occurring **more days than not for at least 6 months**, about a **number of events or activities** (e.g., work or school performance).	A. You worry a lot about multiple things.
B. The individual finds it **difficult to control** the worry.	B. It is hard to stop worrying.
C. The anxiety and worry are associated with **three (or more)** of the following **six symptoms** (with at least some symptoms having been present for more days than not for the past 6 months). **Note:** Only one item is required in children. 1. Restlessness, feeling keyed up or on edge 2. Being easily fatigued 3. Difficulty concentrating or mind going blank 4. Irritability 5. Muscle tension 6. Sleep disturbance (difficulty falling or staying asleep, or restless, unsatisfying sleep)	C. You regularly experience at least three of these: 1. Fidgety/restless 2. Tired 3. Concentration/Focus issues 4. Moody 5. Tight muscles 6. Sleep issues
D. The anxiety, worry, or physical symptoms cause clinically significant **distress or impairment** in social, occupational, or other important areas of functioning.	D. The symptoms make it difficult to function normally (e.g., school, work, social, home, self-care).
E. The disturbance is **not attributable to** the physiological effects of a **substance** (e.g., a drug of abuse, a medication) or another medical condition (e.g., hyperthyroidism).	E. There is no better physical explanation for the symptoms.

Table 10–1. DSM diagnostic criteria for generalized anxiety disorder *(continued)*

DSM-5 text	Condensed version
F. The disturbance is **not better explained by another medical disorder** (e.g., anxiety or worry about having panic attacks in panic disorder, negative evaluation in social anxiety disorder [social phobia], contamination or other obsessions in obsessive-compulsive disorder, separation from attachment figures in separation anxiety disorder, reminders of traumatic events in posttraumatic stress disorder, gaining weight in anorexia nervosa, physical complaints in somatic symptom disorder, perceived appearance flaws in body dysmorphic disorder, having a serious illness in illness anxiety disorder, or the content of delusional beliefs in schizophrenia or delusional disorder).	F. No other diagnosis fits better.

Source. Adapted from American Psychiatric Association: *Diagnostic and Statistical Manual of Mental Disorders*, 5th Edition, Text Revision. Washington, DC, American Psychiatric Association, 2022.

Screening

The U.S. Preventive Services Task Force has recommended that adults younger than 65 years be screened for anxiety. In adults, the self-report Generalized Anxiety Disorder–2 (GAD-2) and Generalized Anxiety Disorder–7 (GAD-7) surveys are commonly used screening tools for GAD. The GAD-2 uses two questions to determine the severity of anxious symptoms and the patient's ability to control worry over the past 2 weeks. Using these questions, it can identify about 86% of people with GAD. The GAD-7 is more extensive: with its seven questions, it identifies up to 92% of people with GAD. In children and adolescents, The Screen for Child Anxiety Related Emotional Disorders (SCARED) may be used. This is a 41-question screening tool for a range of anxiety disorders. Each of these screening tools can indicate if a person is experiencing symptoms of an anxiety-related disorder; however, these tools are not a substitute for a professional diagnosis.

Professional Evaluation

Once someone screens positive for anxiety-like symptoms, a clinician can assess them to determine which diagnosis, if any, is appropriate. This assessment involves a clinical interview, sometimes accompanied by laboratory tests to help rule out other potential causes of the symptoms. However, no laboratory test currently exists specifically for any psychiatric disorder.

Differential Diagnosis

Worry During and After an Actual Threat

Health care providers must consider both what drives worry and how long anxiety symptoms last when they are determining which diagnosis and treatment plan are most appropriate. Fear and anxiety produce a state of heightened alertness, enabling appropriate reactions to danger ("flight or fight"). In these cases, feeling anxious can be a normal and healthy response to address short-term, situational stressors. However, when these symptoms persist after the threat has resolved, trauma- and stressor-related disorders such as adjustment disorder or acute stress disorder may best describe the symptoms. If trauma-related symptoms persist, posttraumatic stress disorder (PTSD) should be considered. Not all stressors resolve. Some individuals living under persistent, long-term stressors such as poverty, self-identification with a marginalized group, or extreme work demands may manifest with symptoms that mimic GAD. Differentiating these chronic stress reactions from GAD can be difficult and may require a professional's opinion.

Chronic Worry About a Specific Concern

When worries cluster around a specific fear (e.g., public speaking, getting sick, dogs) rather than everyday life stressors, a phobia diagnosis that describes that specific fear is optimal. Individuals with social anxiety disorder fret about upcoming social situations in which they believe others will scrutinize or judge them. People with separation anxiety disorder, especially children, worry about the health and safety of attachment figures and fear being apart from them. In illness anxiety disorder and somatic symptom disorder, people worry about real or perceived physical symptoms and their potential significance to their health status.

Chronic Worry About Many Concerns

Chronic anxiety may be a symptom of another medical condition or an effect of a substance (e.g., caffeine, certain medications). Easily testable conditions such as hyperthyroidism and other hormonal imbalances should be ruled out when considering a GAD diagnosis. Other psychiatric disorders that commonly manifest with anxiety include depressive disorders, obsessive-compulsive disorder (OCD), bipolar disorder, attention-deficit/hyperactivity disorder (ADHD), autism spectrum disorder, and sleep disorders. A number of features distinguish the excessive worry of GAD from the symptoms of these other conditions. Particularly, the worry in GAD is about countless perceived future problems, even if they have a low chance of occurring. The theme of worry in other conditions is more distinct. In OCD, for example, obsessions take the form of intrusive and unwanted thoughts, urges, or images, regardless of future concerns. Although OCD-like compulsions may occur in GAD, they serve as a coping mechanism to either avoid negative outcomes or distract oneself from worries. When very stressed, some individuals with GAD may develop bodily sensations that are similar to panic attacks, such as a racing heart, sweating, dizziness, and stomach upset. Many psychiatric disorders can present with nervousness, poor concentration, trouble sleeping, and pessimism. Because of these overlapping symptoms, some patients with GAD are misdiagnosed as having clinical depression. Please consult the appropriate chapters in this text for more details about these other conditions.

Functional Consequences of Generalized Anxiety Disorder

Excessive worrying impairs an individual's capacity to do things quickly and efficiently, whether at home, at work, or at play. Worrying takes time and energy.

The associated symptoms of muscle tension, feeling on edge, tiredness, difficulty concentrating, and disturbed sleep contribute to the impairment. By overwhelming individuals with worries, GAD distracts them from fulfilling their role responsibilities as parents, spouses, coworkers, and so on. GAD is associated with significant disability and distress, and most adults with the disorder are moderately to seriously disabled.

Risk Factors

Similar to other health conditions, many risk factors work together to influence the risk and severity of GAD. In general, any condition that reduces blood flow to a developing fetus can impact brain development and thereby increase the risk of mental disorders such as GAD. Some people tend to negatively interpret and respond to life events. This tendency is a personality trait known as *neuroticism,* and those with higher levels of neuroticism ("neurotic") are at increased risk of developing GAD. Tendencies to avoid harm, to assume defensive positions when exposed to threats, or to hesitate when exposed to novelty are also associated with GAD. Being female, having a history of childhood adversities or parental overprotection, and living in a higher-income country are associated with screening positive for GAD. Genetic factors account for one-third of the risk of experiencing GAD, as discussed later (see "Are Genetics Involved?").

Community Perspectives and Coexisting Conditions

In any 12-month period, approximately 4% of the U.S. population experiences GAD; around 8% will develop GAD at some point in their lifetime. These numbers are twice as high as the global averages. Interestingly, only 5% of African Americans are estimated to screen positive for GAD during their lifetimes. Recent evidence suggests that this may be due to culturally specific interpretations of word choices within three of the seven questions of the GAD-7. As such, African Americans with GAD are more likely to go undetected by the health care system, even when screened.

More than 50% of individuals with GAD are likely to meet criteria for additional anxiety and mood disorders, because many genetic and environmental risk factors are shared among these conditions. Besides these, other psychiatric conditions that often occur with GAD include sleep disorders, ADHD, chronic pain, and OCD. Nonpsychiatric co-occurring conditions include heart failure and stroke.

How Generalized Anxiety Disorder Starts and Progresses

Onset

GAD can present at any stage of life. Many people who develop GAD believe they have been anxious, albeit perhaps subclinically, since childhood. As they become adults, their worries become more generalized and pervasive. Some individuals with GAD and those around them dismiss their symptoms as trivial ("just stop worrying"); others with GAD seek medical care for their anxiety-induced physical symptoms such as dizziness, stomach upset, or muscle pain. Those who seek professional help for anxiety typically first do so between adolescence and their early thirties. The earlier in life that symptoms develop, the more likely other problems such as depression will occur and the more impaired the individual is likely to become. Although there is no cure for GAD, with proper supportive care, many patients find successful ways to manage their symptoms.

Root of the Worry

Individuals with GAD likely have dysfunctional brain circuitries related to processing potential threats. Pathways related to attention, emotion, learning, and memory have been implicated in this disorder. In many cases, this manifests as a discomfort with uncertainty about future events or outcomes. For example, when considering all possible outcomes, someone with GAD fears that any decision could be the wrong one. The key question that leaves them in a state of paralyzing indecision is: "But what if… [insert remotely possible negative outcome]?" The technical term for this is *catastrophizing*. GAD is closely related to desires for perfection, efficiency, and pleasing others. In nearly all cases, individuals either fear the possibility of a bad outcome or experience extreme discomfort with being unable to predict the outcome with certainty.

By Stage of Life

Childhood

Some children who later develop GAD may demonstrate separation anxiety at a young age. Although uncommonly diagnosed in childhood, GAD may manifest as chronic worries or bodily pains. Concerns may include health, safety, and competence in activities such as school or sports. In an attempt to control their environment, affected children may be overly concerned with compliance with rules or may repeatedly ask for reassurance. A child's anxieties often distract and distress them, leading to struggles with daily tasks that may further worsen their insecurities. In many cases, childhood anxiety may manifest as bodily discomfort, such as headaches, upset stomach, and sleep difficulties.

Adolescence

As children with GAD become adolescents, they become more concerned with being accepted by and pleasing others. Coping strategies may include a tendency toward perfectionism, taking extended time to complete tasks, and seeking reassurance. In the teenage years, irritability and depression may accompany GAD.

Early Adulthood

As adolescents with GAD become adults, their worry transitions to adult themes about family, finances, and social and professional endeavors. Going to college or starting their first job can feel overwhelming. They may find socially acceptable ways to mask their symptoms; however, this often comes with increased physical symptoms such as headaches or muscle tension. High levels of estrogen are associated with reduced severity of anxious, depressive, and pain-related symptoms. As such, females with GAD may have more intense symptoms during the last 2 weeks of their menstrual cycles. Behaviorally, adults with GAD may avoid their anxious discomfort by procrastinating and avoiding conflict to an extreme. This may manifest as difficulties with meeting work deadlines, delays in scheduling appointments, taking excessive time to make simple decisions, and interpersonal misunderstandings. In relationships, individuals with GAD tend to misperceive their conflict avoidance as nurturing and caring whereas the other parties interpret this behavior as either emotional distancing or being overly submissive.

Late Adulthood

As adults age into and beyond their forties, the severity of their anxieties tends to decrease somewhat. However, poorer health often accompanies aging. As such, worries about their own or others' safety and health may limit activities. Discomfort with uncertainty may lead to avoidance of acquiring new skills or taking on unfamiliar tasks. This can be particularly difficult as responsibilities shift following the loss of a partner or confidant.

Are Genetics Involved?

Like all psychiatric illness, GAD runs in families partially due to genetic factors. Risk for GAD is about one-third genetic and two-thirds environmental. Compared with a random person in the population, people with first-degree relatives affected by anxiety are four to six times more likely to develop an anxiety disorder. Although a number of genes have been implicated in anxiety disorders, these results require validation. Larger and more diverse study groups and more advanced research approaches are needed before GAD genetics research could become clinically meaningful.

Conclusion

GAD is a condition marked by excessive worry and anxiety that disrupts an individual's daily life. Identification and treatment of GAD require the application of screening tools in primary care such as the GAD-7 and SCARED for early detection. Often, a comprehensive professional evaluation is crucial to distinguish GAD from other psychiatric disorders and health conditions.

Comprehensive understanding of GAD's features, risk factors, and treatment is essential. Such knowledge facilitates a compassionate, informed approach to managing this condition. Recognizing these aspects empowers health care providers, patients, and families to more effectively navigate GAD's challenges, leading to improved management strategies and support.

Recommended Reading

Robichaud M, Dugas MJ, Antony MM: The Generalized Anxiety Disorder Workbook: A Comprehensive CBT Guide for Coping With Uncertainty, Worry, and Fear. Oakland, CA, New Harbinger, 2015

Simon N, Hollander E, Rothbaum BO, et al (eds): The American Psychiatric Association Publishing Textbook of Anxiety, Trauma, and OCD-Related Disorders, 3rd Edition. Washington, DC, American Psychiatric Association Publishing, 2020

11

Specific Phobia

Sydney Parkinson, B.A.
Karen Rowa, Ph.D., C.Psych.

Definition

Many of us have fears of things such as snakes, heights, or enclosed spaces. You may cringe and experience momentary anxiety when you see a spider, but not excessively worry about coming across a spider in your day-to-day life. However, for some individuals, their fears cause intense distress and interfere with everyday functioning. When individuals experience this extreme problematic fear and anxiety of a particular situation or object, they may have a *specific phobia*. When someone with a specific phobia is exposed to their feared object or situation, they experience an immediate and intense anxiety reaction. To cope, they might avoid the phobic object or situation or endure it with intense discomfort.

How Is Specific Phobia Diagnosed?

A specific phobia is usually diagnosed through an interview with a clinician. During this interview, the clinician asks about the severity of the person's fear, how often the fear comes up, and the level of distress and impairment in daily functioning caused by the fear. Once a diagnosis has been established, self-report questionnaires can help the clinician better understand the unique features and level of severity of each person's phobia. For example, two people can both have a specific phobia of dental procedures. However, one person may experience such intense anxiety anticipating a dental appointment that they repeatedly cancel the appointment, whereas the other person attends but their anxiety peaks in a panic attack in the dental chair. Understanding the specific focus of the fear and the types of situations people avoid due to their fear can assist clinicians in developing the most appropriate treatment plan for each person (Table 11–1)

When assessing whether someone has a diagnosis of a specific phobia, it is important to ensure that common fears (which all humans have) are not overdiagnosed as a phobia. For example, Inez dislikes needles, gets anxious on the day of a blood draw, and engages in breathing exercises to cope with having her blood drawn. However, she always follows through with having blood drawn, and the fear does not cause significant distress in her daily life or impair her daily functioning. Therefore, Inez's fear of needles is just that—a fear. On the other hand, Omar has avoided having blood drawn for years (despite his doctor's repeated request for blood work), and he cannot watch others get needles or even see needles on television. In this case, Omar likely has a phobia, because his fear of needles causes intense anxiety and interferes with his ability to follow up on medical advice. Fears are common and normal, but when they are so intense that they cause considerable distress and impact daily functioning, the line between fear and phobia has been crossed.

Risk Factors

Individuals can develop a fear in various ways. For example, someone with a choking phobia may have had a scary experience during which they choked on something. Someone with a fear of enclosed spaces may have been trapped in an elevator for hours. These are examples of phobias acquired through direct experience. However, not all phobias begin because of exposure to a scary event. One can also learn fears by witnessing someone else experience a scary event or seeing someone behave fearfully in a particular situation. For example, watching someone nearly drown may instill a phobia of water in the observer. It is also possible to develop a phobia through messages received from others. Sometimes being warned or receiving repetitive messages about a situation or object's potential danger is sufficient to instill a phobia. For example, being repeatedly warned by a parent about the danger of flying may eventually cause a phobia of flying. All three of these pathways to developing fear share a focus on experience, either directly or indirectly, with the phobic situation or object.

Table 11–1. DSM-5 diagnostic criteria for specific phobia

A. Marked fear or anxiety about a specific object or situation (e.g., flying, heights, animals, receiving an injection, seeing blood).

B. The phobic object or situation almost always provokes immediate fear or anxiety.

C. The phobic object or situation is actively avoided or endured with intense fear or anxiety.

D. The fear or anxiety is out of proportion to the actual danger posed by the specific object or situation and to the sociocultural context.

E. The fear, anxiety, or avoidance is persistent, typically lasting for 6 months or more.

F. The fear, anxiety, or avoidance causes clinically significant distress or impairment in social, occupational, or other important areas of functioning.

G. The disturbance is not better explained by the symptoms of another mental disorder, including fear, anxiety, and avoidance of situations associated with panic-like symptoms or other incapacitating symptoms (as in agoraphobia); objects or situations related to obsessions (as in obsessive-compulsive disorder); reminders of traumatic events (as in posttraumatic stress disorder); separation from home or attachment figures (as in separation anxiety disorder); or social situations (as in social anxiety disorder).

Specify if:

Animal (e.g., spiders, snakes, dogs)

Natural environment (e.g., heights, storms, water)

Blood-injection-injury (e.g., needles, invasive medical procedures)

Situational (e.g., airplanes, elevators, enclosed spaces)

Other type (e.g., fear of choking or vomiting)

Source. From American Psychiatric Association: *Diagnostic and Statistical Manual of Mental Disorders*, 5th Edition, Text Revision. Washington, DC, American Psychiatric Association, 2022.

It is also possible to develop a phobia without any contact with the phobic situation or object. A limited number of fears appear to be determined by biology, meaning no learning is necessary to develop these fears. These innate fears are probably adaptive from an evolutionary perspective. For example, a predisposition to fear snakes can be useful in parts of the world where a snake bite could be deadly. Other factors can increase the risk of developing a phobia. Some people are born with traits that increase the risk. These traits exist on a continuum, meaning some individuals have more of the trait and others have less. For example, the degree to which a person experiences feelings of "disgust" when exposed to certain objects or situations influences their susceptibility to developing certain phobias. People who have a strong disgust reaction to certain situations or objects such as bugs, types of food, or wounds are more likely to develop a specific phobia of that situation or object.

Common Co-Occurring Mental Health Disorders

Specific phobias are often accompanied by the co-occurrence of another anxiety disorder. In this case, the other disorder (e.g., generalized anxiety disorder, social anxiety disorder, panic disorder) tends to be of greater severity than the specific phobia. When someone has one phobia, they often have another phobia. For example, someone may have a specific phobia of heights and also have a secondary specific phobia of snakes. When someone has both a specific phobia and depression, the specific phobia most often exists before the onset of depression.

How Specific Phobia Starts and Progresses

Specific phobia is one of the most common anxiety disorders. Each year, approximately 12.1% of the population will meet diagnostic criteria for a specific phobia, and 18.4% of the population (almost one in five!) can expect to develop a specific phobia sometime in their lifetime. Specific phobias are more commonly experienced by females. However, depending on the specific type of phobia, there is variability across the sexes. For example, females are more likely to experience a phobia of animals, whereas males are more likely to experience a phobia of heights. Most specific phobias develop during childhood, typically before age 15. However, phobias of particular situations, such as flying, heights, or elevators, can develop in adolescence or early adulthood. If left untreated, phobias tend to persist throughout an individual's life. The type of phobia seems to influence the degree of social problems it causes. For example, individuals with a natural environment phobia (e.g., fear of heights or thunder and lightning) experience greater social problems than those with an animal phobia.

Are Genetics Involved?

Genetic factors seem to play a role in the development of specific phobias. If you have a first-degree relative (i.e., parent, full sibling, child) with a specific phobia, you are more likely to develop a phobia. However, the role genetics play in specific phobias may depend on the type of phobia. Genetic factors do not seem to influence the development of situational phobias (e.g., fear of bridges, public transportation, enclosed spaces). In contrast, genetic factors appear to influence the development of blood-injection-injury phobias and animal phobias (perhaps explaining why these types of phobia may develop in the absence of a scary experience).

Conclusion

Fears are very common, but when these fears cause intense distress and impact someone's everyday life, then a specific phobia may be diagnosed. Many complex factors contribute to the development of a specific phobia, including having a history of negative experiences with the phobic object or situation, as well as various psychological and biological factors.

Recommended Reading

Antony MM, Craske MG, Barlow DH: Mastering Your Fears and Phobias: Workbook, 2nd Edition. New York, Oxford University Press, 2006

Castagna PJ, Nebel-Schwalm M, Davis TE 3rd, et al: Specific phobia, in The Cambridge Handbook of Anxiety and Related Disorders. Edited by Olatunji BO. Cambridge, UK, Cambridge University Press, 2019, pp 421–450

12

Eating Disorders

Leslie K. Anderson, Ph.D.
Walter H. Kaye, M.D.

Definition

Eating disorders are complex and severe psychological disorders characterized by maladaptive beliefs and behaviors around eating, weight, and body image. The most common types of eating disorders are anorexia nervosa (AN), bulimia nervosa (BN), and binge-eating disorder (BED). In this chapter, we review the DSM-5 criteria for these eating disorders (Table 12–1), how they are diagnosed, and their risk factors, comorbidities, epidemiology, and genetics.

Eating disorders tend to be defined by three major behaviors: restricting, bingeing, and purging. *Restriction* refers to limiting food intake in terms of the quantity, variety, or frequency of eating. *Bingeing* is defined as episodes of excessive eating during which the individual experiences loss of control. *Purging* refers to recurrent compensatory behaviors to prevent weight gain, such as self-induced vomiting; misuse of laxatives, diuretics, or other medications; or excessive exercise.

Anorexia nervosa is characterized by restriction of food intake resulting in an inability to maintain an appropriate body weight. People with AN also report fear of gaining weight and a distorted perception of their size or the seriousness of their condition. Individuals can be diagnosed with AN if they meet criteria but are not underweight despite significant weight loss. There are two subtypes

Table 12–1. DSM-5 diagnostic criteria for eating disorders

Anorexia nervosa

A. Restriction of energy intake relative to requirements, leading to a significantly low body weight in the context of age, sex, developmental trajectory, and physical health.

B. Intense fear of gaining weight or of becoming fat or persistent behavior that interferes with weight gain, even though at a significantly low weight.

C. Disturbance in the way in which one's body weight or shape is experienced, undue influence of body weight or shape on self-evaluation, or persistent lack of recognition of the seriousness of the low body weight.

Subtypes: Restricting or binge-eating/purging type

Bulimia nervosa

A. Recurrent episodes of binge eating. An episode of binge eating is characterized by both of the following:
   1. Eating, in a discrete period of time (e.g., within any 2-hour period), an amount of food that is definitely larger than what most individuals would eat in a similar period of time under similar circumstances.
   2. A sense of lack of control over eating during the episode (e.g., a feeling that one cannot stop eating or control what or how much one is eating).

B. Recurrent inappropriate compensatory behaviors to prevent weight gain, such as self-induced vomiting; misuse of laxatives, diuretics, or other medications; fasting; or excessive exercise.

C. The binge eating and inappropriate compensatory behaviors both occur, on average, at least once a week for 3 months.

D. Self-evaluation is unduly influenced by body shape and weight.

E. The disturbance does not occur exclusively during episodes of anorexia nervosa.

Binge eating disorder

A. Recurrent episodes of binge eating. An episode of binge eating is characterized by both of the following:
   1. Eating, in a discrete period of time (e.g., within any 2-hour period), an amount of food that is definitely larger than what most people would eat in a similar period of time under similar circumstances.
   2. A sense of lack of control over eating during the episode (e.g., a feeling that one cannot stop eating or control what or how much one is eating).

B. The binge eating episodes are associated with three (or more) of the following:
   1. Eating much more rapidly than normal.
   2. Eating until feeling uncomfortably full.
   3. Eating large amounts of food when not feeling physically hungry.

Table 12–1. DSM-5 diagnostic criteria for eating disorders *(continued)*

4. Eating alone because of feeling embarrassed by how much one is eating.
5. Feeling disgusted with oneself, depressed, or very guilty afterward.

C. Marked distress regarding binge eating is present.

D. The binge eating occurs, on average, at least once a week for 3 months.

E. The binge eating is not associated with the recurrent use of inappropriate compensatory behavior as in bulimia nervosa and does not occur exclusively during the course of bulimia nervosa or anorexia nervosa.

Source. From American Psychiatric Association: *Diagnostic and Statistical Manual of Mental Disorders*, 5th Edition, Text Revision. Washington, DC, American Psychiatric Association, 2022.

of AN: those who only engage in restriction (AN-R), and those who also engage in bingeing or purging (AN-BP).

Bulimia nervosa is diagnosed when an individual engages in binge-eating behaviors and compensatory behaviors at least once a week for 3 months. Typically, this pattern involves bingeing in a way that feels out of control and subsequently purging to get rid of the calories from the binge. Individuals with BN tend to be average weight to overweight.

Binge eating disorder is diagnosed when binge eating occurs at least once a week for 3 months, and the binge eating is not associated with compensatory behavior, such as vomiting or exercise.

Eating disorders are associated with suffering, medical instability, and significantly increased mortality rates. At the same time, patients often lack motivation for and are resistant to treatment, which makes successful treatment very difficult. Long-term follow-up shows that among those with AN, about 40% recover, 25% have a moderate treatment response, and 30% have a poor treatment response. Those with BN fare a bit better, with a 50% treatment response rate and remission rates between 50% and 80%. Overall, however, around half of those with eating disorders may not achieve full remission, and the health consequences of remaining ill can be devastating.

How Are Eating Disorders Diagnosed?

Accurate detection and diagnosis are especially important because earlier age at diagnosis is correlated with improved outcomes. Eating disorders are generally diagnosed by interviewing the patient, gathering a history of eating behaviors, and using DSM-5 criteria. The assessment process also includes evaluating the physical damage that eating behaviors or malnutrition may have caused and ruling out any medical conditions that could cause weight fluctuation. Laboratory tests are conducted to look for physical findings, such as low body mass index (BMI), amenorrhea, bradycardia, gastrointestinal disturbances, skin changes, and changes in dentition. Medical conditions that should be ruled out include hyperthyroidism, malignancy, inflammatory bowel disease, immunodeficiency, malabsorption, chronic infections, Addison's disease, and diabetes.

Risk Factors

Research has identified numerous psychological and biological factors that increase the risk of developing an eating disorder. These include demographic factors, such as being an adolescent or young adult, being female, and the existence of other psychiatric or medical conditions. Familial risk factors include having parents who model eating-disordered behavior or who criticize their child's body shape. There are also broad cultural factors, such as the social pressure in Western societies to fit a certain ideal thin body type. Although everyone experiences this social pressure to some extent, eating disorders develop in only a minority of people, highlighting the importance of biological factors as well. Biologically, various brain imaging methods have been used to advance understanding of brain function in eating disorders.

Common Co-Occurring Mental Health Disorders

Mood disorders are common among individuals with eating disorders. Comorbid major depressive disorder occurs in about 25%–50% of those with AN and 40%–50% of those with BN or BED. This high rate of co-occurrence may be due to the similar underlying psychological and neurobiological factors. The physical and psychological sequelae of eating disorders (e.g., malnutrition, social withdrawal) likely also increase susceptibility to mood disorders.

Anxiety disorders also appear to be closely related to eating disorders. In AN, rates of comorbid anxiety disorders vary from 20% to 75%, and in BN, rates are between 13% and 60%. Studies have shown heightened rates of generalized anxiety disorder, social and simple phobias, agoraphobia, panic disorder, and obsessive-compulsive disorder (OCD) in both those with eating disorders and in their family members. In most cases, anxiety in childhood tended to occur prior the onset of the eating disorder, suggesting that anxiety may be a temperamental trait that plays a role in increasing vulnerability to developing these disorders.

Approximately 50% of individuals with an eating disorder abuse alcohol or illicit substances, which is a much higher rate of abuse compared with those without eating disorders. Research indicates a stronger association between substance use and binge-type disorders (AN-BP, BN, and BED) as opposed to restricting disorders (AN-R). The most prevalent substances abused are alcohol, sedatives, cannabis, and caffeine pills.

Although personality disorders occur in approximately 5%–10% of the general population, they are considerably more common among those with eating disorders. The most frequently diagnosed personality disorder among individuals with AN-R is obsessive-compulsive personality disorder, with a prevalence rate of 22%. For purging disorders, including AN-BP and BN, the most common comorbid personality disorder is borderline personality disorder, with a prevalence rate of 25%–28%. Overall, approximately one-third of eating disorder patients have a diagnosable personality disorder of some kind.

How Eating Disorders Start and Progress

Overall, AN occurs at rates of about 0.5%–1%, BN at about 2%, and BED at 1%–4%. Eating disorders can affect people across the life span, but rates tend to be highest among those who are in adolescence or early adulthood, with an average age at onset of 18 years in AN and BN. Although eating disorders occur most frequently in females, in recent years there has been a noted increase of disordered eating practices among males. There is also emerging evidence that eating disorders occur at a disproportionately high rate in the LGBTQ+ population.

Are Genetics Involved?

Eating disorders may result from a combination of genetic and biological risk factors with environmental stressors. In recent years, studies have suggested that premorbid genetically determined temperament and personality traits render an individual vulnerable to developing an eating disorder.

Eating disorders appear to have substantial hereditary components. Genetic studies have consistently shown increased chances for an eating disorder among female relatives of individuals with eating disorders, and the evidence for a genetic link is stronger for AN than for BN. For example, sisters of individuals with an eating disorder are at six to seven times greater risk of developing an eating disorder than the general population. This genetic link may also be related to shared genes for anxiety. People with eating disorders seem to have an altered gene for the γ-aminobutyric (GABA) system, which is well known to modulate anxiety. This genetic link may also be related to the personality traits found in people with eating disorders that also tend to run in their families, such as perfectionism, high error detection, high anticipatory anxiety, and difficulty feeling or expressing negative emotion. There also appear to be genetic correlations between AN and anxiety, OCD, major depressive disorder, and substance-related disorders.

Several lines of evidence suggest a disturbance in serotonin pathways in the pathophysiology of both AN and BN. This may be why medications that act on serotonin pathways have some degree of efficacy in individuals with eating disorders. Unfortunately, these disturbances tend to persist even after the person has recovered from their eating disorder.

Conclusion

Researchers have made important strides in assessing for and identifying risk factors and comorbidities of eating disorders. Biological and genetic research has helped us gain more understanding of their etiology, and, as a field, our increased knowledge of the presentation and risk factors informs our psychological and pharmacological interventions. However, eating disorders are serious and often treatment refractory, and much work remains to be done to effectively prevent and treat them.

Recommended Reading

Academy for Eating Disorders: https://www.aedweb.org/home

F.E.A.S.T. (Families Empowered And Supporting Treatment for Eating Disorders) support community: https://www.feast-ed.org

13

Body Dysmorphic Disorder

Katharine A. Phillips, M.D.

Definition

Body dysmorphic disorder (BDD) is a common and often severe yet under-recognized disorder. People with BDD worry that there is something wrong with how they look—that they are ugly, unattractive, abnormal, or even hideous. Yet, in the eyes of other people, they look fine or the appearance "flaws" are actually only slight. To differentiate BDD from normal appearance concerns—which are common in the general population—the appearance preoccupations must cause significant emotional distress or significant interference in daily functioning. Table 13–1 shows the diagnostic criteria for BDD from the American Psychiatric Association's *Diagnostic and Statistical Manual of Mental Disorders*, 5th Edition (DSM-5).

Appearance preoccupations can focus on one or many body areas, most often skin (e.g., perceived acne, paleness or redness, scars, lines), hair (e.g., "thinning" hair, "excessive" body or facial hair), or nose (e.g., size or shape), but any aspect of appearance can be a focus of concern (e.g., face or head size or shape, chin, jaw, cheeks, eyes, lips, teeth, breasts, weight, stomach, legs, genitals, height, asymmetry). These preoccupations are intrusive, unwanted, time consuming (3–8 hours/day, on average), and usually difficult to resist or control. Appearance preoccupations trigger repetitive behaviors or mental acts (also called *rituals* or *compulsions*) that aim to check, fix, or hide the perceived defects. These behaviors are not pleasurable, are time consuming, and are difficult to control

Table 13–1. DSM-5 diagnostic criteria for body dysmorphic disorder

A. **Preoccupation** with one or more perceived defects or flaws in physical appearance that are not observable or appear slight to others.

B. At some point during the course of the disorder, the individual has performed **repetitive behaviors** (e.g., mirror checking, excessive grooming, skin picking, reassurance seeking) or **mental acts** (e.g., comparing his or her appearance with that of others) in response to the appearance concerns.

C. The preoccupation **causes clinically significant distress or impairment** in social, occupational, or other important areas of functioning.

D. The appearance preoccupation is not better explained by concerns with body fat or weight in an individual whose symptoms meet diagnostic criteria for an eating disorder.

Specify if: ***With muscle dysmorphia:*** The individual is preoccupied with the idea that their body build is too small or insufficiently muscular. This specifier is used even if the individual is preoccupied with other body areas, which is often the case.

Specify if: *Indicate degree of insight* regarding body dysmorphic disorder beliefs (e.g., "I look ugly" or "I look deformed").

With good or fair insight: The individual recognizes that the body dysmorphic disorder beliefs are definitely or probably not true or that they may or may not be true.

With poor insight: The individual thinks that the body dysmorphic disorder beliefs are probably true.

With absent insight/delusional beliefs: The individual is completely convinced that the body dysmorphic disorder beliefs are true.

Source. From American Psychiatric Association: *Diagnostic and Statistical Manual of Mental Disorders*, 5th Edition, Text Revision. Washington, DC, American Psychiatric Association, 2022.

or stop. Table 13–1 lists common repetitive behaviors; other common behaviors include touching disliked areas to check them, tanning, taking excessive "selfie" photographs, excessively exercising, and seeking cosmetic treatment. Hiding perceived defects (i.e., camouflaging) is a common behavior that may involve repetitive actions (e.g., reapplying makeup or readjusting a hat to hide perceived baldness).

People with the *muscle dysmorphia* form of BDD, who are usually male, are preoccupied with the idea that their body is too small or insufficiently lean or muscular, even though they actually look normal or are even very muscular. Most, but not all, of these individuals diet (e.g., a high-protein, low-fat diet) and exercise or lift weights in excess, sometimes to the point of damaging their body. Some use potentially dangerous supplements and supplements, such as anabolic-androgenic steroids, to try to make their body bigger and more muscular.

Most people with BDD are mostly or completely certain that they really do look ugly or abnormal, even though they actually do not. In other words, most have *poor or absent insight* (see Table 13–1). Their distorted body image is probably caused by aberrations in visual processing—that is, they actually *see* themselves differently than other people see them.

BDD preoccupations are usually very distressing, causing feelings such as depressed mood, anxiety, anger, embarrassment, shame, and suicidal thinking. Daily functioning and quality of life are usually very poor. Nearly everyone with BDD has some impairment in functioning because of appearance concerns, usually ranging from moderate (e.g., avoiding some social situations) to extreme and incapacitating (e.g., being housebound). Most people experience difficulties with relationships and social functioning (e.g., social activities, dating, intimacy, friendships) and in employment, academic, or role functioning (e.g., missing school or work). Impairment is often severe, for example, not working, dropping out of school, or having few or no relationships. These difficulties typically occur because people with BDD do not want other people to see them because they are "ugly" or fear others will reject them or make fun of them because of how they look, or they may occur because the preoccupations and repetitive behaviors are so distressing, time consuming, and distracting.

Most people with BDD have suicidal thinking, and about 25% have made a suicide attempt, often because of their appearance concerns. BDD is characterized by significantly higher rates and levels of suicidal thinking and behavior than other psychiatric disorders with high risk for suicidality. The risk of death from suicide also appears to be very high.

How Is Body Dysmorphic Disorder Diagnosed?

BDD usually begins in early adolescence, beginning before age 18 in two-thirds of individuals. It is usually undiagnosed, often because people with BDD feel too embarrassed and ashamed to reveal their appearance concerns to others or because it has been misdiagnosed. Without the right treatment, BDD is usually chronic and unremitting.

To identify BDD, clinicians usually need to ask specifically about BDD symptoms. The following questions, which reflect the DSM-5 diagnostic criteria in Table 13–1, can be asked to diagnose BDD:

- "Are you very worried about your appearance in any way?" *or* "Are you unhappy with how you look?" *and* "If you add up all the time you spend each day thinking about your appearance, how much time do you think you spend?"
- "Is there anything that you do over and over again in response to your appearance concerns?"

- "How much distress do these concerns cause you?"
- "How do your appearance concerns affect your life?"

Other questions can elaborate on these key issues. A diagnosis of BDD is indicated by answers of spending about 1 hour or more per day in total thinking about appearance flaws that are actually nonexistent or slight, performing repetitive BDD behaviors, and experiencing at least moderate distress or impairment in functioning due to appearance concerns. Repetitive behaviors (e.g., mirror checking, excessive grooming, seeking reassurance about appearance, skin picking) and camouflaging (e.g., excessive tanning, wearing a hat pulled down over one's face) are observable clues that a person may have BDD. Difficulties in functioning, such as avoiding social situations, are also possible clues.

If preoccupation with body fat or weight is present and qualifies for a feeding and eating disorder diagnosis, then these concerns do not "count" toward a BDD diagnosis (see Table 13–1). However, body weight or fat concerns in someone who does *not* have an eating disorder and is *not* significantly overweight can be symptoms of BDD. Some people have both an eating disorder (with weight or fat concerns) *and* BDD (e.g., skin or nose concerns), and clinical expertise may be needed to differentiate BDD with weight or fat concerns from an eating disorder. BDD is often misdiagnosed as another disorder, such as social anxiety disorder, obsessive-compulsive disorder (OCD), agoraphobia, major depressive disorder, a psychotic disorder, or an eating disorder. It is important to not confuse BDD with another disorder because the effective treatment approaches for BDD differ from treatments for other disorders.

Recently, a tsunami of new terms has been spreading through the media and the scientific literature. These neologisms include *body dysmorphia, acne dysmorphia, skin dysmorphia, Zoom dysmorphia, Snapchat dysmorphia*, and *penile dysmorphia*. These terms are not well defined, and it is often unclear whether they refer to BDD or to common, nonpathological body image dissatisfaction. Thus, it is best not to use them.

Common Co-Occurring Mental Health Disorders

Disorders that most commonly co-occur with BDD are major depressive disorder, substance use disorders, social anxiety disorder, OCD, and eating disorders.

How Common Is Body Dysmorphic Disorder?

Approximately 2%–3% of the general population currently has BDD; rates are higher among psychiatric inpatient and outpatient settings and in dermatology

(11%–13%), general cosmetic surgery (13%–15%), rhinoplasty (nose) surgery (20%), and other cosmetic treatment settings. However, BDD is underrecognized in all of these clinical settings.

About 60% of people with BDD are female. BDD affects people from around the world and of all ages, from early childhood to old age. The disorder appears to be most common among adolescents and young adults. Its characteristics are largely similar among adults and youth and among males and females, although there are some differences.

Risk Factors

BDD is associated with having been teased and with childhood neglect, abuse, and trauma, but it is unclear whether these are risk factors for developing the disorder. Use of image-centric social media may possibly increase the risk of developing BDD, but this is not currently known. In addition, the brains of people with BDD have difficulty seeing the "big picture" of what they are looking at (e.g., their face or body) and over-focus on tiny details. This may make minuscule details of appearance look very prominent and flawed to the person with BDD. This aberration in how the brain sees things might increase the risk of developing BDD.

Are Genetics Involved?

About 40%–50% of the risk for developing BDD is related to genetic factors. The disorder shares some genes with OCD, but it also has genetic influences that differ from OCD and are specific to BDD.

Conclusion

BDD is a common, yet underrecognized condition that typically starts during early adolescence. BDD causes significant emotional distress or significant difficulties with day-to-day functioning—usually both. Individuals with BDD frequently have co-occurring major depressive disorder, substance use disorders, social anxiety disorder, and OCD. They also have higher rates of suicidal thinking, suicide attempts, and actual suicide; therefore, it is important to be aware of BDD symptoms and clues that a person may have this disorder. It is also important to obtain mental health treatment from a clinician who is familiar with BDD and its treatment, because treatment significantly improves BDD for most people.

Recommended Reading

Phillips KA: Understanding Body Dysmorphic Disorder: An Essential Guide. New York, Oxford University Press, 2009

Phillips KA (ed): Body Dysmorphic Disorder: Advances in Research and Clinical Practice. New York, Oxford University Press, 2017

14

Prolonged Grief Disorder

M. Katherine Shear, M.D.
Natalia Skritskaya, Ph.D.
Colleen Bloom, M.S.W.

What Is Grief?

The desire and need for close relationships are part of our biology. Our loved ones comfort and support us when things are not going well. They instill confidence and give us the strength and courage to take risks and try new things. They are why we feel that we belong and matter in the world. We also take care of them in return, which is even more important to our well-being.

The death of a loved one is one of life's most significant and painful stressors. Loss changes our lives in dramatic ways. Grief is the natural response to the experience of a meaningful loss. Grief is permanent after we lose someone close, yet it evolves and becomes interwoven into our life as we adjust to the world changed by the loss. We have a natural ability to adapt to even the most painful loss. However, this process can get derailed, which may lead to prolonged grief disorder (PGD). This chapter introduces a way of thinking about grief and adaptation to loss that provides a foundation for understanding PGD.

Grief as a response to loss is not just sadness but a complex mix of thoughts, feelings, actions, and physiological changes. This complexity adds to the stress of early bereavement and the need to find ways to cope with it. Grief is influenced by many factors, such as the circumstances surrounding the death, consequences of the loss, and a person's social, cultural, or religious beliefs. How grief unfolds is unique to each person, and it changes as we adapt to the loss. Additionally, grief can wax and wane in intensity in response to reminders or difficult calendar days.

The days, weeks, and months following an important loss, which is called *acute grief*, almost always include strong feelings of yearning, longing, sadness, anxiety, bitterness, remorse, and guilt. It can be hard to regulate emotions and make decisions. A person may have trouble sleeping and eating. They may question who they are, what they believe in, and what their future holds. Acute grief is painful and preoccupying, making it difficult to concentrate on anything else. However, grief does not persist indefinitely in this severe form.

Why and How Grief Evolves

Loss activates the "psychological immune system," which helps a person adjust over time to changes in one's inner life and outer world. *Coping* is what we do in early grief to help us bear the pain and manage in the moment. Some common ways newly bereaved people cope is by temporarily blocking the knowledge of the loss or avoiding its painful reminders. Instead of confronting the reality of the loss, it is natural to imagine how things could have gone differently or to blame ourselves or others for the death. These coping strategies are useful in the short term, allowing us to pause and obtain respite from pain. However, they can also make adapting more difficult if they persist and come to dominate our minds.

Adapting is different from coping. It unfolds in response to the significant changes a loss brings. It is an ongoing process that differs for each person and each loss. Despite this uniqueness, some common features seem to apply universally. We all must grapple and come to terms with the new unwanted reality which entails 1) accepting that the loss cannot be undone, 2) recognizing the permanence of grief, and 3) learning to live with a changed relationship with the deceased. The other vital piece is restoring our sense of purpose and meaning in life and feelings of belonging and mattering, with possibilities for happiness.

A common misconception is that grief occurs in stages. If this were true, it would mean that grief progresses in a predictable sequence. A more helpful way of thinking about grief is that it changes as we adapt to the loss. Adapting happens naturally and often out of our conscious awareness, but it is not always smooth or easy.

Some common and natural reactions during acute grief can get in the way of or derail the process of adapting if they keep dominating the mind. Early coping responses to a loss such as protesting the death, thoughts and feelings of self-blame or guilt, anger, shame, repeatedly imagining ways things could have gone differently, losing faith in yourself or others, and excessively avoiding reminders of the loss can backfire and interfere with adaptation, thus contributing to development of PGD. When a loved one dies, most people have unsettling thoughts about how things could have been different. We want to protest or block the reality of what happened. There might be strong feelings of anger or bitterness about something someone could or should have done differently. There might be feelings of guilt about something done or not done, or even for being alive. It is also natural for our minds to create different scenarios of how something could have been done to prevent the death, akin to "Monday morning quarterbacking." Such thoughts are natural and even helpful in early grief; however, they can make it more difficult to adapt if they gain a foothold. They can distract us from dealing with the reality of the loss and finding ways to restore our life.

Prolonged Grief Disorder

When symptoms of acute grief are relentless and intense for longer than 1 year, it might be a sign of *prolonged grief disorder*. PGD is now officially recognized as a mental health disorder by the World Health Organization, and it was added to the American Psychiatric Association's *Diagnostic and Statistical Manual of Mental Disorders*, 5th Edition (known as DSM-5) during its 2022 text revision (DSM-5-TR). It is a form of pervasive grief that overwhelms a person's life and makes it difficult to function. For people with PGD, the future seems bleak and empty. They feel lost and alone. Some describe it as being "stuck" in their grief, frozen in time as though the death has just happened. This is a very painful condition that significantly impacts a person's ability to work, socialize, or function in other ways. Sometimes people can manage to function in some way, to take care of essentials such as going to work, but may be impacted by PGD in another way, for example, in their social lives and leisure time.

How Is Prolonged Grief Disorder Diagnosed?

As listed in Table 14–1, the signs of PGD are persistent strong feelings of yearning or longing for a loved one or preoccupying thoughts and memories that get in the way of living life in a meaningful way. A bereaved person with PGD may feel intensely lonely and distance themselves from others. They may be in a lot of emotional pain and try to avoid reminders of their loss, or they may feel emotionally numb and still in disbelief. They may feel unsure of what matters to them and who they are now, and they struggle to reengage with life.

The duration and severity of grief in PGD clearly exceed expected norms in the individual's social, cultural, or religious context. If you are struggling with

Table 14–1. DSM-5-TR diagnostic criteria for prolonged grief disorder

A. Death of a person close to the bereaved at least 12 months ago

B. Persistent pervasive yearning, longing, or preoccupation with the deceased

C. Since the death, at least three of the following are present most days to a clinically significant degree and nearly every day for at least the past month:

   1. Disrupted identity
   2. Marked sense of disbelief
   3. Avoidance of reminders
   4. Intense emotional pain
   5. Difficulty engaging in ongoing life
   6. Emotional numbness
   7. Feeling that life is meaningless
   8. Intense loneliness

D. Significant distress or impairment in personal, family, social, educational, occupational, or other important areas of functioning

Source. From American Psychiatric Association: *Diagnostic and Statistical Manual of Mental Disorders*, 5th Edition, Text Revision. Washington, DC, American Psychiatric Association, 2022.

grief and suspect that you may have PGD, taking the Brief Grief Questionnaire (https://prolongedgrief.columbia.edu/brief-grief-questionnaire) may help. If you score a 4 or higher, an evaluation with a mental health professional to pursue treatment is recommended. There are good evidence-based treatments (see Chapter 28, "Treatment of Prolonged Grief Disorder") that can help invigorate the natural healing process.

Risk Factors

Any death is hard, but certain circumstances, context, and consequences of the loss make some losses more difficult than others and thereby increase the risk of PGD. No one rule fits all; however, a sudden loss is more shocking and more difficult to comprehend. It is also easier after a sudden loss to envision alternative scenarios in which a loved one did not have to die. Other circumstances of the death, such as a violent loss, death of a young person, loss of a particularly close rewarding relationship, or losing multiple important people also increase the likelihood of PGD. Other known risk factors for PGD include a personal history of trauma, anxiety, or depression and dealing with especially challenging financial or social stressors in the aftermath of a death. Approximately 10%

of people bereaved by natural causes develop PGD, and the rate is higher for those bereaved by a violent death, such as an accident, homicide, or suicide.

Common Co-Occurring Mental Health Disorders

PGD shares similarities with major depressive disorder and posttraumatic stress disorder (PTSD), and the conditions frequently occur together. The public and even mental health professionals may confuse these diagnoses, but it is important to differentiate them because they each respond to different treatments. For example, antidepressants do not help with grief. Although both grief and depression are marked by intense sadness, it is not the same. Sadness in depression is generally connected to feeling like a failure in life, whereas in grief it is connected to the absence of the loved one. PGD and PTSD both develop in response to a stressful life event such as the death of a loved one, but PTSD is characterized by fear, whereas PGD is marked by intense yearning for the deceased. PGD, PTSD, and major depressive disorder should not be treated the same; precise and effective help depends on a clear understanding of what a particular person is dealing with. You can learn about effective treatment for PGD in Chapter 28.

Conclusion

Grief is a natural response to a meaningful loss. With time, people typically will adapt to the changes brought by the loss, learning to process their new reality and figuring out ways to rebuild their lives. Although the grief is not completely gone, and it can still become strong for short periods of time, it usually quiets down and recedes into the background of their daily lives.

However, sometimes adaptation to loss and grief becomes derailed, leading to PGD, a condition of persistent and pervasive intense grief that interferes with a person's functioning. PGD may seem similar to major depression or PTSD, but they are distinct conditions requiring different treatments.

Recommended Reading

Heid M: What is complicated grief—and when is it prolonged grief disorder? Everyday Health, April 5, 2022. Available at: https://www.everydayhealth.com/emotional-health/grief/what-is-complicated-grief.

Shear MK: Grief White Paper Series—I. Healing Milestones: What to Expect From Grief With COVID-19 Addendum. New York, The Center for Complicated Grief, 2020. Available at: https://complicatedgrief.columbia.edu/wp-content/uploads/2020/06/HEALING-Milestones_-What-Grievers-Can-Expect-with-Covid-19-Addendum.pdf.

Part II

Treatment of the Disorders

15

Treatment of Major Depression

Charles B. Nemeroff, M.D., Ph.D.
Nicholas Ortiz, M.D.

Introduction

As described by Schatzberg in Chapter 1, "Major Depression," major depressive disorder (MDD) is a common and severe psychiatric syndrome characterized by a number of signs and symptoms including changes in sleep, appetite, and mood as well as the cardinal feature of depression—the relative or absolute inability to experience pleasure. The good news is that evidence-based treatments for depression are available, but the bad news is that there are currently no validated methods to predict which of these treatments will be effective in a given patient. As such, many patients require treatment with a variety of medications, psychotherapies, or neuromodulation techniques before demonstrating clinically significant improvement.

Treatment Options

The gold standard for establishing the efficacy of any treatment for depression is randomized controlled clinical trials in which both patients and raters are "blinded," meaning that they are not aware of the treatments being provided. Placebo-controlled trials are required by the U.S. Food and Drug Administration (FDA) for approval of a new medication for the treatment of depression. The goal of treatment is remission, the return of the mood state the patient enjoyed prior to being depressed, and this is operationalized by using depression symptom severity rating scales such as the Hamilton Rating Scale for Depression (HAM-D) or the Montgomery-Åsberg Depression Rating Scale (MADRS). *Remission* is defined as the fundamental absence of any depressive symptoms, whereas *response* is defined as a 50% improvement in depressive symptom severity. Obviously, the ultimate goal is remission. Unlike a disorder such as schizophrenia, which has a limited number of FDA-approved treatments, a large number of treatments for depression exist, as do treatments approved for use alongside antidepressants to augment the antidepressant effect. In the discussion that follows, we briefly review the evidence-based treatments currently available and describe some new promising investigational treatments. Each of the individual treatments are described in greater detail in individual chapters elsewhere in this volume.

Medication-Based Treatments

Antidepressants

The first antidepressants approved by the FDA were the tricyclic antidepressants (TCAs) and the monoamine oxidase inhibitors (MAOIs). There is no question that these medications are effective antidepressants that, prior to the introduction of the newer-generation agents, were the mainstay of depression treatment. The TCAs, although quite effective, had the major disadvantage of being lethal in overdose, which is an especially problematic property given that suicidal behavior is a major component of the depression syndrome. At one time, the TCAs were responsible for most of the overdose deaths in the United States, but opiates have now far surpassed TCAs in this regard. The TCAs had other troubling side effects as well, including dry mouth, sedation, potential cardiac side effects, constipation, and medication interactions. As with almost all other antidepressants, they also take 3–5 weeks to realize their therapeutic benefit. TCAs are believed to act by increasing availability of the neurotransmitters serotonin and/or norepinephrine in the synaptic cleft, where they can activate their respective receptors. One advantage TCAs have over all other antidepressants is that they have established therapeutic blood levels to guide treatment dosing.

In contrast to TCAs, MAOIs inhibit the breakdown of monoamine neurotransmitters dopamine, serotonin, and norepinephrine, increasing their concentration in the synaptic cleft. Evidence has shown that MAOIs are particularly helpful in patients with so-called atypical depression characterized by increased sleep and appetite and a great deal of anxiety. Unfortunately, these medications are rarely prescribed because of concerns about their interaction with certain foods that contain tyramine, termed the "cheese reaction," and with other medications such as meperidine. These food and medication interactions can result in a medical emergency because of the risk of a high blood pressure "hypertensive crisis" that can lead to a stroke. Such reactions are extremely rare, and patients are counseled as to what foods (e.g., Vegemite, soy sauce) and medications (e.g., pseudoephedrine) need to be avoided. Because of these concerns, many patients who might benefit from the therapeutic effects of MAOIs never receive them.

Selective Serotonin and Serotonin-Norepinephrine Reuptake Inhibitors

Beginning with the approval of fluoxetine (Prozac) in 1999, a series of compounds believed to act by selectively inhibiting the reuptake of serotonin fundamentally changed the treatment of depression worldwide. These drugs, including fluoxetine (Prozac), sertraline (Zoloft), paroxetine (Paxil), citalopram (Celexa), and escitalopram (Lexapro), became the medications of choice for treating depression. They had several major advantages over the MAOIs and TCAs. They were not lethal in overdose and were not sedating. In general, head-to-head comparisons between one or another of these selective serotonin reuptake inhibitors (SSRIs) and a TCA showed the former group to be equal in efficacy, with fewer side effects. SSRIs remain the agents of choice to treat depression, but they are not without side effects, and many patients do not attain remission after treatment with these agents for an adequate duration at an adequate dosage. Although patients often have acute side effects such as headache or nausea, such adverse reactions usually dissipate over time. However, some patients exhibit significant long-term side effects, including sexual dysfunction (e.g., anorgasmia, decreased erectile function and ejaculation), weight gain, and emotional numbing or apathy and experience withdrawal symptoms on abrupt discontinuation. More importantly, it is now clear that only 28%–50% of patients attain remission with SSRIs alone. This is of paramount importance because we know that patients who do not achieve remission are much more likely to become chronically depressed, exhibit increased risk for suicidal behavior, and develop concurrent medical disorders as well as substance and alcohol abuse.

Serotonin-norepinephrine reuptake inhibitors (SNRIs) include venlafaxine (Effexor), desmethylvenlafaxine (Prestiq), duloxetine (Cymbalta) and levomilnacipran (Fetzima). These drugs act by blocking the reuptake of both serotonin and norepinephrine. There is some evidence that these agents are slightly more effective than the SSRIs, but they also have additional side effects including high blood pressure and a withdrawal syndrome after abrupt discontinuation in addition to the side effects of the SSRIs noted earlier.

Several SSRIs and SNRIs are also FDA-approved for treatment of psychiatric conditions that frequently co-occur with major depression, including generalized anxiety disorder, panic disorder, obsessive-compulsive disorder (OCD), and social anxiety disorder.

Other Antidepressants

A hodgepodge of agents that are chemically and pharmacologically unrelated have also been FDA-approved for the treatment of major depression. These include bupropion (Wellbutrin), trazodone (Desyrel), nefazodone (Serzone), vortioxetine (Trintellix), mirtazapine (Remeron), and vilazodone (Vibryd). Many of these medications share some properties with the SSRIs but have additional effects believed to provide some therapeutic benefit. Others, such as bupropion, although effective, act in a manner that is not entirely clear to pharmacologists.

Augmenting Agents and Combination Strategies

As noted earlier, other medications have shown to augment the effects of antidepressants in patients who have not attained remission with monotherapy. Some of these are FDA-approved, such as certain atypical antipsychotics (e.g., aripiprazole, brexpiprazole), whereas others have ample published data of their efficacy but have not been submitted for FDA approval (e.g., lithium, pramipexole, and triiodothyronine [T3], a thyroid hormone). Another common strategy is to combine two antidepressants from two different classes that have presumed different mechanisms of action, such as mirtazapine and venlafaxine or bupropion and sertraline. Space constraints preclude a discussion of the relative merits of augmentation and combination strategies versus the drawback of two medications usually increasing the potential for side effect burden.

Non-Medication-Based Treatments

Psychotherapy

Several psychotherapies have been demonstrated to be effective in the treatment of major depression. The best studied of these is cognitive-behavioral therapy (CBT), developed by Aaron "Tim" Beck at the University of Pennsylvania. Multiple studies have shown its efficacy in the treatment of depression. As discussed in Chapter 54 ("Cognitive-Behavioral Therapy for Major Depressive Disorder"), CBT targets the dysfunctional thinking and cognitive distortions characteristic of depression, in which patients feel hopeless about the future and helpless to do anything about it while they focus on past failures, their own poor self-image, and the notion that they are a burden on their families. Other forms of psychotherapy have been found to be effective in depression as well, including interpersonal psychotherapy and behavioral activation.

Neuromodulation

Three forms of neurostimulation techniques currently have FDA approval for the treatment of depression. The oldest and arguably the most effective treatment of depression is *electroconvulsive therapy* (ECT). This treatment is described in detail in Chapter 48, but, fundamentally, patients are placed under general anesthesia and are given an agent to paralyze their muscles briefly. Then an electric current is applied to the brain to induce a generalized seizure. ECT is usually administered in the hospital two or three times per week for a total of 9–12 treatments. Short-term memory loss is the major side effect. ECT is relatively rapidly acting and lifesaving in patients with severe depressive stupor who are unable to function in daily life.

The second neuromodulation treatment is *repetitive transcranial magnetic stimulation* (rTMS), in which a large magnet is placed on the left side of the head while a patient is sitting in the equivalent of a dental chair or recliner. The stimulation targets the patient's dorsolateral prefrontal cortex. rTMS was initially approved by the FDA for the treatment of depression in 2008. A more accelerated form called *intermittent theta burst stimulation* (iTBS) was approved in 2018. rTMS is administered for approximately 45 minutes per day, 5 days per week, for 6 weeks, and iTBS is administered for approximately 4–10 minutes per day, 5 days per week, for 6 weeks. More recently, the FDA has approved the *Stanford Accelerated Intelligence Neuromodulation Therapy* (SAINT) treatment, in which patients receive 10 minutes of iTBS every hour for 10 treatments over a 5-day period. More than 85% of patients with treatment-resistant depression met criteria for symptom remission at the end of a week of treatment.

The third type of neuromodulation approved by the FDA is *vagus nerve stimulation* (VNS). This is an invasive technique in which a vagus nerve stimulator is surgically implanted under the clavicle by a neurosurgeon or otolaryngologist, with the terminals wrapped around the vagus nerve such that stimulation acts on vagus nerve afferents that enter the brain. Unlike other treatments for depression, this treatment has been shown to work rather slowly over a several-month period. A very large new clinical trial with VNS is currently in progress.

Recently Approved and Novel Investigational Treatments

After a hiatus of a several decades in which no new treatments were developed for depression, recent years have seen a remarkable resurgence. It began with the demonstration that intravenously administered ketamine had an immediate antidepressant effect that persisted for up to 7 days following the initial treatment. There are many problems associated with this database, including the lack of FDA approval, the inability to "blind" the treatment in research studies, and the rapid upsurge in the number of ketamine clinics that are largely directed by nonpsychiatrists who do not routinely screen for past treatment history, substance abuse history, and other important patient background information. In addition, ketamine is, of course, a substance of abuse, known as "Special K." Recent evidence has shown that ketamine may actually act on endogenous opiate systems because its antidepressant effects are blocked by the μ-opiate antagonist naltrexone. On the basis of these findings, intranasal esketamine was studied as a novel antidepressant treatment and, despite considerable controversy regarding the submitted FDA package, it was approved. Because of the need to observe patients for 2 hours in the office following administration and the high cost of the agent, it has not been widely used in the United States. Several ketamine-like compounds believed to act primarily at the *N*-methyl-D-aspartate (NMDA) receptor are currently under investigation including R-ketamine and various formulations of ketamine, such as oral and subcutaneous. Several other NMDA antagonists are under investigation as well.

Other novel antidepressants discussed later in this volume include zuranolone, which is the oral form of brexanolone, a positive allosteric modulator of the γ-aminobutyric acid-A ($GABA_A$) receptor, that is now FDA-approved for treatment of postpartum depression. This compound appears to be particularly effective in patients with depression and comorbid anxiety. Recently, the FDA has approved the combination of dextromethorphan and bupropion, which is also thought to act at the NMDA receptor; clinical trial data suggest this combination has an unusually rapid onset of action. Other investigational compounds under study include ezogabine and esmethadone. The latter compound recently demonstrated clear efficacy after 7 days of treatment in an inpatient setting.

Finally, space constraints preclude a comprehensive discussion of the use of psychedelics in the treatment of depression. The best studied is psilocybin, which despite the difficulty in "blinding" a psychedelic in a clinical trial has shown efficacy in patients with major depression in several studies. Whether other psychedelics such as the dimethyltryptamine series (e.g., 5MeO-DMT), ayahuasca, mescaline, or lysergic acid diethylamide (LSD) may have some benefit is unclear, as is the entire and seminal question as to whether low, nonpsychedelic doses of these compounds have utility in the treatment of depression.

Conclusion

Many individuals will experience major depression during their lifetimes. Fortunately, patients and their psychiatrists have access to a variety of effective treatments, including medications, psychotherapy, and neuromodulation techniques. In addition, there is growing interest among researchers and the public in innovative treatments such as ketamine and psychedelics. With these novel and established therapies, an increasing number of patients can expect relief from their depressive symptoms.

Recommended Reading

Nemeroff CB: The state of our understanding of the pathophysiology and optimal treatment of depression: glass half full or half empty? Am J Psychiatry 177(8):671–685, 2020

Nemeroff CB (ed): The American Psychiatric Association Publishing Textbook of Mood Disorders, 2nd Edition. Washington, DC, American Psychiatric Association Publishing, 2022

16

Treatment of Bipolar Disorder

Gregory H. Jones, M.D.
Rodrigo Machado-Vieira, M.D., Ph.D.
Jair C. Soares, M.D., Ph.D.

Case Vignette

Jonathan has felt depressed since his teenage years. He experienced his first manic episode at age 21 after heading off to college and was effectively treated with quetiapine. However, since that time (several years ago), he has become increasingly depressed and has experienced some weight gain and excess daytime fatigue. After discussion with his psychiatrist, they decide to switch to lurasidone, which has a low risk of weight gain and sedation. After a month, Jonathan feels 30% better and has become more motivated and physically active. However, he still feels depressed about half of the days out of the week and occasionally experiences passive thoughts of suicide. Because of the initial benefit, they decide to add lithium as opposed to switching medications. Several weeks after attaining adequate blood levels of lithium, his suicidal thoughts have gone away. His motivation has also increased enough to attend weekly psychotherapy. After a full 12-week course of cognitive-behavioral therapy (CBT), he still feels a small amount of residual depression. At the next follow-up session, he notes successful remission of his depressive symptoms and has begun making significant lifestyle changes.

Introduction

Bipolar depression is a complex illness that presents several unique challenges compared with other mental health conditions. Each time a patient experiences a manic or depressive episode, the risk for having more frequent and severe episodes in the future goes up. Furthermore, if depressive symptoms are not adequately addressed, they can become harder to treat over time. For some patients, more frequent episodes may also worsen cognitive abilities such as memory, problem solving, and concentration long-term. Prolonged depression has also been associated with increased risk of suicide, disability, hospitalization, and lower overall quality of life. Alternatively, recovery rates are generally higher in patients who start treatment earlier. For these reasons, patients and loved ones should take an active role in finding an effective and tolerable treatment regimen in a timely manner.

A wide range of options is available to address bipolar depression. However, just as every person is unique, each treatment has its own risks and benefits, and it can be hard to predict what will work best for individual patients. A significant proportion of patients will have to try several different medications before obtaining a good response. People with bipolar depression also more frequently are taking multiple medicines simultaneously, although this is not always the most effective strategy. Overall, anticipating some amount of trial and error and working closely with health care providers to develop an individualized treatment regimen are vital to long-term success. In this chapter, we discuss the most common classes of medications used in bipolar depression and provide a general algorithm for treatment.

Treatment Options

Medication-Based Treatments

Second-Generation ("Atypical") Antipsychotics

The second-generation, or "atypical," antipsychotic medications include quetiapine (Seroquel), lurasidone (Latuda), olanzapine (Zyprexa), lumateperone (Caplyta), cariprazine (Vraylar), aripiprazole (Abilify), and asenapine (Saphris). Owing to their superior effectiveness and lower side effect burden, antipsychotics have recently replaced mood stabilizers as the primary initial treatment for bipolar depression. Although each has its own individual properties, as a class, they all help regulate the activity of a chemical called dopamine in the brain.

Originally developed to treat schizophrenia, their properties can also help alleviate a range of bipolar symptoms.

Mood Stabilizers

Mood stabilizers (e.g., lithium [Lithobid, Eskalith], lamotrigine [Lamictal], divalproex [Depakote], carbamazepine [Tegretol, Carbatrol]) work in several different ways, but many are also used to treat seizures because they can calm some of the overactive signals in the brain that may lead to depression or mania. Lithium has its own unique properties and is considered one of the most effective agents to treat mania and help stable patients prevent future depressive/manic episodes. Studies suggest that lithium may also be effective in treating depression (especially when used alongside certain other medicines). It has also shown the ability to reduce suicide risk.

Antidepressants

Numerous medications in each of the antidepressant classes are available and are discussed in more detail in the individual treatment chapters of this volume, but generally, these include the selective serotonin reuptake inhibitors (SSRIs), serotonin-norepinephrine reuptake inhibitors (SNRIs), monoamine oxidase inhibitors (MAOIs), tricyclic antidepressants (TCAs), and norepinephrine and dopamine reuptake inhibitors (NDRIs). The SSRIs and bupropion (Wellbutrin, an NDRI) are generally preferred over other classes. Antidepressants are mainly recommended for certain patients with bipolar disorder, and they should usually be added to an antipsychotic or mood stabilizer (due to their risk of causing [hypo]manic symptoms when used alone). Typically, patients whose illness responds better to these medicines have mild (bipolar II) symptoms, are experiencing "pure depression" (i.e., no current [hypo]manic features), have no alcohol or substance use disorders, and have no history of becoming (hypo)manic after starting these medications previously. The SNRIs are more likely to cause bipolar patients to "switch" into hypomania or mania.

Neuromodulation

Neuromodulation approaches are "non-drug" therapies such as electroconvulsive therapy (ECT) and repetitive transcranial magnetic stimulation (rTMS). ECT uses electrical current to intentionally cause a seizure while patients are under general anesthesia (as in surgery). It is not clear exactly how ECT works, but ECT is considered one of the most effective treatments available for depression and has been shown to reduce the risk of suicide. Although there are always risks associated with general anesthesia (which vary depending on overall state of health), ECT is typically well tolerated and is considered safe enough to use during pregnancy. However, some patients do report memory loss, confusion, or other side effects. With rTMS, patients are awake and receive targeted electrical pulses from a powerful magnet placed near the surface of the head. It works by stimulating specific areas of the brain that are thought to be underactive during depression. Although risk of (hypo)mania has been reported with rTMS, it generally has fewer side effects than ECT but may also be less effective and require more treatments.

Non-Medication-Based Treatments

Psychotherapy

Studies suggest that psychotherapy, or "talk therapy," may be less beneficial in treating the symptoms of bipolar depression than for those of unipolar depression (i.e., major depressive disorder). However, psychotherapy has led to significant improvements when used in combination with medicine, more often in patients with fewer lifetime manic/depressive episodes. Psychotherapy can also help address issues related to personal relationships, past trauma, culture, employment, community, attitudes toward illness and treatment, cognitive function, and other parts of life, which may have long-term benefits not adequately reflected in clinical trials. Although it can be mentally challenging, psychotherapy also has few (if any) serious side effects. Several types of psychotherapy have shown benefit when combined with medicine in bipolar depression:

- *Cognitive-behavioral therapy (CBT)*—focuses on changing thoughts, feelings, and behaviors that lead to depression
- *Family-focused therapy (FFT)*—seeks to improve family communication styles and cooperation with both the patient and family present
- *Interpersonal and social rhythm therapy (IPSRT)*—focuses mainly on repairing sleep and social problems commonly seen in patients with bipolar disorder. Each type requires approximately 10–30 sessions (6–9 months).

Once depression has lifted, any of these styles (in addition to *group psychoeducation* or *formal peer support*) can also help prevent depressive symptoms from returning.

Other Treatments

Other potential treatments include ketamine, stimulants, bright light therapy (with or without sleep deprivation), omega-3 fatty acids (fish/algae oil), coenzyme Q10 (CoQ10), thyroid hormones, and dopamine modulators. These treatments are only recommended as add-on treatments (to antipsychotics or mood stabilizers) in patients whose illness does not respond completely to several first- or second-line treatments (Table 16–1). These are discussed in more detail in the various treatment chapters.

How Treatment Is Decided

The following discussion describes a general algorithm of the treatment options shown in Table 16–1. The brand names or qualifiers for these treatments are provided in parentheses. First-tier therapies include the atypical antipsychotics that have U.S. Food and Drug Administration (FDA) approval for the treatment of bipolar depression and combinations of medications that have a strong level of benefit/tolerability from large, rigorous clinical trials. Second-tier treatments have likewise consistently demonstrated benefit in studies, although not as robust as those in the first tier. Third-tier treatments have either shown a modest benefit or have only been evaluated in a limited number of patients. Except for carbamazepine (which can be used alone), the third-tier approaches are recommended only as add-ons to another treatment (usually another atypical antipsychotic or mood stabilizer, preferably one from the first two tiers). Although each situation is unique, it is generally recommended that patients try multiple treatments from a given tier before selecting from a lower tier.

A Brief Note on Monoamine Oxidase Inhibitors

The MAOIs are listed in the third tier in Table 16–1. These are older medicines, but four of them are approved by the FDA to treat bipolar depression (tranylcypromine [Parnate], isocarboxazid [Marplan], phenelzine [Nardil], and selegiline [Emsam]). Evidence suggests that the MAOIs may be superior to all other antidepressant classes in the treatment of unipolar depression. A number of studies have also found superior response rates in bipolar depression, although more data are needed to confirm this trend. However, the MAOIs are known to interact with a variety of the medication classes and the foods we eat, potentially causing dangerous elevations in blood pressure. The MAOIs and SNRIs also carry a higher risk of transitioning patients into mania. More details on these interactions can be found in the specific treatment chapters of this book. Because of these risks, we have recommended MAOIs as a third-tier treatment. However, for patients who have not experienced relief with other therapies, these agents should be considered a viable treatment option. With careful collaboration between the patient and the mental health care provider, these potential interactions are very manageable for most patients.

Table 16–1. Treatments for bipolar depression ordered by level of supporting evidence (tiers)

Recommended first tier	
Atypical antipsychotics	Cariprazine (Vraylar)
	Lumateperone (Caplyta)
	Lurasidone (Latuda)
	Quetiapine (Seroquel)
Combination treatments	Lamotrigine (Lamictal) + (an atypical antipsychotic or lithium)
	Lurasidone or lumateperone + lithium or divalproex*
	Olanzapine + fluoxetine (Symbyax)
Mood stabilizers	Lithium alone
Recommended second tier	
Atypical antipsychotics	Olanzapine (Zyprexa) alone
Neuromodulation	Electroconvulsive therapy—either alone or in addition to an antipsychotic or mood stabilizer
	Transcranial magnetic stimulation—only in addition to an antipsychotic or mood stabilizer
Mood stabilizers	Divalproex* alone
	Lamotrigine (Lamictal) alone
Combination treatments	Antidepressants (SSRIs or bupropion) + an antipsychotic or mood stabilizer
	Psychotherapy (CBT or FFT) + an antipsychotic or mood stabilizer
Recommended third tier	Antipsychotics (aripiprazole [Abilify] or asenapine [Saphris])
	Bright light therapy (with or without sleep deprivation)
	Carbamazepine (Tegretol)
	Ketamine (anesthetic)
	Other antidepressants (SNRIs or MAOIs)
	Other psychotherapy (interpersonal and social rhythm therapy)
	Pramipexole (Mirapex, a dopamine modulator)
Agents that may be effective but require further study	Celecoxib
	Esketamine
	Gabapentin
	Levetiracetam

Table 16–1. Treatments for bipolar depression ordered by level of supporting evidence (tiers) *(continued)*

Agents that may be effective but require further study *(continued)*	Lisdexamfetamine Memantine N-acetylcysteine Pioglitazone Pregnenolone Riluzole Vagus nerve stimulation
Treatments recommended to avoid (based on negative evidence or safety concerns)	Antidepressants (TCAs, SNRIs) alone, particularly in bipolar I disorder Aripiprazole alone Benzodiazepines Lamotrigine + folic acid Mifepristone Risperidone alone Ziprasidone alone or combination

Note. CBT = cognitive-behavioral therapy; FFT = family-focused therapy; MAOI = monoamine oxidase inhibitor; SNRI = serotonin-norepinephrine reuptake inhibitor; SSRI = selective serotonin reuptake inhibitor; TCA = tricyclic antidepressant.

*Divalproex includes valproate, valpromide, valproic acid, and divalproex sodium

Important Considerations

Switching Versus Adding Another Treatment

Switching treatments is a complex and personalized decision. All things being equal, less medicine is typically better, but it is rarely that simple. For example, patients whose illness responds partially or who like certain aspects of their current treatment may benefit from simply adding something else to target any residual symptoms. Moreover, in addition to a high level of evidence for combining certain antipsychotics (particularly lurasidone or lumateperone) with mood stabilizers (divalproex, lithium, or lamotrigine), this strategy may have the added benefit of preventing future manic and depressive episodes once stability has been achieved. Conversely, if patients become depressed after being stable on any of the antidepressant classes (SSRIs, SNRIs, MAOIs, NDRIs), it is usually better to gradually stop that medication and switch to another type of antidepressant (or to a different treatment class altogether) than to add-on another treatment.

Medication Adherence

Between 20% and 60% of patients with bipolar disorder struggle to consistently take medication as prescribed—often unintentionally. Similar rates are seen for many patients with chronic conditions such as high blood pressure. This can result in abandoning a potentially beneficial treatment prematurely or adding another treatment unnecessarily, on top of other risks (e.g., hospitalization, suicide, nonresponse). Even after successful treatment of depression, it is common to believe the medication is no longer necessary. Patients should be aware that no cures exist for bipolar disorder. Continuing to take medications (unless advised otherwise by your health care provider) is important to reduce the risk of future depression or mania, which is vital to long-term stability. Establishing a positive, open relationship with a health care provider is paramount. Patients should feel comfortable discussing side effects and other reasons for medication nonadherence—free from judgment—so that solutions can be reached together.

Metabolic Syndrome

Metabolic syndrome refers to a collection of medical problems that often occur together, including obesity (high body fat), diabetes (high blood sugar), and heart disease (along with high blood pressure or cholesterol). Patients with bipolar disorder are at much higher risk for developing metabolic syndrome, and it can also develop as a side effect of treatment (particularly with olanzapine and quetiapine). Remember that heart disease is one of the primary contributors to reduced life span for people with bipolar disorder. Making positive lifestyle choices (e.g., a healthy diet, regular exercise, weight loss, diligently treating other medical problems, maintaining adequate sleep, stopping smoking or illicit substance use, and strictly limiting alcohol use) is important for everyone, but particularly for individuals with bipolar disorder. **These behaviors can—and should—be viewed as treatments for bipolar depression themselves.** Beyond increasing the life span, they have been found to significantly improve depression, cognition, and quality of life. Support from their social network (e.g., friends, family, colleagues) has been shown to improve people's ability to adhere to healthy lifestyle goals, so enlist help from those around you. Lastly, when added to diet and exercise regimens, some medicines can augment treatment of metabolic syndrome (or reduce the side effects from other agents). You should always discuss options with your health care provider if appropriate. Some newer diabetes medications (called *incretins*) are very effective for weight loss, even in those who do not have diabetes. They also may improve cognitive function in patients with bipolar disorder, especially those who are obese (although further research is required).

Additional Information

Severe Illness

In patients with severe illness (i.e., needs a rapid response or is suicidal), the use of quetiapine, lurasidone, cariprazine, or the olanzapine/fluoxetine combination seems to lead to some improvement within 1 week. Ketamine brings about improvements within hours (particularly in reducing suicidal ideation), but responses typically do not last more than a few days without repeated dosing. ECT may also be considered earlier for patients who have suicidal thoughts or behaviors. Adding lithium to some regimens (see Table 16–1) may also protect against suicide in the long term. Conversely, lamotrigine requires a slow initiation and may not be appropriate in dire cases.

Co-occurring Anxiety and Depression

When anxiety and depression co-occur, your clinician may consider prescribing quetiapine (alone or with lithium), the olanzapine/fluoxetine combination, or the olanzapine/lithium combination. Evidence from unipolar depression shows lurasidone may be helpful, but it has not been directly investigated in bipolar depression with anxiety.

Mixed Features

For people who have mixed features, meaning they are experiencing depression plus [hypo]manic symptoms simultaneously, treatment with the atypical antipsychotics (particlarly lurasidone, the olanzapine/fluoxetine combination, or asenapine [in combination with other agents]) should be considered first. Antidepressant medications should be avoided.

Rapid Cycling

In *rapid cycling,* the person is switching quickly between (hypo)mania and depression. You should always discuss any illicit substance use with your provider if you are cycling rapidly, and be sure to ask about assessing thyroid function. Lithium, divalproex, olanzapine, and quetiapine all seem to be equally effective in maintaining stability in these cases. Lamotrigine seems to be ineffective, and antidepressants should generally be avoided or discontinued.

Cognitive Problems

Some treatments (lurasidone, cariprazine, pramipexole, liraglutide, cognitive remediation therapy) may have benefits, but far more evidence is needed to solidly establish benefit. Preventing further manic/depressive episodes, avoiding benzodiazepines (used for anxiety/sleep), and making lifestyle changes (e.g., weight loss, regular exercise, adequate sleep, and avoiding alcohol, cannabis, or other illicit substance use) are the most important steps to help improve or preserve cognitive function for all patients.

Psychotic Features

If you are experiencing psychotic features (i.e., hallucinations, paranoia, delusions), your clinician will likely consider treatment with antipsychotics or ECT.

Conclusion

The treatment of bipolar depression is highly personalized and requires a collaborative effort with your health care provider to arrive at the treatment that is best for you. This chapter is intended to provide some general suggestions based on available evidence to assist in those important discussions. For patients with bipolar depression, we want to emphasize the vital importance of healthy lifestyle choices, diet, and exercise. These aspects should be viewed as vital and foundational for any and all patients.

Recommended Reading

McIntyre RS, Berk M, Brietzke E, et al: Bipolar disorders. Lancet 396(10265):1841–1856, 2020 33278937

Yatham LN, Kennedy SH, Parikh SV, et al: Canadian Network for Mood and Anxiety Treatments (CANMAT) and International Society for Bipolar Disorders (ISBD) 2018 guidelines for the management of patients with bipolar disorder. Bipolar Disord 20(2):97–170, 2018 29536616

17

Treatment of Chronic Depression (Persistent Depressive Disorder)

Alexander Grieshaber, M.A.
Dina Vivian, Ph.D.
Daniel N. Klein, Ph.D.

Case Vignette

Linda is a cisgender White female in her late 40s with a bachelor's degree in business administration. She was living with her husband of more than 30 years, had no children, and was self-employed as a consultant. Linda sought cognitive-behavioral analysis system of psychotherapy (CBASP) for depression after her depression failed to respond to antidepressant medications and several courses of "unspecified" talk therapy over the prior few years. Although she had experienced bouts of depression on and off for most of her life, Linda's symptoms had worsened during the past year due to growing dissatisfaction with her professional life and identity. She had also begun avoiding activities she previously enjoyed, including seeing the few friends she had, exercising, and reading. She reported feeling constantly sad, "empty," hopeless, insecure about her professional competence, sensitive about others' opinion of her (i.e., being liked by others), and feeling unsupported and devalued at work. Relatedly, she felt frustrated and irritable when interacting with people at work and avoided confrontations and consequently felt helpless. Her sleep was chronically disrupted due to worrying about work and most other aspects of her life. These feelings of "generalized" anxiety were lifelong but worsened when she was depressed. At intake, Linda did not report feeling suicidal and had never made a suicide attempt, although from time to time she felt that "it would be better if [she were] dead." Linda also felt unhappy in her marriage due a lack of physical closeness with her husband; as such, she had gradually withdrawn from him emotionally, particularly during the past 2–3 years. Likewise, she was not close with members of her family of origin, describing her parents as critical, demanding, and emotionally unavailable—her mother was chronically depressed, and although her relationship with her younger siblings was moderately satisfactory, Linda perceived them as overly dependent on her.

Linda's treatment included a combination of interventions designed to increase her awareness of the relationship between engaging in action (as opposed to the pattern of avoidance she had fallen into) and reducing depression, which led to an increase in her self-efficacy, sense of control, and daily functioning. It was important for Linda to identify how her enduring negative beliefs regarding "the self," particularly her sense of professional and personal competence and "likability," stemmed from the criticism and lack of support she received from her family while growing up, which colored her perceptions of her professional performance and how others saw her. In turn, this led to maladaptive responses toward others (e.g., behavioral avoidance or covert hostility in her interpersonal interactions) and toward herself (e.g., negative self-talk, self-criticism), all of which contributed to her depression. Particularly effective were in-session and out-of-session exercises that helped Linda focus on specific stressful interpersonal events at work and at home wherein she realized that her interpretation of events and her own actions were unhelpful in "getting what she wanted." The more Linda was able to "revise" her negative interpretations and to engage in adaptive, approach-based—rather than avoidant—behavior, the more she felt in control.

In addition to individual work, Linda's treatment also included couples sessions, wherein she and her husband became aware of the maladaptive dyadic patterns that had developed over the years, particularly the emotional distance and alienation that had occurred in the relationship, which were associated with Linda's dissatisfaction with their lack of closeness and her husband's tendency to withdraw or be critical. Both partners were able to engage in more supportive communication and acceptance of each other's needs.

Slowly, Linda's pervasive sense of helplessness, hopelessness, and avoidance of interpersonal and personal activities decreased, as did her depression. Lastly, additional effective interventions included mindfulness practices that enabled Linda to better cope with her excessive worrying and mood dysregulation, and interpersonal effectiveness skills to improve her communication with others at work and in her life (e.g., her siblings). Linda's treatment included approximately 35 sessions over the better part of a year. At completion of treatment, her level of depression was in the nonclinical range. In addition, Linda learned that if her depression recurred, she had the skills to cope adaptively and minimize its impact.

Introduction

Chronic depression, or persistent depressive disorder (PDD) as described in the *Diagnostic and Statistical Manual of Mental Disorders,* 5th Edition (DSM-5), is a mood disorder that includes persistent feelings of low mood (e.g., sadness, depression) accompanied by other symptoms such as changes in eating (poor appetite or overeating) or sleeping (insomnia or excessive sleep), low energy or fatigue, low self-esteem, difficulty concentrating or making decisions, and feelings of hopelessness; these symptoms are present most of the day for more days than not and continue for at least 2 years with little relief (i.e., without a period greater than 2 months without symptoms). PDD symptoms can be consistently mild (*dysthymia*), consistently moderate or severe (*chronic major depression*), or shift between mild and moderate-severe (*double depression*).

To achieve a good response, patients with PDD may benefit more than those with nonchronic depression from a combined treatment that includes antidepressant medication and psychotherapy; in addition, treatment of PDD is typically of longer duration than treatment for nonchronic forms of depression. Importantly, chronic depression is not the same as treatment-resistant clinical depression. In fact, many individuals with PDD greatly benefit from both medication and psychotherapy treatment.

Treatment Options

Medication-Based Treatments

Many antidepressant medications, including tricyclic antidepressants (TCAs), selective serotonin reuptake inhibitors (SSRIs), and atypical antidepressants, are effective in treating PDD. Current research does not provide adequate information to predict which medication will be most effective for a particular patient. Choice of antidepressant is generally based on the pattern of depressive symptoms exhibited by the patient (e.g., energy level, sleep patterns, restlessness or slowed movements), their current medical status, their history (if there is one) of response to antidepressant medications in the past, and the side effect profiles of the medications, which vary considerably.

Some neuromodulatory therapies, such as electroconvulsive therapy (ECT) and repetitive transcranial magnetic stimulation (rTMS) have been shown to be effective in treating depression. These approaches are often used when patients have not responded to multiple trials of pharmacotherapy and psychotherapy. Although many of the patients in clinical trials of these treatments have had PDD, none of these trials have specifically focused on PDD.

Non-Medication-Based Treatments

Psychotherapy is an effective form of treatment for PDD. However, not all types of therapy are equally effective, and the duration of treatment must be sufficient to achieve a good outcome. There is evidence that a minimum of several months of psychotherapy, including 18–20 therapy sessions (or more), are needed for chronically depressed individuals to benefit from psychotherapy. About 50% experience significant improvements in their mood and functioning.

Among various models of therapy, cognitive therapy targets the inaccurate, biased thoughts associated with depression, such as negative thoughts about the self, the world, and the future, to help reduce depressive symptoms and teach patients more adaptive coping strategies. Behavioral activation therapy focuses on helping depressed people increase their involvement in potentially rewarding activities that they currently are doing less of or avoiding, which increases pleasure and a sense of control over mood. Both cognitive therapy and behavioral activation are typically included in cognitive-behavioral therapy (CBT), which is an effective treatment for depression in general. Interpersonal therapy (IPT) is a short-term therapy that has also been found to be effective in treating depression; it centers on improving people's ability to navigate social difficulties, including changes in social roles (e.g., taking a new job, becoming a parent), grief and loss, and problems with social skills. Many therapists also engage in supportive psychotherapy for the treatment of depression, which emphasizes empathy, encouragement, and providing a safe place to talk about difficult topics. Although all these models of treatment for general depression have been found to be moderately and similarly effective, their effectiveness for the treatment of PDD has not been firmly established through well-controlled studies.

CBASP was developed by James P. McCullough specifically for treatment of chronic depression and was designed to address the specific cognitive styles exhibited by people with chronic depression (e.g., maladaptive patterns of self-criticism, low perceived control over life, difficulty in seeing how their actions/thoughts affect others and their own mood), and longstanding interpersonal problems. It integrates behavioral, cognitive, and interpersonal treatment strategies, focusing primarily on social problem-solving and helping patients recognize the consequences of their behavior on others and themselves in attaining outcomes they desire. As such, CBASP increases interpersonal effectiveness, improves patients' satisfaction in their relationships, and strengthens their sense of control and self-efficacy in their interpersonal environments. Clinical trials have shown that CBASP is an effective treatment for reducing depressive symptoms and improving daily functioning in PDD. Unfortunately, the number of psychotherapists trained in CBASP in the United States remains small, but it is growing, and many therapists use CBASP techniques via widely available books and manuals.

How Treatment Is Decided

Comparison of Psychotherapy and Medication

Antidepressant medication may be more effective than psychotherapy for milder forms of PDD (i.e., dysthymia), although the evidence base for this is weak. Medication and psychotherapy are equally effective for moderate to severe forms of PDD (i.e., double and chronic major depression). Antidepressant medication and CBASP are equally effective for PDD, and both appear to be more effective than IPT and supportive therapy.

Combined Approaches to Treatment

Although psychotherapy and antidepressant treatment alone may be effective in treating PDD, the combination of psychotherapy and antidepressant medication appears to be more effective than either alone, and fewer patients drop out before treatment is completed. Nonetheless, for many individuals, psychotherapy or medication alone is sufficient and effective.

Additional Information

Nonresponse to Treatment

PDD responds to treatment in approximately half of patients, and remission of PDD is achieved in approximately one in four patients. PDD that does not respond to one antidepressant medication may respond to the addition or substitution of another medication. Moreover, many individuals whose PDD fails to respond to medication obtain benefit from psychotherapy, and vice versa.

Maintenance Treatment

PDD has a high risk for relapse after recovery. Therefore, continuing treatment after recovery (referred to as *maintenance treatment*) is often useful in consolidating and sustaining treatment gains and reducing the risk of relapse. Maintenance medication and psychotherapy (generally with less frequent sessions) are each effective in preventing relapse. For example, one study showed that as little as one CBASP session per month substantially reduced the risk of relapse.

Conclusion

PDD refers to chronic, longstanding depressions with symptoms that can vary from mild to severe. Antidepressant medications and some forms of psychotherapy (e.g., CBASP) are both effective in treating PDD, and the combination of medication plus psychotherapy is more effective than either treatment approach alone. It is not uncommon for patients' depressions to fail to respond to an initial treatment; however, many will respond after switching to a different treatment. PDD is associated with a high risk of recurrence, but continued (i.e., maintenance) pharmacotherapy and psychotherapy can reduce the probability of developing PDD again in the future.

Recommended Reading

Klein DN, Black SR: Persistent depressive disorder, in The Oxford Handbook of Mood Disorders. Edited by DeRubeis RJ, Strunk DR. New York, Oxford University Press, 2017, pp 227–237

Schramm E, Klein DN, Elsaesser M, et al: Review of persistent depressive disorder: history, correlates, and clinical implications. Lancet Psychiatry 7:801–812, 2020

18

Treatment of Postpartum Depression and Related Disorders

Samantha Meltzer-Brody, M.D., M.P.H.

Case Vignette

Jennifer is a 32-year-old female with a history of postpartum depression after her first baby was born 2 years ago. She delivered her second baby 4 months ago and again developed symptoms of postpartum depression within the first week postpartum. The symptoms consisted of low mood, ruminating thoughts that something bad would happen to the baby, feeling overwhelmed, and having crying spells. She had difficulty sleeping and had lost her appetite and experienced significant weight loss. She was treated with a selective serotonin reuptake inhibitor (SSRI)—sertraline—and psychotherapy. She had previously been treated with sertraline but has been off the medication since becoming pregnant with her second baby. Jennifer stated that she never thought the sertraline helped her very much, and she felt depressed for more than a year until the symptoms resolved. Over the past 2 months, Jennifer reported worsening symptoms, and increasing the dosage of sertraline up to 150 mg did not improve her postpartum depression. She also experienced significant gastrointestinal side effects. She began to feel increasingly hopeless and to experience thoughts that her family would be better off without her.

Jennifer had heard about brexanolone from her postpartum support group and wanted to try this new medication. Her psychiatrist discussed the risks and benefits of treatment with brexanolone. Jennifer understood she would be admitted to the hospital for a 60-hour infusion and that the medication carries a risk of sedation. She had a positive response to the infusion and reported a marked reduction in her symptoms. Her mood was much better, her affect was much brighter, and she was able to sleep well. Her level of anxiety had also improved, and she was able to move past worrying thoughts much easier. Her family noticed a significant change in a positive way and reported she looked like her "usual self." She continued taking sertraline 100 mg throughout her infusion with brexanolone and was discharged home at this dosage.

Introduction

Postpartum depression and anxiety are common conditions that can be treated effectively, so it is important to seek treatment early to prevent unnecessary suffering. Symptoms of postpartum depression and anxiety can include low mood, sadness, feeling unable to enjoy the baby or other activities, anxiety or intrusive thoughts, changes in sleep or appetite, difficulty concentrating, and feeling overwhelmed. In most cases, the symptoms will be present for at least 2 weeks. In the most severe cases, patients can experience suicidal thoughts or changes in perception of reality (i.e., delusional thoughts). Severe symptoms require an urgent visit to the emergency department for evaluation by a medical or mental health professional. The goal of treatment is to have the patient return to feeling "like themselves" and to be able to enjoy their new baby.

Treatment Options

Treatment of Mild Symptoms Consistent With "Baby Blues"

The postpartum period is always a stressful time, even under the best of circumstances. It is vital for new parents to have adequate social support, and help from family and friends is needed. Postpartum women need adequate nutrition and protected sleep. Protected time for sleep is something that should be made a top priority. It is good idea to explicitly ask family and friends to help ensure the postpartum woman can sleep. For example, taking turns with another parent, a grandparent, or another adult to allow for protected sleep of 5–6 hour intervals each night can make a big difference in the postpartum woman's mood, even if they are breastfeeding.

In addition to protected sleep, it is important for postpartum mothers to have time for self-care in small amounts during the postpartum period. Taking walks outside with the baby is a great way to get exercise, be outside of the house, and improve mood. It is also helpful to bring along a friend, a family member, or a partner.

Mild to Moderate Symptoms

Psychotherapy

Psychotherapy (talk therapy) is considered the first-line treatment for postpartum depression and anxiety and requires that the postpartum woman be willing to participate in regular therapy sessions. During psychotherapy, the patient and therapist work together to address the issues causing distress in a safe, supportive way. A number of different types of evidence-based psychotherapy can be effective. Psychotherapy has been shown to decrease symptoms of depression and anxiety and can also improve parent-infant bonding.

When a postpartum mother has mild to moderate symptoms, psychotherapy is usually the preferred treatment option for postpartum depression and anxiety. If possible, it is best to find a clinician who has some experience working with postpartum patients. However, if this is not an option, then the most important thing is to find a therapist who can assist in working through the profound psychosocial changes that occur in the postpartum period. This can involve changes in the relationship with a partner; challenges balancing the needs of caring for a baby with other responsibilities, including other children in the home; career considerations; and other concerns. Engaging in psychotherapy is an important step, and at least six sessions are recommended. Several different forms of psychotherapy have an evidence base in the postpartum period, including cognitive-behavioral therapy (CBT), dialectical behavioral therapy (DBT), interpersonal psychotherapy (IPT), and acceptance and commitment therapy (ACT).

If there are significant psychosocial concerns, it is important to reach out to local social service agencies to get social work support or case management around food bank programs, domestic violence resources, and other vital support services. Postpartum Support International (www.postpartum.net) is an excellent resource providing listings of services in all states in the United States as well as Canada and other countries around the world.

If the birth parent is experiencing moderate symptoms that have begun to interfere with functioning and/or are persistent, lasting more than 2 weeks, treatment of a depressive episode is indicated. A *postpartum depressive episode* is defined as clinical symptoms consisting of mood changes, anxiety, feeling overwhelmed, feeling unable to enjoy things that previously were pleasurable, being unable to sleep even when the baby is sleeping, feeling unable to function as usual, and in severe cases, feeling as though life is not worth living or having suicidal thoughts. It is important that treatment is sought to relieve symptoms and ensure a positive outcome. The Edinburgh Postnatal Depression Scale (EPDS) is a helpful screening test for postpartum depression used around the world. A score of 12 or higher indicates a positive screen usually consistent with a depressive episode. Initiation of an antidepressant or other psychiatric medication is often indicated in addition to psychotherapy. Other forms of treatment, such as transcranial magnetic stimulation (TMS), are also options.

If depressive symptoms persist or become more severe or the patient has thoughts that life is not worth living, then medication treatment will almost always be prescribed. This may include a traditional antidepressant medication or newer antidepressant options (e.g., brexanolone) or, alternatively, electroconvulsive therapy (ECT).

Risk of Harm to Self or Others

The presence of thoughts about harming oneself (suicidal thoughts) or others must be taken very seriously and discussed right away with a mental health clinician. Question 10 on the EPDS screens for suicidal ideation and endorsement of this item should trigger an immediate evaluation with a mental health clinician. In addition, if the postpartum mother has thoughts of homicidal ideation toward the infant, and particularly if there are concerns that they are experiencing postpartum psychosis, emergency mental health care should be sought to ensure safety.

Moderate to Severe Symptoms

Medication-Based Treatments

Psychiatric medications are usually very helpful in decreasing symptoms of moderate to severe depression and anxiety in postpartum patients. When the symptoms are severe, it is imperative to have good psychiatric care and regular monitoring. The medication can be prescribed by the obstetrical provider or a psychiatry provider. The infant's pediatrician should also be included in the discussion about how the postpartum mother is feeling and interacting with the baby. Whenever a pregnant or lactating woman is treated with medications, the risk of any untreated symptoms must be weighed against the risk of medication exposure in breast milk.

If the postpartum woman has a history of depression or anxiety, any psychotropic medication that has been helpful to them in the past (well tolerated and effective) should be prescribed. Usually, an antidepressant medication will be a first-line treatment, but a careful history is always indicated and may guide the treatment plan. In postpartum women, the goal is to use the fewest number of medications to treat the symptoms, and treatment must also include assessment of medication safety in lactation if the mother is breastfeeding.

Prior to starting any psychotropic medication, it is vital to obtain a full psychiatric history to understand the nature of the symptoms of anxiety and depression and to assess the patient for any history of mania, hypomania, or psychosis.

The most commonly prescribed psychotropic medications for postpartum depression and anxiety are SSRIs, including sertraline, citalopram, escitalopram, and fluoxetine; serotonin-norepinephrine reuptake inhibitors (SNRIs), which include duloxetine and venlafaxine; and other types of antidepressants, including bupropion, mirtazapine, tricyclic antidepressants (TCAs), or monoamine oxidase inhibitors (MAOIs). The SSRI sertraline is often a first choice for treatment of postpartum depression and anxiety because it is generally well tolerated, often effective, and has a good safety profile for breastfeeding patients (low transfer of the drug into breast milk). In contrast, venlafaxine has a higher transfer into breast milk because it has very low protein binding and therefore more easily crosses the placental barrier and into breast milk than other antidepressants.

If the postpartum woman does not have relief of symptoms from a traditional antidepressant, or if more severe symptoms are present including suicidality, agitation, or symptoms that are concerning for bipolar disorder, addition of other types of medications may be indicated. For example, medications with mood-stabilizing properties (e.g., lamotrigine, lithium) or atypical antipsychotics with mood-stabilizing properties (e.g., quetiapine, risperidone, olanzapine) can be used to help relieve the symptoms. Valproic acid should be avoided in lactating women and females of reproductive age due to potential adverse effects on the fetus (during pregnancy) and the infant (during lactation).

Using both medication treatment and psychotherapy (combination treatment) is considered a gold-standard approach for postpartum depression and is usually very helpful. The care team should be in communication with each other to monitor the response to treatment (e.g., mood, sleep, appetite, interactions with the baby) so that the best outcomes can be achieved.

Brexanolone. The first psychotropic medication with U.S. Food and Drug Administration (FDA) approval specifically for postpartum depression was approved in March 2019 for severe postpartum depression. Brexanolone is a novel medication that is a proprietary formulation of allopregnanolone (a neuroactive metabolite of progesterone). Brexanolone is administered intravenously over a course of 60 hours and has demonstrated rapid onset of action. It is highly effective in the majority of women with severe postpartum depression. The clinical trials that led to FDA approval demonstrated efficacy and sustained treatment response through the 30-day follow-up of the clinical trial period. Treatment with brexanolone showed statistically significant reductions in symptoms of postpartum depression as compared with placebo, either with or without baseline antidepressant medication. In the 3 years that the medication has been commercially available, it has continued to be an important, efficacious, and well-tolerated clinical treatment tool for patients with severe postpartum depression.

Due to the risk of sedation, brexanolone infusion in the United States must be administered under the Risk Evaluation and Mitigation Strategy (REMS) FDA requirement. The REMS provides specific guidelines that must be followed by health care systems involved in administration of brexanolone.

Overall, brexanolone has been well tolerated, and side effects include flushing or hot flashes, dry mouth, sedation, or somnolence. Sedation can be readily addressed by decreasing the dosage of the medication infusion.

Considerations of Medication Use During Breastfeeding. In postpartum patients who were treated with psychotropic medication during pregnancy, the placental transfer of medication is much more than the transfer into breast milk. Breastfeeding while taking medication can be safely done with thoughtful consideration. Medications with shorter half-lives, greater levels of protein binding, less lipophilicity, and generally larger molecule size are better choices. For infants born prematurely who have low birth weight or other health issues, the pediatrician should be included in the discussion with the psychiatrist or the obstetrical provider when choosing medications and dosages that will be safe for both mother and baby. One excellent resource for clinicians and patients is The National Institute of Health's database LACTMED, which has comprehensive data on medication use during breastfeeding. In general, the monitoring of medication exposure during pregnancy usually *does not* include checking the infant's blood levels. In addition, no data support "pumping and dumping" (discarding breast milk after pumping) for most medications, but doing so could be advised in certain instances of particular concern. In all cases, thoughtful discussion between the patient and the treatment team is needed to ensure the best outcomes for both the postpartum mother and the baby.

Non-Medication-Based Treatments

Repetitive Transcranial Magnetic Stimulation. Repetitive transcranial magnetic stimulation (rTMS) is an effective treatment option and an alternative to medication. rTMS is FDA-approved for major depressive disorder and has shown effectiveness for postpartum depression. This treatment applies targeted magnetic field pulses to the scalp that generate electrical currents in the brain to stimulate neuroplasticity. It is usually well tolerated, and the most common side effects are scalp pain or headache. It requires daily treatments for a few weeks of time, which can be labor intensive and inconvenient for postpartum patients. However, the treatment effects may be more rapid than traditional antidepressant medications, and there is no risk of exposure in breast milk.

Electroconvulsive Therapy. ECT is also a treatment option for more severe illness. ECT is FDA-approved for severe major depression that has been refractory to medication treatment, and it is also used to treat catatonia, bipolar spectrum illness, psychotic disorders, and severe agitation. ECT is performed while the patient is under anesthesia during treatment. During the procedure, electrodes are applied to the patient's skull, and electricity induces a generalized tonic-clonic seizure that is also believed to stimulate neuroplasticity. The benefits of treatment with ECT are a fast response and strong efficacy. The risks include headache, confusion, myalgias, nausea, vomiting, prolonged seizure, and memory loss. ECT is considered an essential treatment for patients with very severe postpartum depression that has not responded to medications. Severe symptoms for which ECT may be a good option include treatment-refractory depression, catatonia, and depression with psychotic features.

Conclusion

The postpartum period is a vulnerable time for anxiety and mood disorders. Multiple effective treatments for postpartum anxiety and depression are available. All postpartum mothers and parents should have routine screening for postpartum mental health symptoms and, if necessary, timely referral should be made for them to receive evidence-based mental health treatment. The goal is always to ensure that the patient returns to feeling "like themselves" so that the patient, the baby, and the family can thrive.

Recommended Reading

Cox E (ed): Women's Mood Disorders: A Clinician's Guide to Perinatal Psychiatry. New York, Springer, 2021

Meltzer-Brody S, Howard LM, Bergink V, et al: Postpartum psychiatric disorders. Nat Rev Dis Primers 4:18022, 2018 29695824

19

Treatment of Seasonal Affective Disorder

Sherri Melrose, Ph.D.

Introduction

Seasonal affective disorder or SAD (also referred to as "seasonal depression") is a type of recurring depression with a seasonal pattern. People living with SAD experience depression that begins and ends during a specific season each year, usually during December, January, and February. As sunlight decreases during the short, dark days of winter, feelings of sadness and low energy can become so intense that people are unable to carry out their normal work, school, social, and family activities. During the winter, cold temperatures make it difficult for people to spend time outdoors in the sunlight. They may wake up and go to bed in darkness and they may be isolated from friends and family. Although SAD can also occur during the summer months, symptoms are most likely to appear each year during late fall and early winter.

Symptoms of winter SAD have two commonly recognized symptoms: an intense craving for sugary, carbohydrate-rich foods and a desire to sleep longer. In turn, an increased appetite, often accompanied by decreased exercise, leads to weight gain. Managing these symptoms is compounded by feelings of sadness and low energy that last most of the day. Concentration and decision-making are difficult. Motivation to engage in activities once enjoyed is decreased. Mood can alternate between feeling sluggish at times and agitated at other times. Importantly, feelings of hopelessness associated with SAD can lead people to consider thoughts of death or suicide.

"Winter blues," is a general term used to describe the sad mood, lack of motivation, and trouble sleeping that some people experience during the winter. Less severe than SAD, people who have winter blues are still able to function and engage in their usual everyday activities.

The symptoms of summer SAD differ somewhat. Decreased appetite, weight loss, insomnia, anxiety, irritability, and agitation can occur. When sunlight increases and people are exposed to longer periods of light, their sleep-wake cycle is disturbed, resulting in sleep deprivation. Periods of blinding sun and summer heat can leave those affected feeling anxious and angry, and their behavior can become aggressive. Like winter SAD, suicidal thinking is a significant concern.

Causes of SAD are related to ways that sunlight affects the body. Decreases and increases in sunlight can disrupt the body's natural circadian rhythm, or biological clock. Decreases in sunlight cause brain levels of serotonin, a brain chemical that regulates mood, to drop. Similarly, less sunlight also results in Vitamin D deficiency, which plays an important role in serotonin levels and has been implicated as a risk factor for depression.

On the other hand, darkness associated with decreased sunlight results in increased production of melatonin, synthesized in the pineal gland and the brain, and regulates sleep. Darkness causes the body to produce more melatonin, and when the sun is shining, the body shuts down production. More melatonin in the body makes people feel sleepy and lethargic.

Those living farthest from the equator in northern latitudes, where long harsh winters offer only a few hours of sunlight each day, are especially susceptible to winter SAD. Conversely, those living closer to the equator are more susceptible to summer SAD. Symptoms in both types of seasonal depression are more common in females and those with a family history of SAD or other forms of depression. For many people, symptoms of SAD decrease with age.

Treatment Options

Medication-Based Treatment

Antidepressants may be necessary when symptoms of SAD become incapacitating and interfere with people's ability to function at work and care for their families. The selective serotonin reuptake inhibitor (SSRI) class of antidepressants significantly enhance mood. Fluoxetine (Prozac) is the SSRI used most often for people with SAD. Citalopram (Celexa), sertraline (Zoloft), paroxetine (Paxil), and escitalopram (Cipralex or Lexapro) are also effective.

The atypical antidepressant bupropion (Wellbutrin), in an extended-release form, can prevent recurrent seasonal depressive episodes when taken early in the season while people are still well. Daily doses are usually started in early fall and continued until spring the following year.

Adverse reactions to antidepressants include drowsiness, fatigue, dry mouth, nausea, diarrhea, vomiting, anorexia, sexual problems, agitation, palpitations, worsening depression, and suicidal thoughts. These reactions usually subside after the first few weeks of treatment. However, any adverse reaction should be reported to the prescribing health professional.

Antidepressant medications typically take several weeks to become fully effective. Early indications that they are working include improved sleep, appetite, and energy. Mood regulation may not be observed until later. Dosages often need adjusting. Antidepressant medications are not addictive, and they must be continued even when people feel better. They must never be stopped suddenly because this may cause symptoms to worsen. When symptoms of SAD are not relieved by one antidepressant, another may be substituted or added.

Non-Medication-Based Treatments

Plan Ahead

Knowing that the distressing symptoms associated with SAD will come back at the same time each year, people can make lifestyle modifications ahead of time. Planning for the lethargy and lack of motivation associated with winter SAD begins in fall. Establishing meaningful connections with people and groups; adjusting family and work commitments if possible; and registering for enjoyable programs and activities need to happen well before winter sets in. Conversely, planning for the sleep deprivation and anxiety of summer SAD can mean reducing commitments and taking advantage of any available breaks or vacations.

Adjust Exposure to Sunlight

Increasing or decreasing exposure to natural sunlight is a simple and effective way to manage SAD. Taking daily walks outside around noon, when the sun is brightest, maximizes exposure to sunlight. When indoors, keeping blinds open and choosing a workspace near a window are effective. Decreasing exposure to sunlight includes avoiding the intense heat and light of midday, seeking shade outdoors, and using blackout blinds to create a cool, dark sleeping environment.

Establish a Realistic Exercise Routine

When people have a realistic and regular exercise routine they follow year-round, they are better equipped to maintain that routine when their mood is altered due to seasonal depression. Effective exercise routines include aerobic activities to stimulate heart and breathing rates and high-intensity resistance training. While engaging in some form of exercise for at least 30 minutes each day is best, three 50-minute sessions each week will make an important difference.

In addition to structured and unstructured gymnasium workouts, sports, yoga, water aerobics, strength training, running, walking, or any other enjoyable movement-oriented activities can be incorporated into exercise routines. Again, exercise done in bright sunlight during winter and shade during summer targets the specific symptoms of SAD related to exposure to sunlight.

Maintain Healthy Dietary Habits

Cravings for sugary, carbohydrate-rich foods can be eased by planning to have regular meals at the same time each day. Including protein with breakfast, lunch, and dinner is important. When people increase their consumption of vegetables, fruits, whole grains, nuts, and seeds, they may be less inclined to turn to high-calorie processed foods.

Add a Vitamin D Supplement

Many people with winter SAD have low levels of vitamin D. Taking 100,000 IU daily may improve symptoms. Adverse effects are rare but can occur from doses of more than 50,000 IU per day.

Bright Light Therapy

Many health professionals believe bright light therapy, or phototherapy, should be the first choice of treatment for winter SAD. Light boxes can be purchased that emit full-spectrum light similar in composition to sunlight. People sit in front of a 10,000-lux light box first thing in the morning for 20–60 minutes from the early fall until spring. Adverse effects include eye strain, increased risk of age-related macular degeneration, headaches, irritability, and difficulty sleeping. Light therapy should not be used in conjunction with photosensitizing medications such as lithium, melatonin, phenothiazine antipsychotics, and certain antibiotics.

Psychotherapy

When people are no longer able to cope with severe symptoms of SAD on their own, psychotherapists offer needed help. One common therapeutic approach, cognitive behavioral therapy for SAD (CBT-SAD), guides people toward thinking differently about problems that seem overwhelming and negative. Therapists help people identify and schedule pleasant, engaging activities to combat feelings of depression and anxiety.

Combining Treatment Approaches

No single treatment approach will alleviate all the symptoms of SAD. Relief is most likely to come from a combination of incorporating lifestyle modifications and antidepressant medications. People can best manage seasonal depression by recognizing the condition and then continuing to try different treatment options until they feel more like themselves again.

Conclusion

People with SAD are unable to function, and the feelings of sadness and low energy they experience have a significant impact on their ability to enjoy life. Some may even consider suicide. Treatment options can include antidepressant medications. Antidepressant medications take several weeks to become effective, may need adjusting, and must never be stopped suddenly. Knowing that the causes of SAD relate to the ways that sunlight affects the body and that the condition will occur at the same time each year, a combination of non-medication-based treatments should also be considered, such as making lifestyle modifications ahead of time, adjusting exposure to sunlight, establishing a realistic exercise routine, maintaining healthy dietary habits, adding a vitamin D supplement, using bright light therapy (light box), and participating in psychotherapy. Living with SAD can feel overwhelming, but recognizing that help is available can provide much needed relief.

Recommended Reading

Melrose S: Seasonal affective disorder: an overview of assessment and treatment approaches. Depress Res Treat 2015:178564, 2015 26688752

Rosenthal NE: What is seasonal affective disorder: answers from the doctor who first described the condition. Norman E. Rosenthal, M.D.: Seasonal Affective Disorder (website), 2023. Available at: https://www.normanrosenthal.com/about/research/seasonal-affective-disorder.

20

Treatment of Posttraumatic Stress Disorder

Barbara O. Rothbaum, Ph.D., ABPP

Introduction

Symptoms of posttraumatic stress disorder (PTSD) are very common following traumatic events. A *trauma* is an event in which survivors thought it was likely they or someone they care about could be killed or seriously injured. Trauma is more than an emotional upset or distress. People with PTSD feel haunted by the event. People often think of PTSD as the war veteran's disease, and it is certainly a huge problem for those who have defended our country, but unfortunately, about 70% of us will be exposed to a potentially traumatic event in our lifetimes, including motor vehicle crashes, natural disasters, physical or sexual assault, abuse or neglect, and industrial accidents. The symptoms of PTSD are part of the natural response to trauma, but for most of us, these symptoms decrease over the first few weeks and months.

The symptoms of PTSD are grouped into four subcategories:

1. *Intrusive symptoms*—These include nightmares, flashbacks, and the feeling of physical reminders in the body that occur both day and night. The haunting nature comes out in the reexperiencing symptoms of PTSD.

2. *Avoidance symptoms*—People with PTSD avoid anything that reminds them of the traumatic event, but unfortunately, this avoidance keeps them from recovering and often results in their lives becoming very narrow.
3. *Negative mood symptoms*—People with PTSD often report feeling emotionally numb.
4. *Hyperarousal symptoms*—These include exaggerated startle response, hypervigilance, and sleep problems. People with PTSD often feel as though danger lurks around every corner, and their bodies must stay on high alert to anticipate and avoid it.

To be diagnosed with PTSD, a person must have symptoms that have lasted for at least 1 month. Someone with chronic PTSD is diagnosed when the symptoms have been present for at least 3 months, and once PTSD has become chronic, it is unlikely to improve without treatment. Treatments for PTSD include medications and psychotherapy.

Several types of providers offer PTSD treatment. Psychiatrists are medical doctors (i.e., have an M.D.) and may prescribe medications and may also provide therapy. Psychologists have a Ph.D. or Psy.D. degree in clinical psychology and are *not* licensed to prescribe medication. Social workers typically have a master's degree in social work (i.e., M.S.W.). In some states, a physician assistant (P.A.) and clinical nurse specialist (C.N.S.) may prescribe medications under the supervision of a physician.

Treatment Options

Evidence-based care means that 1) the treatments have been evaluated in studies and shown to work, and 2) providers are using these proven treatments in the care of their patients.

Medication-Based Treatments

Sertraline (Zoloft) and paroxetine (Paxil) are the only medications approved by the U.S. Food and Drug Administration (FDA) to treat PTSD, although other medications have been shown to be helpful. 3,4-Methylenedioxymethamphetamine (MDMA) is a different kind of medication that is likely to be approved soon by the FDA for PTSD. MDMA does not work by itself for PTSD but is used in combination with psychotherapy.

If someone is already taking these medications and still experiences PTSD, they can continue taking the medication and try adding trauma-focused psychotherapy. Recent research suggests that starting medication and psychotherapy at the same time does not lead to greater benefit. We suggest starting with either approach and only adding the other one based on any remaining symptoms once the first approach has been tried.

Non-Medication-Based Treatments

Psychotherapy

As for psychotherapy, trauma-focused cognitive-behavioral therapy (TF-CBT) is recommended. The trauma-focused therapies that have been shown to be consistently effective in treating PTSD include prolonged exposure (PE), virtual reality exposure (VRE), and other types of exposure therapy; cognitive therapy; cognitive processing therapy (CPT); and eye movement desensitization and reprocessing (EMDR).

Prolonged Exposure

PE has been studied the most for the treatment of PTSD. Because people with PTSD avoid thinking about, talking about, and reminders of the event, PE helps them confront the memory of the traumatic experience and reminders of the event in a safe way to help reduce their distress. PE helps them learn to become more active and socially engaged if they have become isolated. This approach includes education; repeated, real-life exposure (called *in vivo exposure*) to situations, people, or objects that are objectively safe or low risk but that the person is avoiding; and repeated *imaginal exposure* to the trauma memories, followed by talking about the event and the emotions and thoughts they had during the trauma. This helps patients emotionally process their traumatic experiences.

PE typically consists of working one-on-one with a therapist in 8–15 weekly or twice-weekly treatment sessions that are each generally 90 minutes long but can be delivered daily in intensive treatment programs. Thirty years of research have shown that PE is effective in reducing PTSD and other trauma-related problems such as depression, general anxiety, substance use, and anger. Obviously, there are no guarantees about how any one person will respond, but this program has helped thousands of people around the world.

Virtual Reality Exposure Therapy

Virtual reality is an interactive three-dimensional computer-generated immersive environment. Users usually wear a head-mounted display that resembles a helmet and has a small screen in front of each eye, earphones, and a position tracker. As the user moves their head, the position tracker senses the movement and changes the view on the display in real time. Many applications include a handheld sensor or joystick to help users maneuver in the virtual environment.

In VRE, the therapist matches what the patient describes. This is almost exactly like PE, except that the patient's eyes are open so they can see the virtual environment. Most of the virtual environments used for PTSD are for war veterans, although they can also depict motor vehicle crashes, terrorist attacks, and natural disasters.

Cognitive Therapy

Following a traumatic event, some people think they can never be safe again and that danger lurks around every corner. They may feel guilty about what happened during the event or what they did to survive. If others did not survive, they may experience survivor's guilt. They may feel dirty or bad or worthless. Often, they find it hard to trust others. In cognitive therapy, the therapist helps patients with PTSD identify these unhelpful and inaccurate thoughts and then replace them with more helpful and more accurate thoughts. Homework usually involves practicing identifying and challenging these unhelpful thoughts by writing them down.

Cognitive Processing Therapy

CPT is a specific form of TF-CBT based on questioning the assumptions and beliefs arising as a result of traumatic events. Several versions of CPT are available. Some involve writing a *trauma narrative* (a story of what happened) and reading it with the therapist. This narrative is used to identify "stuck points" that usually center around the themes of safety, trust, power and control, esteem, and intimacy. CPT usually takes about 12 sessions and can be done one-on-one or in a group but can also be delivered daily in intensive programs.

Eye Movement Desensitization and Reprocessing

In EMDR, the therapist asks the patient with PTSD to bring up a picture that represents the worst moment in the traumatic event. The survivor and the therapist identify words that go with that picture. These are not necessarily words that were said at the time of the trauma, but rather words that have endured, such as, "I'm not safe." The therapist then asks the patient to identify what emotion they are feeling when they get that picture and to remember those words and where in their body they are feeling the emotion. While the patient keeps this picture in their mind's eye, rehearses the words, and focuses on the feeling in their body, the therapist typically holds up two fingers and moves them from side to side in front of the patient's eyes. The patient is asked to track the therapist's fingers moving back and forth, which produces a back-and-forth eye movement. In between, the therapist checks in with the patient to see if anything about the picture, the words, or the feelings has changed, and then helps them focus for the next set of eye movements. Once the distress associated with the memory decreases, the patient and therapist explore the meaning associated with the event and work on new ways to think about it. EMDR is given one-on-one by a therapist, usually once a week, for approximately 4–12 sessions.

Conclusion

PTSD is a lousy disorder to have. It can interfere with every aspect of a person's life. The good news is that many effective treatments are available to help get them back on track and living their best life. If you or a loved one has PTSD, we encourage you to seek evidence-based care. You are worth it!

Recommended Reading

Rauch SAM, Rothbaum BO: Making Meaning of Difficult Experiences. New York, Oxford University Press, 2023

Rothbaum BO, Rauch SAM: PTSD: What Everyone Needs to Know. New York, Oxford University Press, 2020

21

Treatment of Social Anxiety Disorder

Grace Lethbridge, B.H.Sc.
Beth Patterson, M.Sc.
Michael Van Ameringen, M.D., FRCPC

Case Vignette

Michele was a 32-year-old female who reported experiencing symptoms of social anxiety disorder. She grew up in Malta and recalled struggling with presentations, class participation, and speaking to authority figures. Her symptoms worsened significantly at age 17, when her family immigrated to Canada. While she was studying at university, oral presentations became so anxiety provoking that she would either avoid taking courses that required them or would try to negotiate an alternative assignment. Telephone and one-to-one conversations were extremely difficult, and she began avoiding extended-family gatherings and completely avoided dating. She reported worrying people would think she was stupid and that she would embarrass herself somehow. Nevertheless, she was able to attend law school.

When initially seen in our service, Michele had just quit a job as a lawyer overseas. She could not cope with one-to-one meetings with clients, especially if someone else was in the room. She was living at her aunt's home near Toronto, where she did not know anyone. She had isolated herself from her family in Montreal over a disagreement. Not surprisingly, Michele also reported symptoms of depression. Michele had been taking sertraline 100 mg for 2 weeks. Our first approach was to optimize her sertraline, and she was eventually titrated to 200 mg/day. Her social anxiety disorder partially responded; she was able to reconnect with her family and was starting to look for a job. However, her functioning was still limited by her anxiety, and her symptoms of depression also persisted.

Because Michele's anxiety had responded somewhat to sertraline and she was tolerating it well, we added bupropion, which successfully improved her depressive symptoms. The bupropion was discontinued after 6 months, and Michele's medication was changed to escitalopram and the dosage optimized to 20 mg/day in an attempt to further improve her social anxiety symptoms. Her symptoms improved to the point where she was able to apply for legal jobs and had moved to her own apartment. However, she often avoided job interviews and was still avoiding face-to-face social interactions. She then tried a course of cognitive-behavioral therapy (CBT) for social anxiety disorder in a group treatment setting. This was very effective and seemed to resonate with her.

Following combination group CBT and escitalopram treatment, Michele was able to attend job interviews and found that her discomfort with small talk improved in social situations. She was ultimately successful in obtaining a corporate legal position. At the start of this position, her anxiety was heightened, and she came more frequently to the clinic for support in this new role. With the continued follow-up support from her health care team, Michele also signed up for a dating agency and began dating. She is now a successful lawyer, married with a child, and connected with her family and friends. Although her symptoms were treated successfully, it took time and a few different treatment trials before she achieved a full response. However, with persistence and motivation, she was able to move forward with her life without being encumbered by her social anxiety disorder.

This case illustrates that social anxiety disorder can have a significant impact on the functioning of those who experience it, especially when it co-occurs with disorders such as major depressive disorder. Research has indicated that effective treatments are available for social anxiety disorder; however, not everyone responds in the same way. Sometimes more than one treatment trial or a combination of treatment strategies is required to achieve a full response.

Introduction

Social anxiety disorder, formerly known as *social phobia,* is characterized by dysfunction in daily life due to persistent, intense fear or anxiety about social and performance situations in which the individual perceives the potential to be judged by others. People with social anxiety disorder actively avoid these feared social and performance situations to avoid potential feelings of embarrassment or humiliation. For some people, the symptoms may be restricted to speaking or performing in public, but for most, they may arise in any social setting in which the person may feel noticed, judged, or observed. Treating social anxiety disorder is crucial because it can impair individuals in all areas of their lives, including school or work, social situations, and family relationships. The two main types of evidence-based treatment for social anxiety disorder are psychological treatments and medication.

Treatment Options

Medication-Based Treatments

First-Line Medication Treatments

When choosing an evidence-based medication for the treatment of social anxiety disorder, it is important to consider the strength of the evidence supporting its efficacy, along with potential side effects. The first-line treatments for social anxiety disorder are the antidepressants known as selective serotonin reuptake inhibitors (SSRIs) and the serotonin-norepinephrine reuptake inhibitor (SNRI) venlafaxine (Effexor). Currently, the U.S. Food and Drug Administration (FDA) has approved the SSRIs sertraline (Zoloft), fluvoxamine controlled-release (Luvox CR), and paroxetine immediate- and controlled-release (Paxil, Paxil CR, Seroxat, Seroxat CR, Pexeva), as well as venlafaxine extended-release (Effexor XR), for the treatment of social anxiety disorder. The SSRIs escitalopram (Cipralex, Lexapro) and fluvoxamine (Luvox) do not have an FDA indication for social anxiety disorder but are still considered first-line treatments due to positive results from randomized controlled trials (RCTs) that compared their efficacy with that of a placebo. One meta-analysis reported that treating social anxiety disorder with antidepressants, particularly SSRIs, was associated with a 62% increase in treatment response compared with placebo. Although these SSRIs have all demonstrated efficacy in high-quality placebo-controlled trials, it is not clear whether some medications are more effective than others. These medications typically have a therapeutic effect after 12–14 weeks of treatment, although patients may begin to notice improvements within 2–4 weeks. Because social anxiety disorder is a persistent condition, clinical guidelines suggest that a treatment duration of 6–12 months is ideal for preventing relapses. Treatment guidelines also recommend that patients gradually increase their exposure to feared social and performance situations while taking the medication.

Second- and Third-Line Medication Treatments

If a patient with social anxiety disorder does not respond to two or more adequately dosed trials of SSRI or SNRI medication, the next step involves a second-line medication, which means that either the quality of evidence is less strong (e.g., trials that only include small numbers of patients, or no meta-analyses are available) or there may be concerns about side effects. Citalopram (Celexa), pregabalin (Lyrica), gabapentin (Neurontin, Gralise, Horizant), phenelzine (Nardil), mirtazapine (Remeron), moclobemide (Manerix), bromazepam (Brozam, Lectopam), and clonazepam (Klonopin, Rivotril, Clonapam) are considered second-line medications for social anxiety disorder.

The SSRI citalopram and the anticonvulsant medications pregabalin and gabapentin are supported by positive placebo-controlled trials. SSRIs are usually favored over anticonvulsants because they are also used to treat psychiatric conditions that commonly co-occur with social anxiety disorder, including depression and other anxiety disorders. Phenelzine is an antidepressant medication that belongs to the class of monoamine oxidase inhibitor (MAOI) antidepressants, and moclobemide is a reversible inhibitor of monoamine oxidase. Although phenelzine has shown efficacy in several RCTs, it is only recommended for patients whose illness is unresponsive to first-line pharmacotherapies because phenelzine is often associated with undesirable side effects and interactions with certain foods and medications. One meta-analysis reported a small effect size for moclobemide, suggesting that it was only slightly more effective than placebo. One RCT reported that, when compared with phenelzine, moclobemide demonstrated similar efficacy for the treatment of social anxiety disorder.

The benzodiazepines bromazepam, alprazolam (Xanax, Niravam), and clonazepam have also demonstrated efficacy in placebo-controlled trials. One meta-analysis found these medications to be equal in efficacy to the SSRIs. Clinical guidelines have suggested that these benzodiazepines may be effective when taken with an antidepressant during the first few weeks of social anxiety disorder treatment because their beneficial effects are seen much earlier than those of antidepressants. Although effective, benzodiazepines are considered second-line treatments because they can be addictive if used long-term and should be used with caution in patients with a history of substance use disorders.

Third-line medication treatments for social anxiety disorder include the anesthetic ketamine (Ketalar), which has one double-blind, placebo-controlled trial demonstrating efficacy. Although fluoxetine (Prozac, Sarafem) is an SSRI, the evidence supporting its use is conflicting; only one of three placebo-controlled trials demonstrated efficacy with fluoxetine. Similarly, the antidepressant mirtazapine was effective in one small RCT and not effective in another. Other third-line antidepressants that have shown efficacy in unblinded studies (less-strong evidence) include duloxetine (Cymbalta), bupropion sustained-release, and clomipramine (Anafranil), as well as the anticonvulsants divalproex (Depakote), topiramate (Topamax, Eprontia, Topiragen), and tiagabine (Gabitril) and the anti-Parkinsonian medication selegiline (Eldepryl, Zelapar). The antipsychotic olanzapine (Zyprexa) was found to be superior to placebo in one RCT; however, this medication is associated with significant side effects. Atomoxetine (Strattera) is an antidepressant-like medication used to treat attention-deficit/hyperactivity disorder (ADHD). One large RCT found atomoxetine to be superior to placebo in the treatment of social anxiety disorder, whereas another small RCT did not.

Desvenlafaxine (Pristiq, Khedezla), buspirone (BuSpar, Vanspar), levetiracetam (Keppra, Elepsia), and atenolol (Tenormin) are medications not recommended for treating social anxiety disorder because placebo-controlled trials have shown that they are not effective. Other agents that are not recommended include propranolol (Inderol, Hemangeol), quetiapine (Seroquel), imipramine (Tofranil), and pergolide (Permax).

Non-Medication-Based Treatments

Psychotherapies

Although many psychological treatments have been examined to treat social anxiety disorder, the gold standard is CBT. This approach includes learning information about the disorder (known as *psychoeducation*), gradually entering feared social situations (*exposure*), changing thinking patterns and core beliefs, and learning strategies to prevent relapse. A course of CBT for social anxiety disorder is typically 8–12 sessions. It can be delivered on a one-to-one basis, in a group, or online. RCTs, which are high-quality scientific studies, have consistently shown that CBT for social anxiety disorder is more effective than being on a waitlist for this treatment, but it is not yet clear whether CBT for social anxiety disorder is more effective than another psychological intervention or standard medical care. Notably, one study reported that CBT was less effective than the antidepressant phenelzine.

A *meta-analysis* combines the data collected by a number of RCTs, which enables researchers to attain stronger answers to their research questions because they can analyze the data of a very large number of study participants. One meta-analysis of social anxiety disorder studies reported that all psychological interventions—except supportive therapy, mindfulness training, and interpersonal psychotherapy—were more effective than being on a waitlist for treatment. In descending order of effectiveness, these psychological interventions included CBT, exposure with social skills training, self-help treatment with support from a health care provider, self-help treatment without support, and psychodynamic psychotherapy. Another meta-analysis compared the effectiveness of CBT with that of other psychotherapies (or active control conditions) and revealed CBT to be superior in the treatment of social anxiety disorder, although the difference was small.

Psychodynamic therapy for social anxiety disorder was examined in a large, multicenter RCT and was found to be less effective than CBT. Other studies have compared psychodynamic psychotherapy with active control conditions and also found it to be less effective. This does not mean that psychodynamic psychotherapy should not be used for social anxiety disorder but that research studies have shown other strategies, namely CBT, to be superior.

The evidence for virtual reality exposure (VRE) therapy is conflicting; only two of three studies have suggested it to be superior to being on a waitlist. One study reported that VRE therapy showed similar efficacy as exposure therapy, whereas another reported that it was less effective. Nevertheless, VRE therapy has been demonstrated to be an effective treatment for people who have public speaking anxiety, as described by one waitlist-controlled trial. VRE therapy for public speaking anxiety enables the therapist to control the size and the interest level of the audience, elements that would be difficult to manage in a real-life situation.

Despite some studies having reported that individual CBT is superior to group CBT, meta-analyses have not detected significant differences in efficacy between the two. In addition, RCTs have demonstrated that internet-based CBT (iCBT) is just as effective as face-to-face CBT and is superior to waitlists. However, the methods used in iCBT programs vary quite a bit. Some programs are fully self-administered, whereas others are delivered by online therapists. Treatment guidelines recommend iCBT as an add-on to standard treatments for social anxiety disorder or for use while patients are waiting for face-to-face CBT.

Combination Treatment

It is not standard practice to treat social anxiety disorder with a combination of medications. Combining medications is typically reserved for patients with treatment-resistant conditions that have responded inadequately to first-line medications. Some studies have examined adding antipsychotics, such as aripiprazole (Abilify) or risperidone (Risperdal); antidepressants, such as paroxetine (Paxil, Seroxat, Pexeva); or anxiolytics, such as buspirone, to a first-line treatment. However, these studies did not use a placebo, therefore the evidence is not considered to be strong. Placebo-controlled trials in which clonazepam was added to an SSRI have demonstrated mixed results. One large, multisite RCT found clonazepam added to sertraline to be effective for treatment-resistant social anxiety disorder, whereas another RCT showed that a combination of clonazepam and paroxetine was not superior to a combination of paroxetine and placebo. Pindolol (Visken) added to paroxetine was also found to be inferior to placebo in the treatment of social anxiety disorder.

The evidence supporting combining CBT and various medications for treatment of social anxiety disorder is mixed. One study reported that combining CBT with the second-line antidepressant phenelzine was more effective than either CBT or phenelzine alone. CBT combined with the second-line antidepressant moclobemide was equally as effective as CBT alone but more effective than moclobemide alone. In contrast, an RCT reported that the combination of CBT and the first-line SSRI sertraline was not more effective than either treatment alone.

Combining pharmacotherapies with other psychotherapies, such as psychodynamic psychotherapy and exposure therapy, has also been studied. One study reported that adding psychodynamic psychotherapy to clonazepam was not more effective than clonazepam alone for treating social anxiety disorder. Two of three placebo-controlled trials have reported that D-cycloserine (Seromycin), an antibiotic used for tuberculosis, enhances the therapeutic effects of exposure therapy when added to CBT. D-Cycloserine targets a specific pathway in the brain—the *N*-methyl-D-aspartate (NMDA) receptor—that is involved with extinguishing our responses to fear. It is believed that D-cycloserine increases the brain's ability to extinguish fear.

Conclusion

Social anxiety disorder is a common anxiety disorder that can have a negative impact on individuals' day-to-day functioning and quality of life. Treatments for social anxiety disorder include medication and psychotherapy in the form of CBT. Recommended first-line medication approaches include the SSRIs (e.g., escitalopram, fluvoxamine controlled-release, paroxetine controlled-release, sertraline) and the SNRI venlafaxine extended-release. CBT and exposure therapy are also considered first-line treatments in either individual or group formats. Interestingly, combining CBT and medication does not appear to have any increased benefit as a first-line treatment. When a patient's social anxiety disorder does not respond to several first- or second-line treatments, guidelines recommend reassessing the diagnosis and then trying a third-line agent, which may include adding another medication to a first-line medication or CBT.

Recommended Reading

Caldiroli A, Capuzzi E, Tagliabue I, et al: New frontiers in the pharmacological treatment of social anxiety disorder in adults: an up-to-date comprehensive overview. Expert Opin Pharmacother 24(2):207–219, 2023 36519357

Leichsenring F, Leweke F: Social anxiety disorder. N Engl J Med 376(23):2255–2264, 2017 28591542

22

Treatment of Obsessive-Compulsive Disorder

Wayne K. Goodman, M.D.
Eric A. Storch, Ph.D.

Introduction

The two mainstays of treatment for obsessive-compulsive disorder (OCD) are a form of behavioral therapy called *exposure and response prevention* (ERP) and medications referred to as serotonin reuptake inhibitors (SRIs). The decision whether to start with ERP or an SRI depends on many factors, including the patient's age, other co-occurring disorders, ability to adhere to treatment, past treatment history, and preference. For example, ERP is clearly the first-line preferred option for children and adolescents with OCD, whereas if significant depression is present, SRIs might be indicated because these medications are also antidepressants. Some patients may benefit most from a combination of ERP and SRIs.

Treatment Options

Medication-Based Treatments

The SRIs include both clomipramine (Anafranil), an older medication classified as a tricyclic antidepressant, and the newer selective serotonin reuptake inhibitors (SSRIs), such as fluoxetine (Prozac), fluvoxamine (Luvox), sertraline (Zoloft), paroxetine (Paxil), citalopram (Celexa), and escitalopram (Lexapro). Serotonin is a *neurotransmitter,* a chemical messenger that transmits signals between nerve cells (*neurons*) in the brain. After a neuron releases serotonin, it reabsorbs any serotonin not captured by an adjoining neuron. This process, known as *serotonin reuptake,* acts to recycle serotonin, making it available for later release. SRIs block the reuptake of serotonin, preventing its return to the home neuron, which initially leads to increased serotonin levels in the space between neurons, which is called a *synapse.* After several weeks of medication treatment, these changes in serotonin availability set in motion other changes in brain chemistry that appear to be responsible for the therapeutic effects of SRIs in OCD.

Although SRIs are primarily antidepressants, not all antidepressants are effective in OCD. For example, desipramine, which acts primarily on the neurotransmitter norepinephrine, works well in depression but is ineffective in OCD. The preferential efficacy of SRIs in OCD is one of the distinguishing features between medication treatment of OCD and major depressive disorder (MDD). These observations led to the hypothesis that OCD involves a chemical imbalance in serotonin. However, despite extensive research, no clear evidence has shown that OCD is caused by a deficiency or disturbance in brain serotonin levels or function. SSRIs are generally well tolerated; the most common side effects are nausea, insomnia, daytime drowsiness, and sexual dysfunction (problems with achieving an orgasm).

Another class of antidepressants called serotonin-norepinephrine reuptake inhibitors (SNRIs) may also be beneficial in some patients with OCD but are not considered first-line treatments. They are not usually prescribed unless the patient's OCD has failed to respond to SRIs. Examples of SNRIs include venlafaxine (Effexor), desvenlafaxine (Pristiq), and duloxetine (Cymbalta). SNRIs do not have U.S. Food and Drug Administration (FDA) approval for use in OCD.

Medication treatment of OCD is initiated with an 8- to 12-week trial of an SSRI at an adequate dosage, usually higher than that used in MDD. This starting dosage should be low and increased gradually to usual therapeutic levels through week 8. If improvement is unsatisfactory after week 8, the daily dosage can be increased further as tolerated over the next 4 weeks. Depending on whether the patient's OCD has responded, the next step may either be continuation of the SSRI, switching to a different SSRI, or adding another medication. It is not uncommon to try several different SSRIs before identifying one that produces the best outcome. There is no clear evidence that one SSRI is superior to another; the decision about which to prescribe depends mostly on expected side effects.

A patient's OCD should not be considered resistant to SRI treatment unless the patient has received a trial with clomipramine. Doctors do not start with clomipramine because it tends to have more side effects than the SSRIs. This agent is frequently associated with sedation, dry mouth, constipation, and weight gain. Because it is sedating, it is usually prescribed at bedtime. Clomipramine can also affect heart rhythms and increase risk of seizures, and the daily dosage should not exceed 250 mg/day. Except in research settings, fluvoxamine should not be combined with clomipramine because it elevates the blood levels of clomipramine by interfering with its metabolism (breakdown) in the liver, which can result in serious side effects.

Approximately 35%–50% of patients with OCD experience significant improvement with SRIs. However, response to SRIs is usually gradual and incomplete. Even in "responders," mild to moderate residual symptoms are common. Clinicians can assess the outcome of a treatment trial using an OCD symptom rating scale called the Yale-Brown Obsessive-Compulsive Scale (Y-BOCS). The Y-BOCS measures the impact of obsessions and compulsions on a person's life with respect to how much time they occupy, how much they interfere with the person's functioning, how much distress they cause, and how well they can be resisted and controlled. The score on the Y-BOCS ranges from 0 (no symptoms) to 40 (extreme symptoms). A *responder* is defined as someone who achieves a 25%–35% reduction in their Y-BOCS score from baseline, which translates into clinically meaningful improvement. For example, going from a 23 to a 15 (~35% decrease) on the Y-BOCS may mean spending 2 hours a day on obsessions and compulsions instead of 5 hours a day, accompanied by less distress and functional impairment and greater sense of control. This may allow the individual to return to work or school and resume a relatively normal and fulfilling life. Because depressive symptoms often accompany OCD, the SRIs—which are also antidepressants—may provide additional relief of depression and anxiety. These benefits may also enable patients to better engage in ERP.

For patients whose OCD has shown limited improvement with an SRI alone, another medication can be added to augment response. The augmentation strategy with the strongest evidence-based support is combining a low dose of antipsychotic agent with an SRI. The class of medications known as antipsychotics are not just used to treat psychosis; for example, medicines such as risperidone (Risperdal) or aripiprazole (Abilify) are also used to suppress tics (sudden, repetitive movements or sounds). Patients with OCD and a lifetime history of a chronic tic disorder (e.g., Tourette's disorder) are most likely to show improvement in their obsessive-compulsive symptoms with antipsychotic augmentation of SRIs. There is solid evidence that even patients without tics may derive additional benefit from adding an antipsychotic to an SRI.

Recent research suggests that the neurotransmitter glutamate may play a role in OCD. This has led to trials of medications that act on the brain's glutamate system, such as memantine (Namenda), riluzole, *N*-acetylcysteine, and ketamine. For the most part, these medications were developed for other indications and then repurposed for OCD. Memantine and riluzole have FDA approval for two different neurodegenerative disorders, Alzheimer's disease and amyotrophic lateral sclerosis (ALS), respectively. Based on published case reports, memantine has shown promise in OCD when added to SRIs. So far, these encouraging open-label results have not been confirmed in randomized controlled trials (RCTs), in which patients are assigned either to the active treatment or to placebo in a *double-blind* fashion (i.e., neither patient nor clinician know the identity of the assigned compound). Initial open-label findings of combining riluzole with SRIs for the treatment of OCD were positive; however, RCTs have not found a significant difference between adding riluzole or placebo to SRIs for OCD. A newly synthesized compound related to riluzole, called troriluzole, is currently being tested as an adjunct (add-on) to SRIs in a large-scale RCT for patients with OCD. *N*-Acetylcysteine is a well-tolerated medication available without a prescription. As with riluzole, initial reports of adding *N*-acetylcysteine to SRIs in OCD were positive, but subsequent RCTs proved negative. An intranasal spray form of esketamine (a variant of ketamine; brand name Spravato) is FDA-approved as a rapid-acting treatment for MDD. To date, results of studies with ketamine for OCD have been mixed. At present, it may be best suited for treating OCD with significant secondary depression.

Non-Medication-Based Treatments

Psychotherapy

ERP, which is a specific form of cognitive-behavioral therapy, has demonstrated effectiveness for adults and children with OCD. Studies suggest that approximately 75%–80% of individuals benefit from this approach, with people reporting substantially improved OCD, co-occurring symptoms (e.g., depression, anxiety), and quality of life following successful treatment. Gains tend to persist over time, although many people who benefited from a course of ERP will require additional sessions.

ERP is based on two different theories of how fears are learned and maintained—namely the *habituation* and *inhibitory learning* models. The habituation model suggests that repeatedly confronting distress-provoking triggers without performing compensatory rituals diminishes the emotional response. The inhibitory learning model suggests that patients learn that feared outcomes do not happen if they confront their triggers but do not engage in rituals and that, if the feared outcome *does* occur, they are able to cope with the situation.

ERP typically involves individual therapy sessions and consists of several interrelated components in addition to the core elements of exposure and response prevention. These include education about OCD and treatment (*psychoeducation*), development of fear hierarchy, cognitive exercises, and relapse prevention. Treatment generally starts with psychoeducation about OCD and ERP treatment and involves teaching patients about the nature of OCD, why and how the treatment works, and other key components, such as the need to practice therapy tasks. A strong working relationship between the therapist and person with OCD is critical for successful treatment. Thereafter, therapists and patients collaborate to develop a *fear hierarchy,* which is a list of the triggers that provoke distress and the feared outcome(s) for not engaging in rituals. Triggers are rated on a subjective units of distress scale, usually from 0–10 or 0–100, with higher scores corresponding with greater distress. Once the hierarchy is established, ERP begins with the person confronting distress-provoking triggers in a gradual manner, starting with those that provoke less distress. These exposures are usually to actual stimuli that trigger distress (in vivo), but they can also involve exposure to thoughts or bodily sensations. It is important for individuals to remain exposed to the trigger until their distress reduces and they are able to learn that the feared outcome does not take place or that they can tolerate the discomfort.

As noted, ERP is the core component of effective OCD treatment and is the major element of most sessions after psychoeducation and hierarchy development take place. Learning different cognitive therapy skills is also important to emphasize what has been learned through exposures and how to recognize obsessions and effectively dismiss them. As patients progress in treatment, relapse-prevention planning is used to reinforce approaches and sustain gains. ERP treatment protocols typically include 12–16 weekly sessions, although the duration should be personalized to the individual's needs, and many people participate in substantially more sessions. Intensive treatment programs in which the person receives daily sessions lasting several hours or more have demonstrated effectiveness, especially when more conventional approaches have not been sufficiently beneficial.

Noninvasive Neuromodulation

Transcranial Magnetic Stimulation. Neuromodulation treatments alter neuronal (nerve cell) activity through the use of medical devices that deliver a stimulus tog a specific region or area of the brain. Transcranial magnetic stimulation

(TMS) is a noninvasive procedure that produces electrical impulses in the brain using electromagnetic coils placed near the head and aimed at specific brain regions. The principle is based on Faraday's Law, which states that a fluctuating magnetic field can produce an electrical current within a conductor located perpendicular to its path. In the case of TMS, neurons act as conductors of electricity. A specific form of TMS, called deep TMS (dTMS), can reach deeper brain structures implicated in OCD. dTMS focused on midline structures of the brain has been approved by the FDA for treatment of patients with OCD that has failed to respond to at least one adequate trial of an SRI. An RCT found that 38% of patients in the active group achieved a full response, compared with 11% in the sham group. TMS is safe and generally well tolerated. A full course of treatment requires five daily administrations of TMS for 6 weeks. Despite its FDA approval, some insurance providers do not cover the costs of TMS. Further studies are needed to compare the effectiveness of dTMS with other interventions used for severe and treatment-resistant OCD.

Transcranial Direct Current Stimulation. Transcranial direct current stimulation (tDCS) consists of a medical device that applies a weak electrical current (1–2 mA) between two electrodes placed on the patient's scalp. It acts by changing the excitability of neurons located within the surface of the brain beneath the electrode contacts. These local effects may influence activity of other more distantly located brain regions connected to a broader network. tDCS is safe, well tolerated, and relatively inexpensive. A growing number of reports on tDCS for the treatment of OCD have appeared in the literature; at present, most of these studies involve case reports targeting a variety of brain areas. Larger studies with more rigorous designs are required before its use in OCD can be recommended.

Electroconvulsive Therapy. Electroconvulsive therapy (ECT) involves inducing seizures using electricity under carefully controlled procedures while the patient is under anesthesia. ECT remains a highly effective intervention for severe depression. Repeated administrations are required, typically three times a week, for a total of 6–12 sessions. ECT has not been shown to be effective for OCD except to manage coexisting depression, particularly when suicidal ideation is present.

Neurosurgery

One of the shifts in our conceptualization of OCD is to view it as a brain circuit disorder involving abnormal connections between different brain areas. These connections form an overactive loop that perpetuates the symptoms of OCD. Based on this circuit hypothesis, an intervention acting at *nodes* (or connections) of this loop might interrupt the network responsible for obsessive-compulsive symptoms. This is the rationale for neurosurgical approaches that either create lesions (called *ablative surgery*) or insert an electrical lead (called *deep brain stimulation*, or DBS) in this brain pathway.

Ablative surgery has been used for decades to treat severe and treatment-refractory cases of OCD. The lesions are small and precisely placed, and various techniques can be used to produce them, ranging from radiation to laser beams. Abundant published data suggest that ablative surgery targeting the anterior limb of the internal capsule (ALIC), a white fiber bundle connecting the cortex with deep brain structures, is effective in more than 50% of patients with intractable OCD. The major drawback of ablative surgery is that the effects (i.e., creation of a lesion) are irreversible.

DBS is widely used to treat medication-resistant movement disorders, such as Parkinson's disease and essential tremor. The neurosurgeon places electrical leads in the ALIC (or a related brain region) by inserting them through small openings they create in the skull. The leads are locked in place, and the wires connecting them are tunneled under the skin and connected to a pulse generator inserted in the chest (under the skin), much like a cardiac pacemaker. The DBS device can be programmed using a tablet that communicates wirelessly with the pulse generator to deliver electrical stimulation to the targeted brain area. In contrast to ablative surgery, DBS is reversible (i.e., hardware can be removed without any permanent lesions) and adjustable. Frequent programming visits are required, and it may take 6 months to optimize the stimulation settings. DBS targeting the ventral capsule/ventral striatum has been approved by the FDA for use in adults with severe, treatment-resistant OCD under a Humanitarian Device Exemption. OCD is the only psychiatric disorder for which neurosurgery is an FDA treatment indication. A recent review of the published scientific literature found that 66% of OCD cases respond to DBS. It is intended for adults with severe OCD that has not responded to adequate trials of ERP, multiple SRIs (including clomipramine), and antipsychotic augmentation.

Conclusion

Several highly effective treatments are available for patients with OCD. The two first-line treatments are ERP and SRIs. To be most effective, ERP should be delivered by therapists trained in its use for OCD. By the same token, an adequate trial with medications requires that the prescriber be knowledgeable about dosing and duration of treatment for OCD. Despite the availability of these two treatment modalities, some patients with OCD may not experience significant symptom relief. At present, the only second-line medication option with strong empirical support is adding a low dose of antipsychotic medication. However, emerging research indicates that other medications may prove beneficial when added to an SRI or given on their own. The use of medical devices to treat OCD is gaining traction. dTMS, which is noninvasive, has been cleared by the FDA for use in patients with OCD. For the most severe and treatment-resistant cases, DBS can be a highly effective alternative.

In our collective experience treating thousands of patients with OCD, we have never told anyone that we cannot think of something else to try, whether psychotherapy, medications, or medical devices. Furthermore, there is hope on the horizon as major research is under way with the aim of developing new and even more effective treatments for OCD.

Recommended Reading

Abramowitz JS: Getting Over OCD: A 10-Step Workbook for Taking Back Your Life, 2nd Edition. New York, Guilford Press, 2018

Goodman WK, Storch EA, Sheth SA: Harmonizing the neurobiology and treatment of obsessive-compulsive disorder. Am J Psychiatry 178(1):17–29, 2021 33384007

23

Treatment of Panic Disorder

Isabella G. Spaulding, B.S.
Murray B. Stein, M.D., M.P.H.

Introduction

Many people have experienced strong feelings of panic, fear, or anxiety before, and some may have even experienced one or two panic attacks in their lifetime. It is normal to have these feelings once in a while, but it is not normal to have panic attacks frequently. A *panic attack* is a large surge of extreme fear or discomfort that often comes out of nowhere. It typically does not last for more than 10 minutes and usually hits its worst point within a few minutes. During a panic attack, individuals may feel that their heart is beating very quickly and that they are having difficulty breathing. They may also feel dizzy, sweaty, and shaky and become afraid that they are "going crazy" or might die. Although these attacks are not life threatening, people feel very scared during them, and they can have large effects on people's day-to-day lives.

Individuals who have frequent panic attacks and who feel very worried about having another attack for longer than 1 month have *panic disorder*. They may also change their behavior and avoid certain things to try to prevent having another attack. This means panic disorder is not only the state of having panic attacks but also involves worrying frequently about having another panic attack. If you are experiencing panic attacks, it is important to see a doctor. They can conduct a medical evaluation to make sure no physical conditions are causing your attacks, such as thyroid disorders or cardiovascular issues. Panic attacks can also be brought on by excessive substance use, such as consuming too much caffeine or using stimulant drugs such as cocaine. Individuals experiencing withdrawal symptoms after they stop drinking alcohol may also have panic attacks.

About 2.8% of people in the United States have panic disorder in a given year, with a lifetime prevalence of 4.7%. Most people develop panic disorder as adults and often deal with the condition for a long time, especially if they do not seek treatment. Many individuals who have panic disorder experience other psychological disorders, such as depression, or other anxiety disorders, such as agoraphobia. *Agoraphobia* is when someone avoids multiple places or situations because they are afraid they might have a panic attack. Although there is no cure for panic disorder, many treatments are available that are highly effective at reducing symptoms, including psychotherapy, medication, and a combination of both treatments.

Treatment Options

Medication-Based Treatments

Several classes of medications have been shown to be safe and effective in the treatment of panic disorder, including antidepressants and benzodiazepines. Several others are sometimes used but have less evidence supporting their use. These medications may be prescribed by primary care practitioners, psychiatrists, or by any licensed medical provider.

Antidepressants

Selective serotonin reuptake inhibitors (SSRIs) and serotonin-norepinephrine reuptake inhibitors (SNRIs) are considered first-line agents for the treatment of panic disorder. SSRIs include fluoxetine (Prozac), sertraline (Zoloft), paroxetine (Paxil), fluvoxamine (Luvox), citalopram (Celexa), and escitalopram (Lexapro). SNRIs include venlafaxine (Effexor), desvenlafaxine (Pristiq), and duloxetine (Cymbalta). Most guidelines and reviews recommend SSRIs as the initial pharmacological treatment for anxiety disorders. Antidepressants are useful in the treatment of panic disorder even in the absence of major depression, but they are also useful in individuals who have both panic disorder and major depression. There are many antidepressants to choose from, and any of them may be used initially in the treatment of panic disorder. When one antidepressant proves to be ineffective or to have intolerable side effects, a switch to another antidepressant—sometimes from an SSRI to an SNRI, but sometimes from one SSRI to another—is usually the next step.

Treatment with antidepressants for panic disorder is started at low dosages—often half the starting dosage for major depression—to minimize an early effect of worsening anxiety, which is common but usually short lived, lasting a few days after each dosage increase. (Sometimes a benzodiazepine such as lorazepam [Ativan] or clonazepam [Klonopin] is started simultaneously to prevent or minimize this initial increase in anxiety and is then tapered and stopped after a month or two.) The antidepressant dosage is slowly increased, typically over several weeks, until a therapeutic dosage is achieved. Although an initial response may be seen as early as 2–4 weeks into treatment, a trial of up to 8–12 weeks at a therapeutic dosage is necessary to assess efficacy. The antidepressant is usually continued at the full therapeutic dosage for a year before the physician will consider slowly lowering the dosage (over several weeks or months) and then discontinuing the medication. During this time, the patient may also engage in a course of cognitive-behavioral therapy [CBT] to learn skills that may reduce the likelihood of relapse.) Abrupt discontinuation is not recommended and, in fact, may be dangerous.

SSRIs and SNRIs are generally well tolerated, although some individuals may experience diarrhea, headaches, dizziness, or other side effects. These usually dissipate over time, but dosage reduction or a switch to a different antidepressant is sometimes needed. Sexual dysfunction is not uncommon, and sexual side effects do not usually get better with time; reducing the dosage, switching to another antidepressant, or adding other medications to help with sexual function may be helpful. The U.S. Food and Drug Administration (FDA) issued a "black box warning" for all antidepressants, cautioning their use in children and young adults because of concern about increased suicidality in these individuals, particularly during the first few weeks and months of treatment. Accordingly, patients in this age group should be monitored more closely by their treating clinician, but that should not prevent the use of these medications for those who are in need and likely to benefit, especially patients who have tried and whose illness has not responded to psychotherapeutic approaches.

Benzodiazepines and Other Antianxiety Medications

Benzodiazepines such as lorazepam (Ativan), alprazolam (Xanax), and clonazepam (Klonopin), are considered second-line treatments for panic disorder. Although they are effective, and their onset can be rapid, they have the potential for misuse and abuse and, as such, are not suitable for patients with a history of substance abuse. Common side effects of benzodiazepines include sedation, tiredness, and dizziness; these effects tend to diminish with time. When benzodiazepines are started, patients should exercise caution when driving or using heavy machinery, and the medications should not be combined with alcohol, marijuana, or other potentially sedating substances.

As noted in the previous section, benzodiazepines are sometimes used concurrently with the start of antidepressants to provide some anxiety symptom relief while waiting for the anti-panic effects of the antidepressant medication to develop, which can take weeks. They are also used when an individual obtains some benefit from their antidepressant but is still having breakthrough panic attacks. In such instances, a benzodiazepine that is taken regularly, for example, two or three times a day (rather than as-needed) for lorazepam, may be added to the antidepressant and continued for as long as that antidepressant is prescribed. Rarely, benzodiazepines may be used as the sole treatment for panic disorder for patients who have experienced intolerable side effects with antidepressants. When benzodiazepines are to be stopped, they must be discontinued gradually, usually over several weeks or months, under the supervision of a physician or other licensed provider.

Gabapentin (Neurontin) and pregabalin (Lyrica) are sometimes utilized as alternatives to benzodiazepines in the treatment of panic and other anxiety disorders, although research support for their utility is limited. Beta-adrenergic-blocking drugs such as propranolol (Inderal) are sometimes prescribed for the treatment of panic disorder, but evidence for their usefulness and safety in this context is lacking.

Non-Medication-Based Treatments

Psychotherapy

Psychotherapy typically involves meeting with a mental health professional over a series of sessions to discuss your thoughts, behaviors, and emotions. One of the best treatments for panic disorder supported by research is CBT. When used for panic disorder, CBT teaches patients about the panic response and helps them learn skills to change their thinking and behavior to reduce panic symptoms. One of the ways it does this is through *exposure therapy,* in which patients work with clinicians in a safe environment to slowly expose themselves to some of the situations or behaviors they may have been avoiding. One kind of exposure is called *in vivo exposure,* in which the patient and clinician create a hierarchy of potential exposures from least to most distressing. Together, they go through each of the exposures in person, gradually progressing to those that cause the patient the most distress. Another type of exposure that is often specifically used for panic disorder is *interoceptive exposure.* Many individuals with panic disorder worry about experiencing the physical sensations they associate with having a panic attack and, as a result, might avoid activities that trigger these sensations. Interoceptive exposure works to challenge the idea that physical sensations will lead to negative events, such as having a panic attack, by exposing the patient to these physical sensations. Such exposures may include intentionally increasing the patient's heart rate or breathing so that they will gradually learn to no longer associate these physical sensations with panic attacks.

In addition to exposure therapy, CBT also teaches patients skills to help reduce bodily symptoms of panic, such as breathing exercises or techniques for muscle relaxation. Research supports CBT, suggesting it is the best type of psychotherapy for patients with panic disorder. The length of CBT treatment can vary, but typically patients meet with a mental health professional for 10–12 sessions lasting 1 hour each week. These sessions can be one-on-one or in a group setting with other individuals also receiving treatment for panic disorder.

Another evidence-based treatment modifies face-to-face CBT so it can be delivered by computer or mobile device. For some patients, internet-based CBT (iCBT) may be a more accessible option, especially for those who have difficulty attending weekly treatment sessions in person or who prefer the format of virtual treatment. CBT delivered via computer or mobile phone is supported by research as an effective treatment for panic disorder.

Combined Treatment

For many patients with panic disorder, clinicians will suggest combination treatment using both medication and psychotherapy to treat panic symptoms. This is often the case for patients for whom one treatment alone was not helpful. In fact, some research suggests that combined pharmacological and psychological treatment has better results than either treatment alone. Other studies have found that combining CBT with an SSRI was most effective during the active treatment period, whereas combination treatment or CBT alone was effective during the period following active treatment. In addition, combined treatment with CBT and an SSRI or SNRI may be best for patients with panic disorder and agoraphobia. Ultimately, the process of finding the right treatment is unique to each individual, and patients should work with their clinicians to find out what treatment works best for them. For example, consider the following patient:

> Jessica, a 22-year-old college student, had been experiencing daily panic attacks for several months and had also become depressed. She started a course of CBT for panic disorder with an experienced therapist but found it difficult to concentrate in her sessions with the therapist. She was so anxious that doing the home reading and assignments was not possible. After a few weeks of weekly psychotherapy, the therapist recommended that Jessica see her primary care physician about starting an antidepressant. Jessica was started on 25 mg/day of sertraline, and this was increased to 50 mg and then to 100 mg over the ensuing 2 weeks. She continued to see the CBT therapist during this time and was able to better engage in therapy as the antidepressant improved her depressive symptoms and reduced the frequency and intensity of her panic attacks. After completing the

full course of CBT and a number of "booster" sessions, and continuing to take 200 mg/day of sertraline, Jessica had become both panic- and depression-free.

Conclusion

Panic disorder is a serious mental health condition that can cause significant distress and difficulties for individuals who have symptoms. However, many options are available for people with panic disorder to help them reduce their symptoms, including psychotherapy and medication. Although there is no single right treatment, and different treatments may work well for some that do not work well for others, research suggests that CBT is the best psychotherapy treatment to try first, and SSRIs are the best medication treatments. These two treatments can also be used together, especially when one treatment alone is not helpful. If you think you may be experiencing symptoms of panic disorder, you should talk to a doctor, nurse, psychologist, or other health care provider about your treatment options.

Recommended Reading

Rabasco A, McKay D, Smits JA, et al: Psychosocial treatment for panic disorder: an umbrella review of systematic reviews and meta-analyses. J Anxiety Disord 86:102528, 2022

Stein MB, Craske MG: Treating anxiety in 2017: optimizing care to improve outcomes. JAMA 318:235–236, 2017

24

Treatment of Generalized Anxiety Disorder

Jonathan E. Alpert, M.D., Ph.D.
Simon A. Rego, Psy.D., ABPP

Case Vignette

Daniel is a 32-year-old attorney who was referred to a psychiatrist by his primary care doctor for "work stress." On evaluation, it became clear that he worried daily not only about whether he is doing a good enough job at work but also whether his rent will be raised beyond his means, his car will break down on the way to a weekend trip, his mentor will leave his firm, and his parents and significant others will get ill. Although his anxiety has worsened in recent years, Daniel is no stranger to anxiety. For as long as he can remember, his grandmother has referred to him as "Nervous Nellie."

Daniel now finds himself constantly stressed and unable to relax. He frequently paces and wrings his hands. In bed at night, his mind races to worst-case scenarios. He experiences a constant "knot" in his stomach and frequent headaches. Although clearly distressed, he says he is more anxious than depressed. When not preoccupied by worry, he still enjoys social activities, exercise, and practicing the guitar. He drinks sparingly and uses cannabis about one or two times per month. Although his anxiety has been longstanding, the uptick of anxiety during the past year makes him think that he is destined for a "nervous breakdown." He is thinking about leaving his job and wondering about hospitalization. The psychiatrist rules out other diagnoses such as major depressive disorder

(MDD), bipolar disorder, substance use problems, and psychotic disorders. She believes the most likely diagnosis is generalized anxiety disorder (GAD).

Given the severity of his current symptoms, the psychiatrist initiates a short-term prescription of the benzodiazepine lorazepam (Ativan) at 0.5 mg up to twice a day as needed and prescribes escitalopram (Lexapro) at 5 mg/day. At his follow-up appointment 2 weeks later, Daniel reports that the lorazepam has been helpful to "take the edge off" his anxiety and insomnia but that he uses it only intermittently because it makes him feel "dull." The psychiatrist increases the Lexapro prescription to 10 mg/day. Over the next 6 weeks, Daniel reports ongoing anxious thoughts and physical symptoms but relief from more severe and constant "dread." The psychiatrist increases the Lexapro again to 20 mg/day. Three months into treatment, Daniel reports feeling 40% better, which is very welcome, but he still experiences frequent anxious ruminations about anticipated catastrophic events and continues to miss deadlines because he avoids activities that make him anxious, such as drafting court filings.

Daniel and his psychiatrist discuss possible options, including switching his Lexapro to another serotonergic agent, such as venlafaxine (Effexor); augmenting the Lexapro with another agent, such as pregabalin (Lyrica); or trying cognitive-behavioral therapy (CBT). They decide to try CBT, and the psychiatrist refers Daniel to a psychologist experienced with this approach. With the psychologist, Daniel constructs a hierarchy of worries and starts regular mood and anxiety charting, which they review together at his weekly sessions. He embarks on cognitive restructuring and relaxation training. As he acquires these skills, he becomes increasingly able to engage in exposure, at first during his CBT sessions involving imagined situations, and then in actual activities in his outside life.

In the final weeks of CBT, Daniel and his therapist acknowledge his substantial progress. They agree he is in a significantly better place than when he first entered treatment and, indeed, he feels more confident and less anxious than he can recall since early adolescence. Given the prior chronicity and severity of his GAD, they continue his Lexapro for now because it has been only 7 months, but they agree to reevaluate this at regular intervals for a possible taper later, perhaps in conjunction with a CBT "booster session." They also anticipate future times when anxiety will reoccur and develop strategies for addressing it. They conclude their work but leave the door open for occasional booster sessions in the future.

Introduction

GAD is a common and distressing clinical condition that all too often goes untreated. According to a survey by the World Health Organization, only about one in three people with GAD report ever receiving treatment. However, of those who sought treatment, most were helped. Our goal in this chapter is to help readers become familiar with the growing range of safe and effective medication and non-medication treatment options for GAD and how these are used in current clinical practice. Treatment for GAD can substantially improve the health and quality of life of individuals who experience the persistent and excessive fear and worry that characterize the disorder.

Studies on GAD treatments have demonstrated the benefit of selected pharmacotherapies (medications) and psychotherapies (talk therapies). These approaches, whether used alone or in combination, are the mainstay of current treatment for GAD. Although less robust evidence exists for the effectiveness of complementary or integrative approaches for GAD, such as yoga, individuals with mild forms of stress and anxiety may wish to discuss these approaches with their clinicians. Neurostimulation treatments for GAD also show promise, such as transcranial magnetic stimulation (TMS), but more research is needed.

Very few direct head-to-head studies of pharmacotherapy versus psychotherapy for GAD have been conducted. Research to date suggests that they are probably roughly equivalent in their effectiveness. For this reason, the choice of initial treatment is often based on patient preference and feasibility. Most patients with GAD express a preference for psychotherapy. However, some prefer medications or may find psychotherapy initially impractical due to the time commitment or their limited access to expert psychotherapists or because their anxiety symptoms need to be lessened first with medications before they feel able to make full use of psychotherapy. A combination of pharmacotherapy and psychotherapy may offer the most relief for patients with moderate or severe GAD or for those whose GAD has already not responded adequately to either approach alone.

In clinical practice, decisions regarding initial treatment are also influenced by the presence of co-occurring conditions such as MDD, which is common among people with GAD and other anxiety disorders. Fortunately, many of the medications and psychotherapies known to be effective for GAD are also effective for some of these co-occurring conditions. When contemplating treatment, relevant lifestyle and general health measures should always be discussed. For some people with GAD, addressing these measures may be sufficient to reduce their anxiety to tolerable levels. For others, targeting these factors helps set the stage for better treatment outcomes with psychotherapy or medications.

Treatment Options

Medication-Based Treatments

Just as CBT is the preferred initial psychotherapy treatment for GAD based on the substantial evidence base demonstrating its effectiveness, medications that inhibit the reuptake of serotonin within nerve terminals are the preferred initial pharmacological treatments for GAD. Other medications that may have a role in the treatment of GAD include the benzodiazepines and buspirone, as well as certain anticonvulsants, antihistamines, and antipsychotics, particularly when initial treatment has not worked well enough. Broadly speaking, all medications that treat anxiety may be called anxiolytics (agents that "lyse" or break up anxiety). However, the term *anxiolytic* is used in various ways, sometimes referring to all of the medications we discuss here, sometimes referring only to the serotonergic medications and benzodiazepines, and sometimes referring to the benzodiazepines alone.

The optimal duration of medication treatment for GAD is unknown. However, because GAD is typically a chronic condition, most individuals treated successfully with medications remain on their medication for at least 9–12 months, both to achieve symptom reduction and to protect against relapse. For individuals with significant and long-term distress and impairment from GAD, it is not unusual to continue taking medication for years. Patients and clinicians often make decisions concerning the duration of medication treatment based on the prior severity and persistence of GAD as well as the degree to which the medications remain helpful, tolerable, and feasible. Although more studies are needed, many clinicians believe that adding CBT to medications provides additional protection against relapse, even when medications are eventually discontinued.

Serotonergic Medications

The serotonergic medications include the selective serotonin reuptake inhibitors (SSRIs) and the serotonin-norepinephrine reuptake inhibitors (SNRIs). These medications are classified as antidepressants. However, numerous studies have shown their efficacy for the treatment of GAD even in the absence of depression. The SSRIs best studied for the treatment of GAD are sertraline (Zoloft), paroxetine (Paxil), citalopram (Celexa), and escitalopram (Lexapro). Other SSRIs, including fluoxetine (Prozac) and fluvoxamine (Luvox), are less studied for GAD but likely to have similar benefit. The SNRIs best studied for GAD are venlafaxine (Effexor) and duloxetine (Cymbalta). Desvenlafaxine (Pristiq) and levomilnacipran (Fetzima) are also likely to be effective, although they are also less studied and are less commonly used as first-line treatment.

Common possible side effects of SSRIs and SNRIs include initial jitteriness, activation, or insomnia that usually subsides over a short time. Individuals with anxiety disorders may be particularly sensitive to these side effects and may therefore be started on lower-than-usual dosages for the first days or weeks, with the plan to continue to gradually increase the dosage to a therapeutic range over time.

Although equivalently safe when compared with the SSRIs and SNRIs, the newer, "atypical" serotonergic antidepressant medications, including vilazodone (Viibryd) and vortioxetine (Trintellix), have not been utilized or studied widely enough in GAD to recommend them as an initial treatment, but they are reasonable considerations when SSRIs or SNRIs have not worked well or have not been well tolerated. Mirtazapine (Remeron) is also an atypical serotonergic antidepressant that has been effective in individuals with GAD in preliminary studies. Because it causes drowsiness, mirtazapine is often given at bedtime and can be helpful for the insomnia that often accompanies GAD.

Older serotonergic agents include the tricyclic antidepressants (TCAs), such as imipramine (Tofranil) and amitriptyline (Elavil), as well as the monoamine oxidase inhibitors (MAOIs), such as phenelzine (Nardil), tranylcypromine (Parnate), and isocarboxazid (Marplan). These medications played an important role in the treatment of depression and anxiety in the 1960s through the 1980s, before the discovery of the SSRIs and SNRIs. Because these medications are associated with more serious potential cardiovascular side effects as well as some dangerous interactions with certain medications and foods, they are no longer used as first-line treatment. Although the TCAs and MAOIs are probably no more effective than the SSRIs or SNRIs for most people, GAD in some patients appears to respond better to them than to the newer agents. Experienced clinicians may, therefore, consider TCAs or MAOIs for select patients with GAD whose illness has not responded to other treatments.

Benzodiazepines

Beginning with agents introduced in the 1960s, such as chlordiazepoxide (Librium) and diazepam (Valium), the benzodiazepines are among the oldest contemporary psychiatric medications, along with the TCAs and MAOIs. The most common benzodiazepines used for GAD are clonazepam (Klonopin), lorazepam (Ativan), and alprazolam (Xanax). The benzodiazepines do not have a direct effect on serotonin; thus, they have minimal or no antidepressant benefits. Instead, they interact with specialized benzodiazepine receptors on nerve cells that produce another neurotransmitter, γ-aminobutyric acid (GABA), and their most specific use is for the treatment of anxiety or insomnia, as well as other conditions such as alcohol withdrawal symptoms or seizures (convulsions).

There are some other notable differences between the serotonergic medications and the benzodiazepines. To be effective, serotonergic medications must be taken daily and may take several or more weeks to begin to work. In contrast, the antianxiety effects of benzodiazepines are usually experienced within minutes to an hour of the very first dose. Like antidepressants, benzodiazepines may be taken on a daily basis. However, unlike antidepressants, they also may be taken on an as-needed basis to address only periods of particularly severe anxiety or insomnia. Finally, unlike serotonergic antidepressants, benzodiazepines are associated with a risk of dependence or addiction. Most patients who have no history of problem substance use and who receive benzodiazepines in a clinical context with monitoring do not develop addiction symptoms, such as having cravings for benzodiazepines or urges to misuse them for recreational or other purposes.

Patients who take benzodiazepines daily over months or years and wish to discontinue their treatment will likely need to taper the medication gradually to avoid "rebound" anxiety, insomnia, or even seizures. In addition, it is hazardous to mix benzodiazepines with other substances, particularly alcohol and opioids, because they can promote more severe intoxication when used in combination and may result in life-threatening *respiratory depression* (diminished breathing rate). Overall, benzodiazepines are the most rapidly acting and effective medication treatments available for anxiety, and they represent an important potential component in the pharmacological treatment of GAD. However, because of the associated risks, clinicians typically prescribe these agents for the shortest time and at the lowest effective dosages. For patients with mild to moderate GAD, the SSRIs and SNRIs may suffice, and benzodiazepines may not be needed. For individuals with more severe GAD, benzodiazepines may offer meaningful relief initially while they wait for their serotonergic medications, such as SSRIs and SNRIs or other treatments, to kick in. A subset of individuals with severe, persistent GAD may benefit from ongoing benzodiazepine treatment in addition to their serotonergic medication and psychotherapy, such as CBT.

Other Medications

In addition to the serotonergic antidepressants and benzodiazepines, which are the most widely prescribed and well-studied medications for GAD, other agents have been found to be effective for GAD symptoms. Buspirone (Buspar) interacts with a serotonin receptor called 5-hydroxytryptaminc-1A (5-HT_{1A}). It is not an antidepressant but, rather, has primarily antianxiety effects. Like other serotonergic medications, it needs to be taken daily in order to work and often takes several weeks to demonstrate benefit. Although buspirone is safe and usually well tolerated, its initial side effects can include nausea or dizziness. Buspirone is often less noticeably effective than the benzodiazepines but may be a useful alternative to them for individuals who have current or prior substance use problems or who do not tolerate the drowsiness or other side effects of benzodiazepines. Like benzodiazepines, buspirone can be used as a stand-alone medication or in conjunction with SSRIs or SNRIs, whose effects it may help augment.

Antihistamines such as hydroxyzine (Vistaril) are sometimes helpful to treat some of the symptoms of GAD, particularly restlessness or insomnia. Like benzodiazepines, they can be used on an as-needed basis and do not need to build up over time. Unlike benzodiazepines, they carry no risk of respiratory depression or addiction and, like buspirone, can be used in patients with substance use problems. The primary side effects of antihistamines include drowsiness and dry mouth. Other potential effects include weight gain, urinary retention, constipation, and a rare "paradoxical" agitation. Antihistamines should be used with care in older individuals, who are more likely to experience memory problems and other cognitive side effects with these agents.

Antiepileptic medications, particularly pregabalin (Lyrica) and gabapentin (Neurontin), have been used in the treatment of GAD symptoms, particularly as adjuncts to SSRIs or SNRIs. When these medications are prescribed, they are generally taken daily. Unlike the benzodiazepines, they carry low risk of addiction; however, like the benzodiazepines, they should not be stopped abruptly due to the risk of rebound seizures, even among individuals without a seizure disorder. Gabapentin and pregabalin have other uses as well, including treatment of pain syndromes such as diabetic neuropathy. They are generally safe but may cause drowsiness.

The *second-generation* or *atypical* antipsychotics were developed for treatment of schizophrenia; however, over the past two decades, they have emerged as effective treatments for some mood and anxiety disorders such as bipolar disorder, MDD, and GAD. Examples of these medications studied but not yet approved by the U.S. Food and Drug Administration (FDA) for treatment of GAD are quetiapine (Seroquel), aripiprazole (Abilify), risperidone (Risperdal), olanzapine (Zyprexa), and ziprasidone (Geodon). Antipsychotic medications are associated with potential metabolic effects, such as weight gain and elevated blood sugar (glucose) or serum lipids (e.g., triglycerides), and motor effects such as *akathisia* (physical restlessness that can resemble anxiety) or *tardive dyskinesia* (involuntary movements of the face or other body parts). Given the comparative safety and well-documented efficacy of the SSRIs and SNRIs, atypical antipsychotics are generally reserved for individuals with severe GAD that has not responded fully to other agents alone. Fortunately, when used for the treatment of GAD, the atypical antipsychotics can often be used as adjuncts to other treatments, such as SSRIs and SNRIs, at dosages that are lower than those needed to treat other conditions such as schizophrenia or bipolar disorder, thus reducing side effects and risks.

Non-Medication-Based Treatments

Lifestyle and General Health Measures

Insomnia is often a symptom of GAD. Reciprocally, poor sleep can worsen anxiety. Behavioral steps that improve sleep hygiene often reduce sleep disruption and may help decrease anxiety. These include avoiding light-emitting screens (e.g., smartphones or laptops) before sleep; maintaining a regular sleep/wake schedule and avoiding naps; increasing daytime exercise; taking a warm bath or shower before bedtime; engaging in calming activities about 30 minutes before bedtime, such as listening to soothing music or meditation applications; and promoting a cool, dark, quiet, and uncluttered bedroom environment that is not used for activities that cause stress or mental activation, such as paying bills or studying for exams.

Caffeine can promote anxiety symptoms in anyone. People with GAD and other anxiety conditions may be biologically prone to even greater sensitivity to the effects of caffeine. Therefore, anyone who struggles with anxiety and insomnia should consider reducing their intake of caffeinated beverages. Although many individuals with anxiety disorders self-medicate with alcohol, cannabis, or nicotine, the effects of these substances on anxiety and sleep are, in fact, quite complex. For some individuals, they may promote a welcome sense of relaxation in the short-term but produce uncomfortable activation over the ensuing hours or days. Because these substances may worsen sleep and anxiety, clinicians often recommend minimizing their use by individuals with GAD.

A range of medical conditions can contribute to anxiety symptoms. Among the most common of these conditions are hyperthyroidism, diabetes, and hypertension. All individuals with severe, persistent anxiety should be screened for common medical conditions. The optimal treatment of GAD requires a holistic framework that includes good overall health care. Although treatment of previously untreated or poorly controlled conditions may not eliminate GAD symptoms, improved general health will likely enhance the chances of successful treatment.

A wide range of medications and supplements also may cause or worsen anxiety symptoms, including over-the-counter decongestants such as phenylephrine (Sudafed), corticosteroids such as prednisone, inhalers such as albuterol, psychostimulants such as dextroamphetamine, thyroid medications such as levothyroxine (Synthroid), and a range of weight-loss supplements such as bitter orange. Some medications, such as the antihistamine diphenhydramine (Benadryl), cause drowsiness in most people but cause paradoxical anxiety and activation in others. Individuals with GAD should discuss with their clinician whether any of their medications or supplements may be contributing to their anxiety symptoms. If so, it is important to explore whether those agents can be reduced, eliminated, or replaced by medications or supplements less likely to worsen anxiety.

Psychotherapies

Many forms of psychotherapy appear to help reduce symptoms of GAD. However, the majority of studies on psychotherapy for this condition have focused on cognitive-behavioral therapy (CBT), which is, therefore, often considered the psychotherapy of choice for GAD. CBT can be delivered in a range of formats, including group therapy, internet-based therapy, telephone-based therapy, or self-guided readings (bibliotherapy) but is most typically provided in weekly (or biweekly) individual sessions with a qualified mental health professional. An initial evaluation often includes an interview and the completion of self-report questionnaires that identify particular areas of worry (e.g., academic performance, finances, health, safety of loved ones); other potentially related symptoms such as irritability, muscle tension, and insomnia; and other possible conditions such as depression, trauma, or substance use.

Although treatment is tailored to the individual, a usual course of CBT for GAD extends over approximately 12–16 sessions and may involve a written manual as a guide to structure the sessions as well as a workbook to provide education and tools for patients. CBT also often involves homework assignments between sessions. The assignments may include using monitoring logs such as a mood diary and worry record that provide a format for individuals to keep track of their daily moods and episodes of heightened anxiety as well as the contexts in which anxiety emerges and the thoughts and behaviors that accompany them. The therapist may also assign behavioral exercises between sessions with the aim of enhancing the patient's skills to successfully engage in and tolerate anxiety-generating situations.

CBT for GAD generally targets the thoughts and behaviors most commonly associated with the disorder, including

- Overestimating the likelihood that future negative events will occur, "catastrophizing" the imagined consequences of these events, and underestimating one's ability to cope (e.g., "I will fail the exam, drop out of school, and never achieve a meaningful career")
- Perfectionism, intolerance of uncertainty, and fear of making the wrong decision (e.g., "How can I know for sure their classmate's house is safe enough for a sleepover?")
- Repeatedly worrying (*ruminating*) about current problems rather than engaging in problem solving (e.g., continuously worrying about finances rather than meeting with a financial advisor)
- Avoidance and procrastination related to anxiety-generating situations, tasks, thoughts, images, and emotions, thereby unnecessarily constricting one's life activities or exacerbating problems (e.g., not opening emails and thereby missing important deadlines).

This approach draws upon several, well-studied core cognitive and behavioral techniques including

- *Cognitive restructuring:* Identifying and modifying inaccurate appraisals that contribute to anxiety. This may include highlighting a person's bias toward interpreting neutral or ambiguous events as threatening or otherwise negative while exploring ways to test alternative hypotheses regarding these events. It may also include encouraging individuals to consider available evidence when overestimating the probability of dire outcomes and underestimating their ability to cope so they can develop more realistic assessments of risk and more accurate assessments of their own capacity to manage challenging situations.

- *Relaxation training:* Providing patients with skills, including breathing and muscle relaxation exercises, to reduce their overall level of anxiety and help them cope better with anxiety-provoking situations when they arise.
- *Exposure:* Helping people gradually tolerate anxiety-related thoughts and situations while using their cognitive restructuring and relaxation skills to generate alternative hypotheses and more realistic assessments and to reduce the physical symptoms of anxiety, such as muscle tension or heart palpitations. Exposure may include imagery, such as compiling a hierarchy of worries and then imagining worst-case scenarios and a realistic range of alternative outcomes. It may also include explicit assignments that expand the range of real-life activities the person has avoided, such as starting a first draft of a résumé and entering situations that involve increasing levels of uncertainty (but are still safe), such as planning a weekend trip away from home.
- *Other strategies:* May include designating specific, circumscribed "worry time" rather than leaving anxiety to consume most of an individual's day, as well as planning more pleasurable and meaningful activities to occupy the time freed up from continuous worrying.

Although they are often combined together and used in conjunction with exposure, cognitive restructuring and relaxation training have each shown significant benefit for GAD when used alone. Depending on the individual, CBT may emphasize one of these core techniques over another.

The final sessions of CBT for GAD usually focus on *relapse prevention.* This phase typically includes education about the likelihood that worries and anxiety will occasionally resurface as a routine part of the condition (and a consequence of living in today's stressful world!) and should not be considered evidence of failure or catastrophe. This phase of treatment also includes a plan to draw upon cognitive restructuring, relaxation, and exposure skills again when worries and anxiety return.

Other forms of psychotherapy also show promise in the treatment of GAD, but more study is needed. Some of these psychotherapies integrate mindfulness approaches, which emphasize making nonjudgmental observations about moment-to-moment experiences (e.g., "I notice my muscles are clenched") and recognizing that thoughts, including catastrophizing worries (e.g., "my presentation will be awful"), are "just" thoughts, not realities. *Mindfulness-based stress reduction* (MBSR) incorporates a mindfulness approach with meditation skills. *Acceptance and commitment therapy* (ACT) combines skills that foster acceptance while focusing on and taking intentional actions toward valued life goals.

Another approach is *psychodynamic psychotherapy*. Based on psychoanalytic theory, psychodynamic psychotherapies for GAD generally focus on expanding psychological insight and addressing "insecure attachment" style as a potential underpinning of anxiety. While psychodynamic psychotherapies have traditionally involved long-term treatment, often over years, several short-term versions have been developed that resemble CBT, MBSR, and ACT, with a more structured and time-limited format that can be completed in a few months.

In clinical practice, some people connect more naturally with and make better use of some psychotherapy approaches than others. As research on psychotherapies for GAD proceeds, the range of evidence-based psychotherapies for this condition will inevitably continue to expand. At the same time, researchers are trying to learn what factors can predict who will respond best to which therapies.

Neurostimulation

The potential value of approaches other than medications or psychotherapy for GAD, such as brain stimulation, remains largely to be explored. One emerging area relates to repetitive transcranial magnetic stimulation (rTMS), a noninvasive form of brain stimulation approved by the FDA for treatment-refractory MDD and obsessive-compulsive disorder (OCD). Its use for GAD is still considered investigational. rTMS treatment typically involves placement of an electromagnetic coil on the scalp to deliver a series of stimulating pulses that indirectly affect neurons at the surface of the brain. Treatment is usually repeated once a day on weekdays for up to 4–5 weeks. Although it is not yet a recognized treatment for GAD, preliminary studies suggest that rTMS and other forms of neurostimulation may hold promise as an additional therapeutic avenue in the future.

Complementary and Integrative Approaches

People with GAD and other anxiety disorders frequently express an interest in complementary and integrative approaches, and these methods clearly deserve more research. The National Center for Complementary and Integrative Health (NCCIH) is a federal agency that funds research in this area. The NCCIH website (www.nccih.nih.gov/health/anxiety-at-a-glance) is a reliable resource for emerging knowledge in this area.

Several complementary approaches, including therapeutic massage, yoga, and acupuncture, have shown some benefit in individuals with GAD and other anxiety disorders. As with other conditions, such as depression, exercise appears to be helpful for some people with anxiety and obviously yields other potential health benefits as well. Some supplements, including chamomile extract, have shown promise in individuals with GAD. Kava extract also appears to have some antianxiety benefit, but its association with rare but severe liver toxicity has precluded its use.

Conclusion

GAD is a common and treatable condition affecting approximately 6.8 million adults, or 3.1% of the U.S. population. Unfortunately, it is an often chronic condition that causes distress and impairment over years. Fortunately, effective psychotherapy and medication treatments are available, and most people who are treated experience substantial benefit. Current evidence suggests that medications and psychotherapies are equally effective for GAD, so either avenue offers a reasonable starting point.

CBT is the psychotherapy approach with the most evidence to date. It focuses on reevaluating maladaptive ways of thinking and behaving while providing tangible skills to help patients more realistically appraise the situations that cause anxiety and learn ways to relax. Patients are also helped to expand the range of activities they previously avoided due to their anxiety. Serotonergic medications, particularly the SSRIs and SNRIs, are typically the first-line medication treatments for GAD, although benzodiazepines may also play a useful role for some patients because of their rapid onset of action.

Neurostimulation approaches such as rTMS are not yet approved for GAD but have shown promise in some studies. Complementary and integrative treatments such as yoga are often of interest to individuals with anxiety and deserve more study; at present, they are used as initial steps for people with relatively mild anxiety or may be combined with medication or psychotherapy treatment for those with more prominent GAD symptoms.

For individuals whose GAD does not respond to initial medication or psychotherapy, good options are available, including augmenting SSRIs or SNRIs with other classes of medications or switching psychotherapies from a CBT focus to another approach such as psychodynamic psychotherapy. Moreover, although additional studies are needed, based on widespread clinical experience, the combination of psychotherapy and pharmacotherapy appears to be an effective and more comprehensive approach for many individuals with GAD.

Recommended Reading

DeMartini J, Patel G, Fancher TL: Generalized anxiety disorder. Ann Intern Med 170(7):ITC49–ITC64, 2019 30934083

Szuhaney KL, Simon NM: Anxiety disorders: a review. JAMA 328(24):2431–2445, 2022 36573969

25

Treatment of Specific Phobia

Arij Alarachi, B.Sc.
Randi E. McCabe, Ph.D., C.Psych.

Introduction

Specific phobia is one of the most treatable of all the anxiety disorders. Compared with other anxiety disorders, treatment also typically requires less time to drastically reduce or even eliminate all symptoms. Unfortunately, individuals with specific phobia may not receive the professional support they need because they may be embarrassed to discuss their symptoms and ask for help or may not be aware of available treatments or where to access them. This chapter provides an overview of treatments to inform those with specific phobia and their loved ones about available options and encourage them to seek care.

Treatment Options

Non-Medication-Based Treatments

Cognitive-Behavioral Therapy

Cognitive-behavioral therapy (CBT) is the most effective and researched treatment for specific phobia. *Cognitive-behavioral therapy* is a general term for various psychological treatment strategies used to change the unhelpful thoughts and behaviors that contribute to excessive fear and avoidance. CBT may be provided by a therapist or be self-guided (e.g., using a workbook or internet-based program). It is typically offered for five to eight 90-minute sessions, depending on the severity of the phobia and the treatment response. Research shows that some phobias can be effectively "cured" with one prolonged treatment session. CBT strategies most often used for specific phobia include psychoeducation, exposure therapy, cognitive therapy, and, in the case of very severe symptoms, anxiety management (e.g., to reduce distress and support participation in exposure therapy).

Psychoeducation. Psychoeducation involves learning about the nature of specific phobia and how it is treated. This key information enables a person to have a better understanding of the symptoms they are experiencing and the strategies used to reduce their fear and avoidance. It may also help reduce feelings of embarrassment as they learn that they are not alone in their fear.

Exposure therapy. Exposure therapy is the most effective ingredient in treatment for specific phobia and may be used on its own or combined with the other CBT strategies as needed. Exposure involves facing the feared situation in a gradual and manageable way to reduce fear, promote new learning, and increase feelings of self-confidence. Treatment is guided by an *exposure hierarchy*, a list of the situations a person fears that is organized from least fear-inducing to most fear-inducing, typically rated on a scale from 0 (no fear) to 100 (extreme fear). The individual decides where they want to start on the list and then practices being in the feared situation repeatedly (often daily or multiple times a day) until their fear level reduces. Then the person can move up the hierarchy to tackle a more challenging situation. As they move up their exposure hierarchy, their confidence to tackle situations increases and their fear associated with higher items decreases.

Different types of exposure can be used, depending on the phobia and the availability of resources. *In vivo* (or "live") *exposure* involves confronting the feared situation in real life (e.g., seeing a pet mouse in a cage in the case of a mouse phobia). *Imaginal exposure* involves confronting the feared situation through imagination, usually guided by a script. It is used when it is difficult to recreate the feared situation (e.g., imagining oneself vomiting in the case of vomiting phobia) or when the situation may be too costly or infrequent (e.g., imagining flying in an airplane in the case of flying phobia). *Virtual reality exposure* involves immersing the individual in their feared situation using a virtual platform. Due to its costliness, virtual reality equipment is not commonly available outside of research clinics. *Interoceptive exposure* involves the practice of experiencing feared physical sensations, which is often a feature of those with situational phobias, such as fear of enclosed places. For example, interoceptive exposure for someone with claustrophobia may involve spinning in a chair to evoke the dizzy feeling they may get when in small, enclosed spaces. Studies show that although all exposure types are associated with fear reduction, in vivo exposure is the most effective.

Exposure hierarchies also integrate safety behaviors, which are avoidance or coping strategies that are used to reduce anxiety but ultimately maintain unhelpful beliefs about the fear. For example, a person with a specific phobia of driving may avoid being a passenger so they can maintain control when driving, take long driving routes to get to their destination to avoid driving on the highway, or only drive at times when the roads are not busy. To incorporate these safety behaviors in exposures, a hierarchy may include being a passenger while someone else is driving on a slow, empty street (fear rating 25), watching a point-of-view highway driving video (40), driving on a busy street (55), being a passenger while someone else drives on a busy street (70), driving on the highway (80), and being a passenger while someone else is driving on the highway (90).

Depending on the specific phobia type, exposure therapy may be combined with other treatment strategies to maximize effectiveness. For example, individuals with a specific phobia of blood, injury, or injections tend to have a fainting response when exposed to their feared situation. In this case, exposure therapy is combined with a technique called *applied tension* in which individuals repeatedly tense their muscles during exposure to temporarily increase blood pressure and prevent the fainting response.

Cognitive therapy. Cognitive therapy involves recognizing and challenging unhelpful, anxiety-provoking thought patterns that amplify fear and emotional distress. It can be conducted while doing exposure therapy or prior to exposure to increase receptiveness to the therapy if the patient is very apprehensive. In cognitive therapy, individuals develop awareness of their anxious thought patterns and learn to consider other, less fear-provoking perspectives of the feared situation. Cognitive therapy promotes helpful self-talk that allows the individual to approach and stay in a phobic situation as well as reduce their safety behaviors. For example, a patient with a snake phobia who is approaching a live snake during an exposure may tell themselves, "The snake is only testing the environment when its tongue is out, it is not a sign it wants to eat me; in fact, it is more afraid of me than I am of it."

Anxiety management. Anxiety management involves using breathing and relaxation techniques to relieve high levels of distress. This is typically only used if individuals are so fearful that they cannot engage with the other treatment techniques.

Family/Partner Involvement

Family and partners can actively support their loved one through treatment by providing encouragement and acting as a helper for some exposures. For example, being a passenger for a loved one with driving phobia supports recovery efforts so the loved one can practice driving in more anxiety-provoking situations that may be harder to tackle on their own. In addition, family and partners may engage in behaviors to alleviate their loved one's anxiety, such as providing reassurance or reinforcing avoidance behaviors that may contribute to maintaining the phobia. Family and partners can increase awareness of these behaviors and reduce them to help support treatment progress.

Medication-Based Treatments

Psychiatric medications are not typically used in the treatment of specific phobia because research does not support their effectiveness as a first-line intervention. However, medications may be prescribed to those who seldom encounter their phobic situation or object (e.g., an infrequent flyer with a flight phobia), do not have access to CBT with exposure, or refuse or have unsuccessfully engaged in exposures. A class of medications called *benzodiazepines* may be used when the feared situation is seldom encountered and necessary or unavoidable. Benzodiazepines are taken prior to entering the phobic situation and provide a short-term reduction in anxiety. For example, a person with a specific phobia of medical procedures who refuses to undergo a necessary dental treatment may benefit from taking a benzodiazepine (e.g., lorazepam) so they can undergo the procedure. Benzodiazepines can be highly addictive, may interact with alcohol or drugs, and have a sedating effect, so they should not be used if the person has a risk of substance use disorder or will be operating a vehicle or machinery. Another class of medications that may be prescribed is selective serotonin reuptake inhibitors (SSRIs; e.g., sertraline). SSRIs may be helpful for individuals who experience panic-like symptoms in relation to their phobia, which is commonly reported among those with situational phobias (e.g., claustrophobia) and those who repeatedly encounter the phobic situation over a prolonged period. Ideally, if a medication is used, it should be in conjunction with exposure therapy to maximize benefit.

Additional Information

Fears may return if a person does not regularly encounter the feared situation, so individuals should keep an eye out for increased anxiety or avoidance of the feared situation that might trigger a relapse. They may want to find ways of exposing themselves to the feared object or situation in their everyday life, even after treatment is completed, to maintain the gains they achieved. For example, individuals with a phobia of flying might regularly travel to prevent the symptoms from returning or someone with a snake phobia might keep a picture of a snake on their refrigerator.

Conclusion

Specific phobia causes significant distress and leads individuals to go to great lengths to avoid their feared situation. Treatment is both highly effective and accessible. If interested in seeking treatment, you can start with self-guided treatment by working through a workbook (see "Recommended Reading"). If you need more support, look for a therapist who has specialized training in CBT for specific phobias. Ask your family physician or visit www.adaa.org/find-help to find a therapist near you.

Recommended Reading

Antony MM, Craske MG, Barlow DH: Mastering Your Fears and Phobias: Workbook, 2nd Edition. New York, Oxford University Press, 2006

Bourne EJ: The Anxiety and Phobia Workbook, 7th Edition. Oakland, CA, New Harbinger, 2020

26

Treatment of Eating Disorders

B. Timothy Walsh, M.D.
Deborah R. Glasofer, Ph.D.

Introduction

Eating disorders are defined by problems people have with their eating behaviors that can lead to emotional distress and potentially serious medical complications. The four major eating disorders are:

- **Anorexia nervosa (AN).** This disorder, which primarily (but not exclusively) affects young females, is characterized by severe voluntary restriction of food intake, leading to substantial weight loss.
- **Bulimia nervosa (BN).** In this disorder, which also primarily (but not exclusively) affects young females, individuals frequently eat large amounts of food ("binges") and then get rid of the calories consumed via some inappropriate method, such as inducing vomiting.
- **Binge-eating disorder (BED).** Individuals with this disorder frequently eat large amounts of food while experiencing a distressing loss of control over their eating, but do not attempt to get rid of the food afterward.

- **Avoidant/restrictive food intake disorder (ARFID).** People with ARFID avoid some or many foods because of the nature of the food or eating experience. Unlike those with AN, individuals with this eating disorder are not overly concerned with their body weight or shape.

The goal of treatment for any eating disorder is for affected individuals to learn to eat in a healthy manner. Both psychological treatments and medications can be helpful, but the most helpful interventions vary by disorder.

Anorexia Nervosa

Treatment Options

Medication-Based Treatments

Olanzapine (Zyprexa) is used to treat several serious psychiatric disorders, including schizophrenia. Olanzapine stimulates the appetite, and people taking it often gain substantial weight. Several studies have found that olanzapine can help people with AN gain some weight, but the effects are not dramatic. Therefore, it should be used only in conjunction with psychological treatment.

Non-Medication-Based Treatments

Weight Restoration. Treatment for AN emphasizes weight restoration (or for youth, a return to the expected growth milestones) and normalization of eating behaviors. The physician will evaluate the severity of the problem and the patient's prior treatment history and, based on treatment availability, make recommendations regarding treatment type and setting. Target weight-goal ranges (and the reason for these recommendations) are typically a part of the treatment plan, along with clear expectations about the rate of weight gain and plans for weight monitoring. Once the patient has achieved the recommended weight, the physician will reassess their physical and psychological symptoms and reevaluate goals to include maintaining a stable weight range.

Because AN is a complex disorder, a team approach involving medical and psychological providers can be quite useful in helping people meet treatment goals. Nutritional counseling—although not "required" for renourishment to occur—is often quite helpful as individuals work to tolerate the challenges of weight restoration while fearing unending weight gain. The dietitian's role and responsibilities vary depending on the treatment setting. Sometimes, nutritional counseling extends to experiential exercises, including practice with grocery shopping, food preparation/cooking, or dining out. Nutritional counseling is also commonly used alongside psychotherapy to support weight maintenance and normal eating patterns in patients stepping down from intensive inpatient treatment to an outpatient setting. It can be an especially useful addition to talk therapy when patients have a diet-related medical condition, such as Type 1 diabetes, celiac disease, or food allergies, or have co-occurring psychiatric disorders that may need to be prioritized in the psychological treatment.

Nonspecific, Supportive Psychological Treatments. Psychological treatment of adults with AN can be challenging and complicated. Ambivalence about recovery and denial about the seriousness of the problem are symptoms of the illness. Unlike other eating disorders, AN lacks clear, data-driven support for any specific psychological treatment approach.

Both cognitive-behavioral therapy (CBT) and nonspecific, supportive outpatient interventions are helpful for those with AN as they normalize eating and reach an optimal weight range. If patients are unable to make progress in outpatient therapy, structured treatment settings such as residential or inpatient programs—which can provide more mealtime support and supervision—have a good track record of helping people recover from the starved state.

Following weight restoration, psychotherapy tends to focus on preventing relapse (including weight loss). This may include continuing to challenge restrictive or rigid food choices, addressing poor body image, and enhancing non-appearance-related aspects of identity.

Family-Based Therapy. Family based therapy (FBT) is a psychotherapy that has been well studied in adolescents with AN. The theory underlying FBT is that normal adolescent development has been interrupted by the eating disorder, and therefore parent involvement is as essential in treatment as it would be for any kind of serious illness. The therapist helps parents, siblings, and caretakers identify and change patterns that are contributing to or arising from the disorder, open the lines of communication, and provide skills for dealing with the illness. The first phase of FBT emphasizes renourishment. Parents take control of areas of the patient's life that may be impacted by the eating disorder, specifically eating and exercise, and prepare and supervise all meals. In the second phase, parents gradually hand control back to the adolescent. The third phase emphasizes returning to a balanced life, which, for a family with an adolescent, includes the typical developmental struggles that may have been ignored due to the eating disorder.

In a handful of scientific studies of FBT, the results have been encouraging. FBT appears best suited to patients younger than 18 who live at home with their families and whose families are able and willing to set aside other issues in the service of treating AN. Firm and consistent parental involvement is likely the essential feature of treatment. In those for whom this approach is a good fit, the benefits appear to hold up in the long term. In one FBT study, for example, most adolescents no longer met criteria for AN 3 years after treatment. As a result of such promising findings, FBT has been applied in other eating disorders as well.

Atypical Anorexia Nervosa

Atypical anorexia nervosa is a term used to describe individuals who have lost significant amounts of weight and developed the core psychological symptoms of AN but whose weight remains statistically within or above the normal range. Research on atypical AN has only recently begun, but it is clear that individuals with this problem can have significant medical and psychological problems. Current treatment approaches follow similar principles to those that guide the treatment of "typical" AN.

Bulimia Nervosa

Treatment Options

Medication-Based Treatments

It is well established that the medications used to treat depression—antidepressants—also help individuals with BN reduce or eliminate their binge eating and purging. Surprisingly, antidepressants are useful even for those who are not depressed. The class of antidepressants most frequently used is the selective serotonin reuptake inhibitors (SSRIs). The first SSRI introduced in the United States was fluoxetine (Prozac), and the U.S. Food and Drug Administration (FDA) has officially approved its use in the treatment of BN. However, very good evidence indicates that other SSRIs are also helpful.

Non-Medication-Based Treatments

Cognitive-Behavioral Therapy. The model underlying CBT—a well-studied psychotherapy for many different psychiatric problems—for treatment of eating disorders emphasizes the role of biased beliefs and problematic behaviors in maintaining the problem. In BN, overvaluing one's appearance is considered a primary reason why individuals establish strict dietary rules. Dietary restriction makes people more likely to binge eat and to then use behaviors, such as self-induced vomiting, to "counteract" the effects of eating. Instead, these behaviors perpetuate the cycle, disrupting normal fullness and hunger signals and reinforcing guilt about eating and concern with appearance.

A present-focused approach, CBT targets the cycle rather than the origin of symptoms. Treatment includes education about the risks of rule-bound eating and of purging behaviors, prescribes a regular eating pattern and gradual reintroduction of "difficult" foods, teaches strategies for coping with high-risk situations, and helps patients evaluate the thoughts perpetuating the disorder. It is designed to be a short-term, skills-based psychotherapy.

CBT is a first-line treatment for BN and can be delivered one-on-one or in a group. It has been found to help people completely stop or significantly reduce binge eating and purging over the course of approximately 6 months (typically about 20 sessions). Studies suggest that CBT is a superior stand-alone treatment to medication, but combining CBT with antidepressants can also be useful. People receiving CBT seem to experience improvements not only in eating disorder symptoms but also in their mood, relationships, and self-esteem.

Family-Based Therapy. Given the helpfulness of FBT for adolescents with AN, the treatment has been adapted for youth with BN. The primary distinction is that in FBT for BN, a more collaborative approach is taken between the adolescent and their caregivers to work toward recovery; this is thought to be possible because youth with BN are likely to be distressed by their binge eating and purging.

Binge-Eating Disorder

Treatment Options

Medication-Based Treatments

A number of medications are helpful in the treatment of BED. As with BN, antidepressants, especially SSRIs, help patients with BED reduce their binge eating. Surprisingly, however, people do not automatically lose weight.The only medications that help people both stop binge eating and lose weight are those known to be associated with weight loss. The best example of these is lisdexamfetamine (Vyvanse), which is a stimulant used to treat attention-deficit/hyperactivity disorder (ADHD). Lisdexamfetamine is the only medication approved by the FDA for the treatment of BED. Recently, a new class of medicines has been introduced that stimulate the release of hormones normally released after eating a meal, and these have been found to lead to impressive amounts of weight loss among individuals who are overweight or obese. Whether these medicines (e.g., tirzepatide [Mounjaro]) would help with binge eating has not been studied, but it would not be surprising.

Non-Medication-Based Treatments

Cognitive-behavioral therapy. As with BN, CBT is a first-line treatment for BED and is delivered similarly to the description given earlier for treatment of BN. However, in BED, the emphasis is on binge-eating episodes and their precipitants rather than on purging, which is absent in BED. Studies have shown that CBT is helpful for people trying to abstain from or significantly reduce binge eating behaviors and can improve mood, anxiety, relationships, and how these individuals feel about themselves overall.

CBT targeting BED is *not* meant to be a weight-loss treatment. Results from several trials underscore that no more than modest weight loss should be expected from the treatment.

Interpersonal psychotherapy. Interpersonal psychotherapy (IPT), developed as a short-term treatment for adults with depression, has been adapted for individuals with eating disorders and as a preventive intervention for youth at risk for loss-of-control eating. IPT is recognized as a helpful approach for adults with BED. In contrast to CBT, IPT does not directly focus on eating behaviors or on body shape and weight concerns. Disturbances in eating behavior, including binge eating, are thought to happen in response to relationship stressors and low mood. The emphasis in IPT is therefore on identifying and addressing the interpersonal problems that maintain or worsen symptoms.

IPT can be delivered on an individual or group basis. A group setting provides a means to reduce social isolation, develop new relationships, and practice communication skills. It can also be a unique refuge for patients who may have previously hidden their symptoms from others out of guilt or shame.

Avoidant/Restrictive Food Intake Disorder

Treatment Options

Medication-Based Treatments

No medications have been identified that are clearly helpful for ARFID.

Non-Medication-Based Treatments

Research on ARFID, including how best to treat it, has only just begun. What we know so far is that, among young people, it is important to involve parents and to focus directly on the eating behavior. CBT has been adapted to specifically address issues that frequently arise in this clinical population, including the use of exposure and response prevention (ERP) principles. Elements of ERP, a first-line treatment for obsessive-compulsive disorder (OCD), are built into CBT for social anxiety disorder, specific phobia, and posttraumatic stress disorder (PTSD). In ERP, patients work during and between sessions to confront feared their stimuli without using "safety" behaviors. In CBT for ARFID, a patient with a fear of choking on food may be asked to put a lot of dry crackers in their mouth and let them sit there. If food avoidance is related to texture, the therapist may coach the patient to "taste-test" a number of foods with the aversive texture in order to gain experience with it. The aim is to provide people with a chance to learn through experience that what they fear is unlikely to happen and that even if it does, they will be able to manage it. A pilot study of CBT for ARFID suggested that this approach can help underweight youth gain weight and can help all patients make clinically meaningful progress (e.g., improving the repertoire of food eaten, reducing the social impact of food avoidance).

Additional Information

Third-Wave Psychotherapies

Third-wave psychotherapies refers to treatments developed in recent years that have evolved from CBT and include a greater focus on mindfulness, emotions, acceptance, values, and meta-cognition. These approaches include dialectical behavior therapy (DBT), acceptance and commitment therapy (ACT), compassion-focused therapy, mindfulness-based interventions, and others. Many clinicians have found these therapies helpful in the treatment of eating disorders, but because neither DBT nor ACT has been proven to be better than CBT, it remains the front-running psychological treatment.

Conclusion

Eating disorders are serious problems defined by the presence of abnormalities in eating behavior and are associated with significant psychological distress and potentially serious medical problems. They can be successfully treated with psychological interventions and/or with medication, but the treatments vary with the disorder.

Recommended Reading

Lock J, Le Grange D: Help Your Teenager Beat an Eating Disorder, 2nd Edition. New York, Guilford, 2015

Walsh BT, Attia E, Glasofer DR: Eating Disorders: What Everyone Needs to Know. New York, Oxford University Press, 2020

27

Treatment of Body Dysmorphic Disorder

Jasmine Kim, M.D.
Katherine Chemakin, B.S.
Eric Hollander, M.D.

Case Vignette

Debra is a 40-year-old female with body dysmorphic disorder (BDD). She has had feelings of bodily defect regarding her body shape since age 8. Her primary concerns are the size of her thighs and abdomen in relation to those of her peers. She checks her image in mirrors repetitively, and her concerns have persisted throughout adulthood. She has stopped attending events because she feels judged by others, which has led to social and professional impairment. Her mood symptoms have worsened, including feelings of tiredness, hopelessness, self-loathing, anhedonia, increased appetite, and diminished libido. She has begun to think about ending her life via overdose on prescription medication.

Because her symptoms are so severe, Debra is admitted to the hospital, where she is first treated with a selective serotonin reuptake inhibitor (SSRI). She attends group therapy, receives exposure and responsive prevention (ERP) therapy, and cognitive-behavioral therapy (CBT) intervention and is given psychoeducation about distress tolerance skills and behavioral activation. She uses painting as her coping method when experiencing stress. She is also introduced to the rubber band technique to help break habitual behaviors and stop her negative thoughts. In this technique, the person places a rubber band on their wrist and then lightly snaps it whenever they start to feel anxious or develop negative thoughts. The idea is that the brain will subconsciously start avoiding the stimulus (in this case, being anxious or having negative thoughts) in order to prevent the unpleasant snapping of the rubber band. Debra is discharged home following 1 week of inpatient treatment, and she is then seen at an outpatient clinic for follow-up care. She continues taking her SSRI and other medications added later to help with other symptoms, including prazosin (an α_1-antagonist that helps with nightmares associated with posttraumatic stress disorder [PTSD]) and trazodone (a serotonin antagonist/reuptake inhibitor that helps with depression and sleep). She also continues attending psychotherapy.

Introduction

As discussed in Chapter 13 ("Body Dysmorphic Disorder"), BDD is a chronic and disabling psychiatric disorder characterized by a preoccupation with one or more perceived defects or flaws in one's physical appearance that are not observable or appear slight to others. Patients believe that they look or have a feature that is abnormal, deformed, or unattractive, when objectively they look normal. These perceived flaws lead to hyperfixation and repetitive behaviors (i.e., checking self in mirror) or even to having repetitive cosmetic procedures in order to fix the perceived defect. These behaviors are usually difficult for patients to resist and are not pleasurable. BDD is classified as one of the obsessive-compulsive and related disorders (OCRD) in the *Diagnostic and Statistical Manual of Mental Disorders,* 5th Edition (DSM-5).

BDD is quite common, occurring in 2%–3% of the general population and up to 7% of psychiatric patients, with an even higher rate of occurrence among certain subgroups with comorbid anxiety disorders, obsessive-compulsive disorder (OCD), depressive disorders, and eating disorders. BDD is frequently underrecognized and can lead to significant distress and functional impairment, with an increased risk of suicidal ideation and behaviors. Patients often seek nonpsychiatric, cosmetic treatments (most commonly dermatological or surgical) for their perceived physical defects. These approaches are ineffective for most people with BDD and can be risky for both the patient and their clinician if the patient is unhappy with the outcome. In contrast, pharmacotherapy and CBT have been found to be efficacious treatments for individuals with BDD, and patients usually receive a combination of both approaches. Although currently no treatments for BDD have received U.S. Food and Drug Administration (FDA) approval, a number of studies have demonstrated that the psychiatric medications commonly utilized to treat OCD can provide great relief and significant BDD symptom improvement.

Treatment Options

Medication-Based Treatments

The first-line pharmacological treatment of BDD is centered around the use of SSRIs. These agents are commonly used for other mental illnesses, such as OCD, depression, anxiety, and PTSD, to name a few. They are known to be efficacious, tolerable, and generally safe. Some examples of SSRIs are escitalopram (e.g., Lexapro), fluoxetine (e.g., Prozac), paroxetine (e.g., Paxil), and sertraline (e.g., Zoloft). In a placebo-controlled study of fluoxetine in patients with BDD, it was shown to be safe and more effective than placebo. In a study of escitalopram, patients' depressive symptoms, delusionality, functioning, and quality of life significantly improved, suggesting that it is also safe and efficacious for individuals with BDD. Most BDD patients improved with a serotonin reuptake inhibitor (SRI), and all SRIs appear to be well tolerated in this population. This study also showed that when SRIs are discontinued, patients are likely to relapse, and that continuation-phase escitalopram delays time to relapse. Patients may start with a lower dosage of one of these medications and slowly titrate up to a higher dosage every few weeks depending on symptom improvement and tolerability.

In patients whose BDD does not respond to SSRI treatment, clomipramine, a tricyclic antidepressant (TCA) with potent serotonergic effects, is an effective second-line treatment option. Clomipramine is reserved for cases in which the SSRIs have not proven to be of benefit, because the side effect profile of SSRIs tends to be milder than that of TCAs. A crossover study showed that clomipramine was effective in the acute treatment of BDD symptoms, as measured by assessment of patients' obsessive preoccupation with perceived body defects, repetitive behaviors in response to this preoccupation, and global ratings of symptom severity. Clomipramine helps to decrease obsessional preoccupation, compulsive behaviors, distress, anger, hostility, and somatic symptoms and to improve mental health–related quality of life and functional impairment. SSRIs and clomipramine also work well to address other psychiatric comorbidities that are common in patients with BDD, such as depression, anxiety, and suicidal ideation. First-line, second-line, and third-line medication, psychosocial, and neurostimulation treatments for BDD are depicted in Figure 27–1.

Other types of medications, such as atypical antipsychotics and serotonin-norepinephrine reuptake inhibitors (SNRIs), are available when the previous medications are not effective. Case studies have found that atypical antipsychotics are effective as an augmentation strategy in treatment-resistant BDD. These third-line treatments overall have a lower level of confidence. More studies are

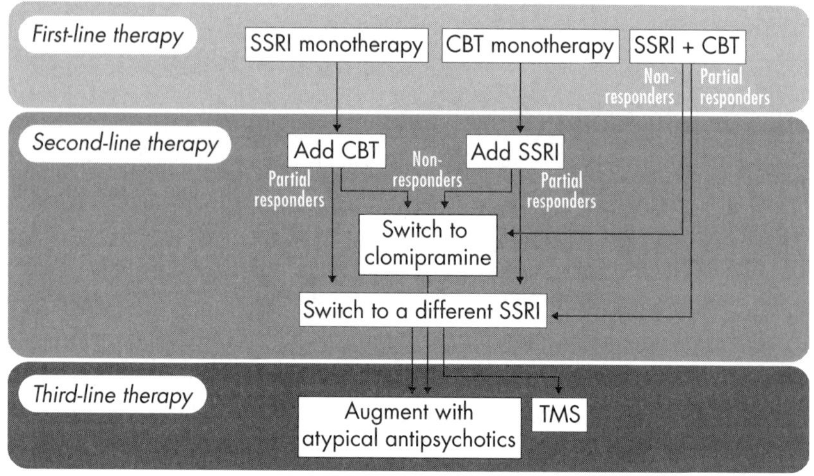

Figure 27–1. Stepwise pharmacotherapeutic and CBT approach to body dysmorphic disorder.

Note. CBT=cognitive-behavioral therapy; SSRI=selective serotonin reuptake inhibitor; TMS=transcranial magnetic stimulation.

warranted to evaluate the effectiveness of atypical antipsychotics for BDD. A trial of the SNRI venlafaxine revealed that it may be effective in lessening the specific symptoms and global severity of BDD (i.e., obsessions and compulsions scores). Repetitive transcranial magnetic stimulation (rTMS) is a neurostimulation technique that is FDA-approved for treatment of major depression and OCD and may be effective in OCRD such as BDD. A recent study showed that patients with BDD who received a newer form of rTMS—intermittent theta-burst stimulation (iTBS)—showed improvement in their evaluative/affective experiences of their physical appearance.

Non-Medication-Based Treatments

Cognitive-Behavioral Therapy

CBT involves exploring, analyzing, and changing the ways individuals think. This type of therapy is widely used for various mental illnesses, including OCD, depression, anxiety disorders, alcohol and drug use problems, and eating disorders. The cognitive-behavioral model of BDD (Figure 27–2) explores the experience of excessive self-focused attention on an image or felt impression of the self. This consequently creates assumptions about the importance of one's ap-

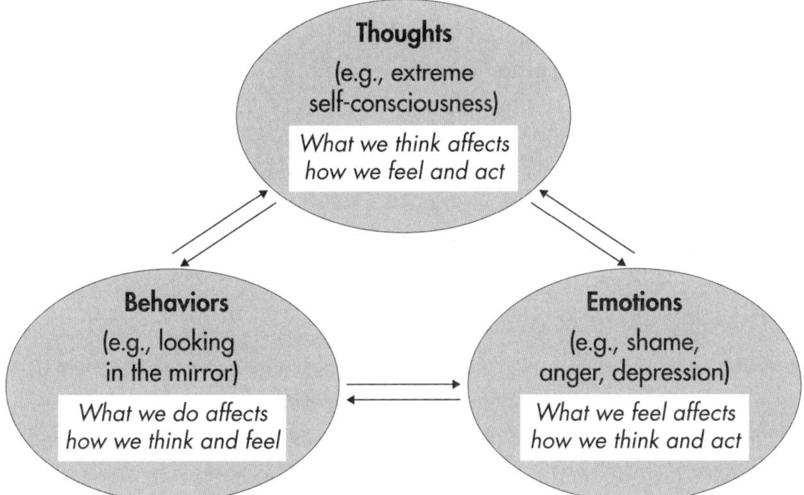

Figure 27–2. Cognitive-behavioral therapy model in body dysmorphic disorder.

pearance in defining the self and the various ways of responding (e.g., avoidance and safety-seeking behaviors, ruminating, and comparing). Several exercises can be done with the therapist in which the patient goes through their thought processes and reflects upon them. Therapists may ask questions such as

- "Describe a recent typical situation in which you were attacking yourself. Did it start with an intrusive thought, image, memory, or someone that you compared yourself to? What were you doing at the time?"
- "What did you tell yourself? Did you then become withdrawn?"
- "Is there a pattern to the situations that are typically linked to self-attacking that you could change? For example, can you do anything to prevent such situations from occurring? Do you need to buy that celebrity magazine? Can you put old photographs back in an album?"

Once a patient identifies the costs and benefits of their self-defeating thoughts, they can go through these ideas with the therapist to find ways to be compassionate toward themselves.

CBT will also help patients set valued goals, conduct exposure and ritual prevention, modify self-defeating assumptions about the importance of appearance, and enhance self-acceptance, self-esteem, and self-compassion. CBT for BDD has been proven effective through multiple clinical studies. In one recent clinical trial, adults with BDD received weekly treatments for 24 weeks, followed by 3- and 6-month follow-up assessments. This study showed that BDD severity and associated symptoms appeared to improve with both CBT for BDD and supportive psychotherapy, although CBT was associated with more consistent improvement in symptom severity and quality of life.

In clinical trials, CBT for BDD typically involves 12–22 weekly sessions, with a key therapeutic strategy being exposure and response prevention (ERP). ERP involves the patient gradually confronting a feared situation (e.g., bright lights, mirrors, social situations) and resisting the urge to perform safety-seeking behaviors (e.g., camouflaging, applying excessive makeup, focusing attention internally) to neutralize their distress, with the goal of achieving anxiety habituation.

Supportive Psychotherapy

Supportive psychotherapy focuses on maintaining, improving, and restoring self-esteem and adaptive coping skills, as well as on reflecting and expressing emotions about current life issues. The intent of this nondirective treatment is to help patients learn to cope with external and psychological challenges, emphasizing therapeutic relationships and self-esteem as vehicles for improvement. A supportive psychotherapy manual was enhanced with BDD-specific psychoeducation and treatment rationale to improve treatment engagement, quality, and credibility.

Conclusion

In this chapter, we began with a case vignette that illustrates the clinical presentation and course of treatment of a woman with BDD. We described BDD, highlighted *Diagnostic and Statistical Manual of Mental Disorders* (DSM-5) criteria, and discussed its epidemiology. We then reviewed current available treatments, including both pharmacological and nonpharmacological modalities, that can be used on their own or in combination, at the discretion of the medical provider, and in accordance with the patients' preference.

BDD can be severely debilitating and is often accompanied by depression and suicidal thoughts. When patients experience distress and functional impairment, we recommend that they obtain mental health treatment from a professional with expertise in treating BDD. Patients can greatly benefit from optimal treatment.

Recommended Reading

Hollander E, Allen A, Kwon J, et al: Clomipramine vs desipramine crossover trial in body dysmorphic disorder: selective efficacy of a serotonin reuptake inhibitor in imagined ugliness. Arch Gen Psychiatry 56(11):1033–1039, 1999 10565503

Wilhelm S, Phillips KA, Greenberg JL, et al: Efficacy and posttreatment effects of therapist-delivered cognitive behavioral therapy vs supportive psychotherapy for adults with body dysmorphic disorder: a randomized clinical trial. JAMA Psychiatry 76(4):363–373, 2019 30785624 (Published correction appears in JAMA Psychiatry 76[4]:447, 2019)

28

Treatment of Prolonged Grief Disorder

Donald J. Robinaugh, Ph.D.
Naomi M. Simon, M.D.

Introduction

Grief is the psychological response to the loss of a loved one: a collection of emotions, perceptions, cognitions, and behaviors that commonly arise together following bereavement. For many, grief subsides over the initial weeks and months following the loss. For others, it remains intense, distressing, and impairing for years afterward. Distressing and impairing grief that persists for at least 1 year may represent *prolonged grief disorder* (PGD), a condition recently included in the text revision of the American Psychiatric Association's *Diagnostic and Statistical Manual of Mental Disorders,* 5th Edition (DSM-5-TR; see Chapter 14 for more detail on PGD). This chapter is for people who are struggling with grief or prolonged grief and is intended to introduce the types of supports and evidence-based treatment options available and to identify some indications that care may be helpful.

Treatment Options

Medication-Based Treatments

As described elsewhere in this book, evidence-supported medications for depression and anxiety disorders are available, but no psychiatric medication is yet U.S. Food and Drug Administration (FDA)-approved for treatment of PGD. In health care settings, medications such as selective serotonin reuptake inhibitors (SSRIs)—a widely used class of antidepressants—may be offered as a potential treatment, and clinicians may prescribe medication to target specific symptoms that persist or that do not respond to psychotherapy (e.g., depression, anxiety, insomnia). A large, randomized controlled trial showed that patients receiving the SSRI citalopram exhibited reductions in grief severity over time, but no more so than those who received a placebo pill. There was, however, some evidence that citalopram was better than placebo in reducing co-occurring depression symptoms. Notably, in this study, citalopram was significantly less effective than psychotherapy for treating prolonged grief, suggesting that, where available, evidence-based psychotherapies specifically targeting prolonged grief are the preferred treatment.

Non-Medication-Based Treatments

Acute Grief: Support and Treatment

Family members and loved ones are deeply interwoven into our social worlds, daily routines, and sense of selves. It is thus not surprising that the death of a loved one is among life's greatest stressors and will typically require a period of adaptation to adjust to life after the loss. The experience of acute grief varies among individuals and across different losses in one's life. Nonetheless, it often includes a common set of experiences, including a sense of disbelief, intense yearning for the deceased, waves of emotional pain, dysregulation of deeply embedded routines, and a perceived loss of purpose or meaning in life. This period often includes positive emotions as well—opportunities to reflect on the lives our loved one led and to connect with and be supported by others. Indeed, bereavement often initiates a natural process of adaptation, oscillating between confronting the painful reality of the loss and restoring a sense of meaning and purpose in life after the loss.

During their acute grief, some people find comfort and strength in support groups, religious groups, or community organizations whose mission is to support the bereaved. Others either do not feel the need to join such activities or do not find the format of such groups helpful. The choice of whether to join grief support groups should be guided by the desires and goals of the bereaved individual. Grief support groups may be especially helpful for gaining a greater understanding of grief, recognizing that the bereaved person is not alone in their experiences, confronting the reality of the loss in a supportive environment, and finding opportunity for social connection and sense of purpose among a community of other bereaved people.

Although grief is a near-universal experience that most manage without professional intervention, there are times such intervention is helpful or even needed. No simple guide exists for determining when treatment with a mental health professional is appropriate, but there are several factors to consider. The most important is safety. Bereaved adults often question whether life is worth living without their loved one or have thoughts about wishing to die so that they may be reunited with their loved one. If these thoughts include the consideration of taking one's own life, consultation with a health professional is warranted; help is also available through the National Suicide Prevention Lifeline (9-8-8), or the local emergency department. Similarly, if acute grief is resulting in severe and persistent difficulty with routine functioning and self-care, health professionals, including primary care doctors, can play the critical role of helping connect bereaved people with appropriate resources and support. Severe or persisting depressed mood, global loss of interest and pleasure, high levels of persistent anxiety, or worsening of preexisting mental health problems may also indicate intervention would be helpful.

A final consideration is change over time. It is not uncommon that grief may be very distressing during the initial weeks or months following the loss and then subside considerably in intensity over the next year. For some, drawing on internal resources and informal supports during these initial months, ideally in communication with existing professional caregivers, may be sufficient to navigate even this intense period of acute grief. However, if grief is persistently severe and impairs day-to-day functioning, additional support may be helpful.

Prolonged Grief: Support and Treatment

For individuals experiencing prolonged grief, evidence-supported treatments are available to help. The strongest evidence is for short-term psychotherapies that are rooted in well-established cognitive-behavioral principles and aimed specifically at helping people process their loss and adapt to life without the deceased. These treatments may include cognitive components that focus on how people think about themselves and about the loss; behavioral components that focus on activities that support processing the loss and engaging in an enjoyable life; and meaning-based components that focus on building or restoring a sense of meaning or purpose in one's life following the loss. These treatments have been tested in multiple randomized clinical trials by multiple research groups and have consistently reduced prolonged grief severity to a greater extent than comparison conditions (e.g., supportive counseling).

Prolonged Grief Disorder Therapy

Among this family of cognitive-behavioral psychotherapies for grief, the most widely studied is called *prolonged grief disorder treatment* (PGDT; previously called *complicated grief treatment*). In three randomized clinical trials, PGDT resulted in better outcomes than the psychotherapeutic (i.e., interpersonal psychotherapy) and medication (i.e., the antidepressant citalopram) interventions with which it was compared. Furthermore, most participants (~70%) showed sufficient reduction in grief severity with PGDT to be considered treatment responders.

PGDT is grounded in the theory that adaptation to loss requires an oscillation between confronting the painful reality of the loss and restoring a sense of meaning or purpose in life; a framework known as the *dual-process model*. Importantly, the aim of PGDT is not the eradication of grief; rather, the aim is to encourage the natural process of adaptation and, in doing so, change the role that grief plays in one's life. This includes reducing the severity of grief-related distress and impairment and helping people move toward a place in which they are able to honor their loved one while regaining meaning and purpose in life after the loss.

PGDT includes three broad sets of activities. The first focuses on understanding grief. Therapists work with patients to come to a shared understanding of their experience and the things that are keeping them stuck in their intense grief. Patients also complete daily diaries, recording the ebbs and flows of their grief and the situations and times in which grief tends to be most severe, providing them insight into their own experience. The second set of activities focuses on confronting the reality of the loss in a compassionate and supportive environment. These activities include retelling the story of the loss ("imaginal revisiting") and approaching reminders of the loss in day-to-day life ("situational revisiting"). Together, these activities help patients move toward acceptance of the loss and strengthen their confidence in their ability to navigate the distressing emotions of grief. The third set of activities focuses on restoration, connection to others, and reestablishing a sense of meaning or purpose in one's life. Patients work with therapists to identify "aspirational goals," find support from a friend or significant other, and share memories of the deceased, with the aim of honoring and finding strength in their memory.

Conclusion

There is robust evidence that a family of psychotherapies rooted in the principles of cognitive-behavioral therapy can provide considerable support to those struggling with prolonged grief. These therapies help people change the role that grief plays in their lives, providing a foundation for moving forward with a life of meaning and purpose.

Recommended Reading

The Center for Prolonged Grief: Prolonged Grief: What It Is. New York, Columbia University, 2023. Available at: https://prolongedgrief.columbia.edu/what-it-is.

Shear MK, Reynolds CF 3rd, Simon NM, et al: Optimizing treatment of complicated grief: a randomized clinical trial. JAMA Psychiatry 73(7):685–694, 2016 27276373

Part III

The Treatments

Pharmacological

29

Selective Serotonin Reuptake Inhibitors

Amit Chopra, M.D.
Jerrold Rosenbaum, M.D.

Introduction

Selective serotonin reuptake inhibitors (SSRIs) are the most widely prescribed first-line antidepressant medications for depression and anxiety disorders due to their overall efficacy, safety, and tolerability. SSRIs act by blocking the reabsorption (*reuptake*) of serotonin into neurons, which enhances the availability of serotonin to improve the transmission of signals between neurons. SSRIs currently have FDA-labeled indications for several psychiatric conditions, including major depressive disorder, generalized anxiety disorder, panic disorder, social anxiety disorder, obsessive-compulsive disorder (OCD), premenstrual dysphoric disorder, posttraumatic stress disorder (PTSD), and bulimia nervosa. SSRIs are typically taken once daily to improve the targeted mood and anxiety symptoms. SSRI treatment typically takes 4–6 weeks to achieve expected benefits. These agents can be safely used in special populations, including children, adolescents, and elderly patients. Their use in pregnancy must be based on the relative risks and benefits of the treatment compared with nontreatment.

The SSRIs are generally safe and well-tolerated antidepressants, but they are associated with both transient and enduring side effects. Many common side effects, such as nausea, are short-lived and improve within a few weeks of treatment. Although they are not addictive, abrupt discontinuation or missed doses of certain SSRIs can cause SSRI discontinuation syndrome. With their improved safety and tolerability profile over older antidepressants, the SSRIs are rarely the cause of fatal toxicity in overdose.

Before the discovery of SSRIs, medication treatment for major depression was limited mainly to monoamine oxidase inhibitors (MAOIs) and tricyclic antidepressants (TCAs), agents first identified in the 1950s. However, some pharmacological actions of those medications accounted for therapeutically unnecessary and undesirable adverse effects profiles and a potential for toxicity, including mortality with overdose, thus limiting their risk/benefit profile. Consequently, researchers pursued development of alternative medications with similar efficacy but fewer adverse effects, which culminated in the discovery of the SSRIs. The development of SSRIs, by making medication treatment more acceptable, has been an important milestone in the treatment of depression and other psychiatric disorders.

In 1987, the first SSRI, fluoxetine (Prozac), was approved for the treatment of depression by the U.S. Food and Drug Administration (FDA), and other agents, including paroxetine (Paxil), sertraline (Zoloft), citalopram (Celexa), escitalopram (Lexapro), fluvoxamine (Luvox), vortioxetine (Trintellix), and vilazodone (Viibryd), were subsequently introduced. The SSRIs can be used safely in many patient populations, including elderly patients, children, and people with medical comorbidities who are more sensitive to the adverse effects of older antidepressants. As a result, more people are now successfully treated for depression and anxiety disorders than ever before.

How Do They Work?

Whereas earlier medications were discovered by serendipity, SSRIs are the first class of psychiatric medications identified due to their specific mechanism of action in the brain and rationally designed to produce a medication as efficacious as, but safer and better tolerated than, older medications. They work by increasing the duration of serotonin signaling in brain nerve synapses. *Serotonin* is one of the chemical messengers (*neurotransmitters*) that carry signals between the nerve cells (*neurons*) in the brain. Serotonin deficiency in the brain was initially thought to play a role in the causation of depression and anxiety disorders, based on the therapeutic action of these medications, but the delay in benefit and the observation of other treatment consequences, including enhanced neuroplasticity, suggest that how these medications relieve depression is still an open question for neuroscience research. SSRIs are called *selective* because they mainly affect serotonin and not the other neurotransmitters, such as norepinephrine and acetylcholine. The effect of SSRIs on serotonin reuptake in the brain is immediate; however, it takes about 2–4 weeks to observe the emergence of their therapeutic benefit.

What Are Selective Serotonin Reuptake Inhibitors Used to Treat?

The SSRIs currently approved by the FDA for use in the United States are fluoxetine, sertraline, paroxetine, fluvoxamine, citalopram, escitalopram, vortioxetine, and vilazodone. As mentioned earlier, they currently have FDA-labeled indications to treat various psychiatric conditions. In addition, their off-label use includes, but is not limited to, treatment of binge-eating disorder, body dysmorphic disorder, fibromyalgia, and vasomotor symptoms associated with menopause.

The efficacy of SSRIs, as compared with placebo, has been demonstrated in several randomized, placebo-controlled clinical trials for acute and maintenance treatment of major depression and other psychiatric indications. SSRIs that are FDA-approved for depression include all of those listed at the beginning of this section except fluvoxamine. Similarly, the FDA has approved paroxetine and escitalopram for generalized anxiety disorder; sertraline, fluoxetine, and fluvoxamine for OCD; fluoxetine, paroxetine, and sertraline for panic disorder; sertraline and paroxetine for social anxiety disorder; fluoxetine, paroxetine, and sertraline for premenstrual dysphoric disorder; sertraline and paroxetine for PTSD; and fluoxetine for bulimia nervosa.

Standard Dosing and Treatment Regimen

SSRI medications are only available orally and come in multiple forms, including tablets, capsules, or liquid suspension/solution. Typically administered as once-daily medication in the morning or nighttime, they are usually prescribed at the lowest effective dosage to improve the target mood and anxiety symptoms. Most agents start to help within 2 weeks of treatment initiation; however, it usually takes at least 4–6 weeks to notice the full effect and, in some cases, may take as long as 12 weeks. A course of SSRI treatment usually continues for 6–9 months following improvement in depression symptoms in order to prevent relapse, and longer courses of treatment may be advised based on clinical factors. *Remission* from depression is defined as being free or nearly free of symptoms for the current episode. It is noteworthy that the response rate following first-line treatment with SSRIs is moderate, varying from 40% to 60%, and remission rates vary from 30% to 45%. In case of poor response to SSRIs, the prescribing clinician should consider a dosage increase before exploring alternative treatments of depression.

Use in Special Populations

Children and Adolescents

SSRIs are the most commonly prescribed antidepressants in children and adolescents for the treatment of depression and anxiety disorders. The Treatment for Adolescents and Depression Study (TADS) showed that SSRIs were effective in approximately 80% of adolescents who improved over 9 months in terms of depression outcomes. Currently, four SSRI medications—fluoxetine, escitalopram, sertraline, and fluvoxamine—are FDA-approved for use in children and adolescents. Both fluoxetine and escitalopram are FDA-approved for acute and maintenance treatment of depression in youth. Strong evidence suggests that SSRIs are effective for treating pediatric anxiety disorders, including social anxiety disorder, generalized anxiety disorder, and OCD. The FDA issued a "black-box warning" for the SSRIs in 2004 due to a possible increased risk of suicidal thoughts among pediatric and young adult (up to age 25) populations. According to the FDA, this heightened risk of suicidal thoughts occurs within the first 1–2 months of SSRI treatment. The risk and benefits of initiating SSRI therapy in patients who are acutely suicidal must be weighed because depression itself is a significant risk factor for suicidality and requires treatment. Younger patients prescribed SSRIs should be regularly monitored for suicidality and advised to seek help immediately if experiencing suicidal thoughts.

Pregnancy

The decision to use SSRIs during pregnancy must be based on the balance between the risks and benefits of the treatment. Although SSRIs are not risk-free, the absolute risks are low and may be outweighed by the risks of untreated depression for childbearing patients and their offspring. The biggest concern is typically the possible risk of birth defects or impact on fetal development from exposure to antidepressants. However, studies that found effects from SSRI use on offspring during gestation failed to account for the effects of the childbearing parent's psychiatric illness. Untreated mental illness itself poses risks to a developing fetus; for example, untreated depression may increase the risk of preterm birth or cause low birth weight. Overall, the risk of birth defects and other problems for babies whose birth parent took antidepressants during pregnancy is very low. Patients taking SSRI medication who are considering becoming pregnant should talk with their physician about the possible risks and benefits and should not stop taking their medication without consulting the prescribing clinician first, because this might pose increased risk of significant worsening of depression.

Elderly Patients

When considering antidepressant medication to treat elderly patients, it should be noted that older adults have response rates comparable with those of younger adults. In addition, antidepressants have similar efficacy when used to treat elderly patients with and without multiple medical comorbidities. The SSRIs that are considered to have the best safety profile and lowest potential for medication interactions in elderly patients are citalopram, escitalopram, and sertraline. The starting dosage of SSRIs should be half the dosage prescribed for a younger adult in order to minimize side effects. Elderly patients are prone to increased side effects due to changes in metabolism with aging, concurrent medical conditions, and medication interactions. People taking SSRIs rarely may experience a severe fall in sodium levels known as *hyponatremia.* SSRIs can cause this side effect by blocking the effects of a hormone that helps regulate levels of sodium and fluid in the body. Hyponatremia may lead to a buildup of fluid inside the body's cells, which can be potentially dangerous. Mild hyponatremia can cause symptoms including feeling sick, headaches, muscle pain, reduced appetite, and confusion. Severe hyponatremia can cause disorientation, agitation, and even seizures. Thus, patients' sodium levels should be checked 1 month after beginning SSRI treatment, especially in those who are taking other medications that have a propensity to cause hyponatremia, such as diuretics. Although starting low and going slow is the guide for dosing in the elderly population, ultimately, many patients require standard dosing to achieve optimal benefit.

Medication Interactions

For people taking SSRIs, the use of any other prescription or over-the-counter agents, including herbal or other types of supplements, should be discussed with the prescribing clinician. Some SSRIs can interfere with the effectiveness of other medicines, and some can lead to dangerous reactions when they are combined with certain medications or herbal supplements. For example, SSRIs may increase the risk of bleeding, especially if taken with other agents that also increase this risk, such as the nonsteroidal anti-inflammatory drugs (NSAIDs), aspirin, warfarin, and other blood thinners.

Side Effects

SSRIs are generally safe and well tolerated but are not devoid of side effects. The most common of these are dry mouth, nausea, diarrhea, headaches, dizziness, drowsiness, fatigue, insomnia, weight gain, and sexual problems such as low sex drive and erectile dysfunction. Many common SSRI side effects are temporary and improve within a few weeks of treatment. Strategies to improve outcomes include adjusting the dosage or timing of the medication and adopting a treatment approach for specific side effects. These side effects can negatively impact the treatment adherence, response, and quality of life of patients taking SSRIs, but their successful management enhances adherence, improves patient comfort and function, and prevents premature discontinuation of SSRI therapy.

SSRIs can interact with other medications that increase serotonin levels in the brain, such as other antidepressants, prescription opioids, migraine medications, and St. John's wort (an herb used to treat depression). Sudden and high increases in serotonin transmission in the brain can result if one or more of these medicines are used with an SSRI, potentially leading to *serotonin syndrome.* Signs and symptoms of serotonin syndrome include anxiety, agitation, high fever, sweating, confusion, tremors, restlessness, lack of coordination, major changes in blood pressure, and a rapid heart rate. This syndrome is a medical emergency requiring urgent medical attention for treatment.

Compared with other antidepressant classes, mortality from SSRI overdose is rare, and overdose usually does not have serious consequences. Among the SSRIs, citalopram and escitalopram present more significant risk in overdose due to their increased risk of cardiac toxicity, which can progress to serious heart rhythm abnormalities.

As mentioned at the beginning of this chapter, the SSRIs are not addictive; however, abrupt discontinuation of the antidepressant or missing several doses can cause symptoms of SSRI discontinuation syndrome, including lethargy, nausea, dizziness, and flu-like illness. These are generally mild, begin within 1 week of discontinuing SSRI therapy, and typically resolve within 3 weeks. Temporary reinstatement of the SSRI helps resolve symptoms. Not surprisingly, discontinuation symptoms are more common with SSRIs that have the shortest duration of action, such as paroxetine and fluvoxamine. The discontinuation syndrome is best avoided by employing a slow medication taper when stopping SSRI therapy. Therefore, patients should seek the advice of their prescribing clinician to gradually and safely decrease their SSRI medication.

Conclusion

Because of their overall efficacy, safety, and tolerability, the SSRIs are widely prescribed as the first-line antidepressant treatment for depressive and anxiety disorders. SSRIs act by blocking the reuptake of serotonin into neurons to enhance its availability, thus improving the transmission of signals between neurons. These agents are typically administered as once-daily medication, and they require 4–6 weeks to achieve expected treatment benefits. They can be safely used in special populations, including children, adolescents, and elderly patients, but their use during pregnancy must be based on the relative risks and benefits of treatment compared with nontreatment. Although safe and well tolerated, the SSRIs have been associated with both transient and enduring side effects, many of which are short-lived and improve within a few weeks of treatment. These side effects can negatively impact the treatment adherence, response, and quality of life of patients taking SSRIs; however, successful management of these effects enhances medication adherence, improves patient comfort, and prevents premature discontinuation of SSRI treatment.

Recommended Reading

Mayo Clinic Staff: Selective Serotonin Reuptake Inhibitors (SSRIs). Rochester, MN, Mayo Clinic, 2019. Available at: https://www.mayoclinic.org/diseases-conditions/depression/in-depth/ssris/art-20044825.

National Health Service: Overview: Selective Serotonin Reuptake Inhibitors (SSRIs). London, National Health Service, December 2021. Available at: https://www.nhs.uk/mental-health/talking-therapies-medicine-treatments/medicines-and-psychiatry/ssri-antidepressants/overview.

30

Serotonin-Norepinephrine Reuptake Inhibitors

Fatma Ozlem Hokelekli, M.D., Ph.D.
Manish Kumar Jha, M.B.B.S.

Introduction

Serotonin norepinephrine reuptake inhibitors (SNRIs) such as desvenlafaxine (Pristiq), duloxetine (Cymbalta), levomilnacipran (Fetzima), milnacipran (Savella), and venlafaxine (Effexor, immediate- and extended-release formulations) are commonly used first-line treatments for a number of mental illnesses. These medications resemble the widely used selective serotonin reuptake inhibitors (SSRIs) in blocking the reuptake of serotonin at the synapses of neurons in the brain but differ by additionally blocking the reuptake of norepinephrine. Therefore, these medications potentially affect brain regions that are regulated by both neurotransmitters. Members of this class of medications have been approved by the U.S. Food and Drug Administration (FDA) for the treatment of major depressive disorder (MDD), generalized anxiety disorder (GAD), social anxiety disorder, panic disorder, fibromyalgia, diabetic peripheral neuropathic pain, and chronic musculoskeletal pain.

Individual SNRI medications differ in the frequency of daily administration, anticipated side effects, and proportionate effects on serotonin versus norepinephrine reuptake at dosages used in clinical practice. They are usually well tolerated, with certain side effects more common early in the course of treatment (e.g., nausea and abdominal discomfort) and other potential effects that may occur with longer-term treatment (e.g., sexual dysfunction). Because these medications are often similar in efficacy, their use in clinical practice should include a shared decision-making process that incorporates factors such as cost, anticipated side effects, and risk of discontinuation symptoms.

Psychiatric disorders such as MDD are widely prevalent and affect functioning across many aspects of life, including physical health, emotional well-being, interpersonal relationships, productivity in work- and non-work-related daily activities, and overall quality of life. Systematic screening for depression and anxiety in outpatient clinics is now universally recommended to promote early identification of these illnesses. Because more than one-third of the U.S. population resides in an area where mental health providers are scarce, access to psychotherapy for these conditions is limited, and treatment with medications may often be the preferred approach. Among medications for MDD and anxiety disorders, the SNRIs are widely used and often the first-line treatment. These medications have some properties that overlap with those of the SSRIs, which are discussed in Chapter 29, "Selective Serotonin Reuptake Inhibitors." In this chapter, we briefly discuss the mechanisms of action of SNRIs, their indications for use in clinical practice, and considerations while using them, such as dosage, side effects, and interactions with other medications.

How Do They Work?

As the name indicates, the SNRIs rapidly inhibit reuptake of both serotonin and norepinephrine into presynaptic nerve terminals. These *neurotransmitters* are important chemical messengers in the brain that exert widespread control over regions involved in the processing of emotions, response to threat, cognition, and alertness/wakefulness. To produce these effects, SNRIs bind to proteins on the surface of neurons that transport serotonin (*serotonin transporters*) and norepinephrine (*norepinephrine transporters*) and block the action of these transporters. All SNRIs have stronger affinity for binding to serotonin transporters than to norepinephrine transporters; thus, they predominantly act by inhibiting serotonin reuptake at lower dosages, with greater inhibition of norepinephrine reuptake at higher dosages. It is now well established that this inhibition occurs soon after the initiation of SNRI treatment, but the therapeutic effects (i.e., improvement in depression or anxiety symptoms) may take weeks to months. The reasons for this delay between treatment initiation and maximal effect are not well understood but indicate that SNRIs must be used at an adequate dosage for 6–8 weeks before any determination can be made about their efficacy.

What Are Serotonin-Norepinephrine Reuptake Inhibitors Used to Treat?

The treatment indications for which the SNRIs have FDA approval are listed in Table 30–1. All medications of this class, except milnacipran, are FDA-approved for the treatment of MDD in adults. Milnacipran is approved by the FDA solely for the treatment of fibromyalgia. Levomilnacipran, an enantiomer of milnacipran, is approved for treatment of MDD. Venlafaxine is available in two formulations: immediate-release and extended-release (venlafaxine XR). Although the immediate-release formulation is FDA-approved only for MDD treatment, venlafaxine XR is also approved for treatment of GAD, panic disorder, and social anxiety disorder. Desvenlafaxine, an active metabolite of venlafaxine, is FDA-approved for treatment of MDD. Duloxetine is approved for treatment of MDD and GAD as well as chronic pain conditions including fibromyalgia, diabetic peripheral neuropathic pain, and chronic musculoskeletal pain.

The SNRIs have often been utilized for other indications as well. For example, venlafaxine XR is one of the few antidepressants recommended by practice guidelines for the treatment of posttraumatic stress disorder (PTSD). Venlafaxine has also been used off-label for treatment of attention-deficit/hyperactivity disorder (ADHD), chronic pain conditions (e.g., fibromyalgia, diabetic peripheral neuropathic pain, complex pain syndromes), obsessive-compulsive disorder (OCD), and premenstrual dysphoric disorder. Off-label uses of duloxetine include chemotherapy-induced peripheral neuropathy and stress urinary incontinence.

Standard Dosing and Treatment Regimen

Information about standard dosing for SNRIs from the FDA prescribing label are also presented in Table 30–1. Please note that the starting, target, and maximum daily dosages for the same agent may differ based on the indication for use. For example, the maximum daily dosage of venlafaxine XR for treatment of MDD, GAD, and panic disorder is 225 mg, but for the treatment of social anxiety disorder it is only 75 mg. The dose frequency of SNRI medications also varies. The immediate-release formulation of venlafaxine should be administered in two or three divided doses per day, whereas venlafaxine XR is typically administered once a day. Similarly, milnacipran is administered in two divided doses per day, whereas levomilnacipran is dosed once daily. Desvenlafaxine and duloxetine are both also dosed once daily. We recommend the use of a prescribed SNRI for at least 6–8 weeks at or above the target daily dosage listed in Table 30–1 to evaluate whether the medication is effective. In cases of suboptimal improvement, increasing to the maximum daily dosage should be considered.

Table 30–1. Serotonin-norepinephrine reuptake inhibitors and their FDA-approved indications

	Indication	Daily dosage, *mg*		
		Starting	Target	Max
Desvenlafaxine	MDD	50	50	100
Duloxetine	MDD	40–60	60	120
	GAD	60	60	120
	Fibromyalgia	30	60	60
	Diabetic peripheral neuropathic pain	60	60	60
	Chronic musculoskeletal pain	30	60	60
Levomilnacipran XR	MDD	20	40–120	120
Milnacipran	Fibromyalgia	12.5	100	200
Venlafaxine*	MDD	75	150	375
Venlafaxine XR	MDD	37.5–75	75	225
	GAD	37.5–75	75	225
	Social anxiety disorder	75	75	75
	Panic disorder	37.5	75	225

Note. FDA=U.S. Food and Drug Administration; GAD=generalized anxiety disorder; Max=maximum; MDD=major depressive disorder; XR=extended-release.

*Immediate-release formulation of venlafaxine.

The duration of treatment after clinical improvement may need to be individualized based on the patient's course of illness. For example, the persistence of residual symptoms, such as insomnia, following clinical improvement increases the likelihood of future relapse and may warrant strategies that target these residual symptoms. A more treatment-refractory course of illness, as indicated by multiple prior episodes or a larger number of treatment steps needed to attain clinical improvement, may indicate the need to continue treatment for a longer period. In the absence of factors that increase the risk of future relapse, we recommend continuing SNRI treatment for 6–9 months following initial improvement.

A measurement-based care approach is best for selecting the optimal dosage of SNRIs. This approach uses systematic assessment of symptom severity, side effects, and adherence at regularly scheduled (every 2–3 weeks) treatment visits, which facilitates timely dosage increases and allows for detection of burdensome side effects that may limit such increases. It also prevents use of these medications at low dosage strengths at which their benefit has not been demonstrated. In addition, because some patients may require higher-than-usual dosages of these medications, the measurement-based care approach facilitates prompt attainment of a therapeutic dosage.

Use in Special Populations

Children and Adolescents

None of the SNRIs (i.e., desvenlafaxine, duloxetine, milnacipran, levomilnacipran, venlafaxine, and venlafaxine XR) are approved by the FDA for use in pediatric populations. According to the FDA, in two clinical trials that enrolled 766 pediatric patients with MDD, use of venlafaxine XR did not result in any significantly greater reduction in depression than placebo. Similarly, in two clinical trials that enrolled 793 pediatric patients with GAD, no difference in improvement was seen with venlafaxine XR compared with placebo. Therefore, use of venlafaxine XR in pediatric patients is not supported by extant data. Similarly, three large clinical trials of duloxetine in pediatric patients with MDD did not find any significant improvement compared with placebo. Both venlafaxine and duloxetine were associated with higher rates of adverse effects than placebo in these trials; therefore, use of SSRI medications that have demonstrated efficacy in pediatric patients should be preferred over these SNRI medications.

Pregnancy

As with SSRIs, decisions regarding the use of SNRIs in pregnant patients should be based on the risks associated with these medications versus the risk of continued or worsening mental illness during pregnancy. Studies from population-based registries have shown that discontinuing antidepressant treatment during pregnancy increases the risk of psychiatric emergencies following the birth. Because fetal exposure can occur during the early weeks of pregnancy, individuals of childbearing potential should consider using birth control methods to avoid unintended fetal exposure to these medications. Individuals taking SNRIs who are considering pregnancy should talk to their prescribing clinician about the risks versus the benefits of continuing their medications during pregnancy. Interested readers should see Chapter 18, "Treatment of Postpartum Depression and Related Disorders" for information on treatment during pregnancy and in the postpartum period.

Elderly Patients

Studies of venlafaxine XR have found it to be effective in treating GAD in elderly individuals, with rates of discontinuation due to burdensome side effects that were similar to those in adults younger than 60 years of age. Similarly, venlafaxine XR has been found to be effective in treating MDD as well as depression with accompanying anxiety in elderly patients.

Use of SNRIs in elderly patients requires careful consideration of the risks and benefits. The SNRIs may be associated with a reduction in sodium levels (hyponatremia) in this population; thus, caution is necessary when prescribing these agents, and sodium levels should be checked after initiating treatment and periodically thereafter. Dosage adjustment based on the age of the patient is not required for SNRIs; however, due to age-related declines, checking patients' renal function prior to initiating these medications is recommended. In addition, monitoring of blood pressure is recommended because several SNRI medications may increase blood pressure. Use of desvenlafaxine is associated with increased incidence of *orthostatic hypotension*, a sudden decline in blood pressure that can lead to loss of consciousness, in elderly individuals.

Other Special Populations

Dosages of desvenlafaxine should not exceed 50 mg/day in patients with moderate impairment of kidney functioning (i.e., moderate renal impairment). In patients with severe renal impairment or end-stage renal disease, the recommended dosage of desvenlafaxine is 50 mg every other day. Dosages of desvenlafaxine higher than 100 mg/day are not recommended for people with impaired liver function (i.e., hepatic impairment).

Use of duloxetine and milnacipran is contraindicated in patients with uncontrolled narrow-angle glaucoma. The daily dosage of levomilnacipran should not exceed 80 mg in patients with moderate renal impairment and 40 mg in those with severe renal impairment.

The dosage of venlafaxine should be reduced by 25%–50% in patients with renal impairment, by 50% in those with mild or moderate hepatic impairment, and by more than 50% in patients with severe hepatic impairment or liver cirrhosis.

Medication Interactions

All SNRIs have the potential to interact with other medications that increase levels of serotonin in the brain, such as other antidepressants, prescription opioids, migraine medications, and St. John's wort (an herb used to treat depression) and the potential to cause serotonin syndrome. Signs and symptoms of serotonin syndrome include anxiety, agitation, high fever, sweating, confusion, tremors, restlessness, lack of coordination, major changes in blood pressure, and a rapid heart rate. Serotonin syndrome is a rare medical emergency requiring urgent medical attention. If used in close proximity with monoamine oxidase inhibitors (MAOIs), SNRIs can also cause increases in blood pressure that rarely can be life threatening. Certain medications such as ketoconazole can reduce the breakdown of levomilnacipran, and the dosage of levomilnacipran should not exceed 80 mg/day when these agents are used together. Duloxetine inhibits liver enzymes that can affect levels of other medications, and the levels of duloxetine can be affected by other medications as well, so the risk of such interactions should be carefully considered when duloxetine is used with other medications. All of the SNRIs can interfere with bleeding, and caution should be exercised when they are used with other medications that increase risk of bleeding, such as nonsteroidal anti-inflammatory drugs (NSAIDs).

Side Effects

Side effects associated with SNRIs include nausea, abdominal discomfort, insomnia, increased sweating, constipation, and reduced appetite or weight loss. Use of these medications can also cause nervousness or worsening of anxiety (especially with venlafaxine and desvenlafaxine) and sleep impairments such as abnormal dreams or daytime somnolence. Use of SNRIs also may be associated with sexual dysfunction, including abnormal ejaculation and erectile dysfunction. They can also raise blood pressure, especially when used at higher dosages. Duloxetine has also been associated with dry mouth and fatigue. Certain side effects may be bothersome early in the course of treatment, such as nausea and abdominal discomfort, whereas others may emerge with longer-term use, such as sexual dysfunction. Because mental illnesses such as depression may also be associated with sexual dysfunction, these symptoms should be systematically assessed prior to treatment initiation in order to distinguish those attributed to the disorder itself from those related to the medication.

Additional Considerations

Discontinuation Symptoms

Abrupt discontinuation of antidepressants, including the SNRIs and SSRIs, after having taken them for several weeks to months can be associated with the emergence of *discontinuation syndrome*. This includes flu-like symptoms, worsening of mood, irritability, agitation, dizziness, anxiety, confusion, headache, lethargy, disturbances in sensation (e.g., tingling, electric shock sensations, ringing in ears) and insomnia. These symptoms typically start soon after the discontinuation and resolve with reinitiation of the medication. Among SNRIs, the highest rate of discontinuation symptoms has been reported for the immediate-release formulation of venlafaxine. The presence of these discontinuation symptoms does not mean that these medications are addictive. Individuals taking SNRIs should consult their prescribing clinicians to discuss discontinuation and use strategies such as gradual tapering of the dosage.

Selecting Among the Antidepressant Medications

There is limited evidence that any one antidepressant medication is better than any others. So, when using antidepressants, such as SSRIs and SNRIs, the decision may have to be based on prior experience (poor tolerability in the past may lead to avoidance of that medication), anticipated side effects, and evidence for efficacy for that specific indication. For example, among SNRIs, only duloxetine and venlafaxine XR have an FDA-approved indication for treatment of GAD. Emerging evidence suggests that some biological features may be able to guide selection of one antidepressant over another. Obesity may be one such factor; individuals with moderate or severe obesity do not respond well to SSRI antidepressants (e.g., escitalopram) and are more likely to benefit with venlafaxine XR or with a combination of bupropion and escitalopram.

Shared Decision-Making

Because no one unequivocally superior option exists among the multitude of antidepressant medications, clinicians and patients (along with other health professionals, friends, and families) should use a shared decision-making approach to make the optimal treatment decision. This includes exchanging information between clinicians, who may share information about available options, including the risks and benefits, and with the patients, who convey their specific preferences or values. Specific questions include whether antidepressant treatment is indicated and, if so, which medication should be used. Common considerations when selecting antidepressants include the cost; availability; anticipated side effects, including weight gain and sexual dysfunction; potential for interaction with other medications; and risk of discontinuation symptoms. This approach has been demonstrated to improve the relationship between individuals with mental illnesses and their clinicians and to promote patient adherence to treatment.

Conclusion

Medications in the SNRI class are commonly used and have been shown to be efficacious in patients with a range of mood and anxiety disorders. These agents, specifically duloxetine, have also been shown to help in chronic pain conditions. Their use may be associated with risks and should be considered in the context of other illnesses that the patient may have or other medications that they may be taking. The utility of SNRIs in pediatric patients has not yet been established, and therefore they should be avoided as first-line treatment. Abruptly stopping these medications can lead to discontinuation symptoms, and people who are taking SNRIs should consult their prescribing clinician if they want to stop using them.

Recommended Reading

Cipriani A, Furukawa TA, Salanti G, et al: Comparative efficacy and acceptability of 21 antidepressant drugs for the acute treatment of adults with major depressive disorder: a systematic review and network meta-analysis. Lancet 391(10128):1357–1366, 2018, 29477251

Shelton RC: Serotonin and norepinephrine reuptake inhibitors. Handb Exp Pharmacol 250:145–180, 2019 30838456

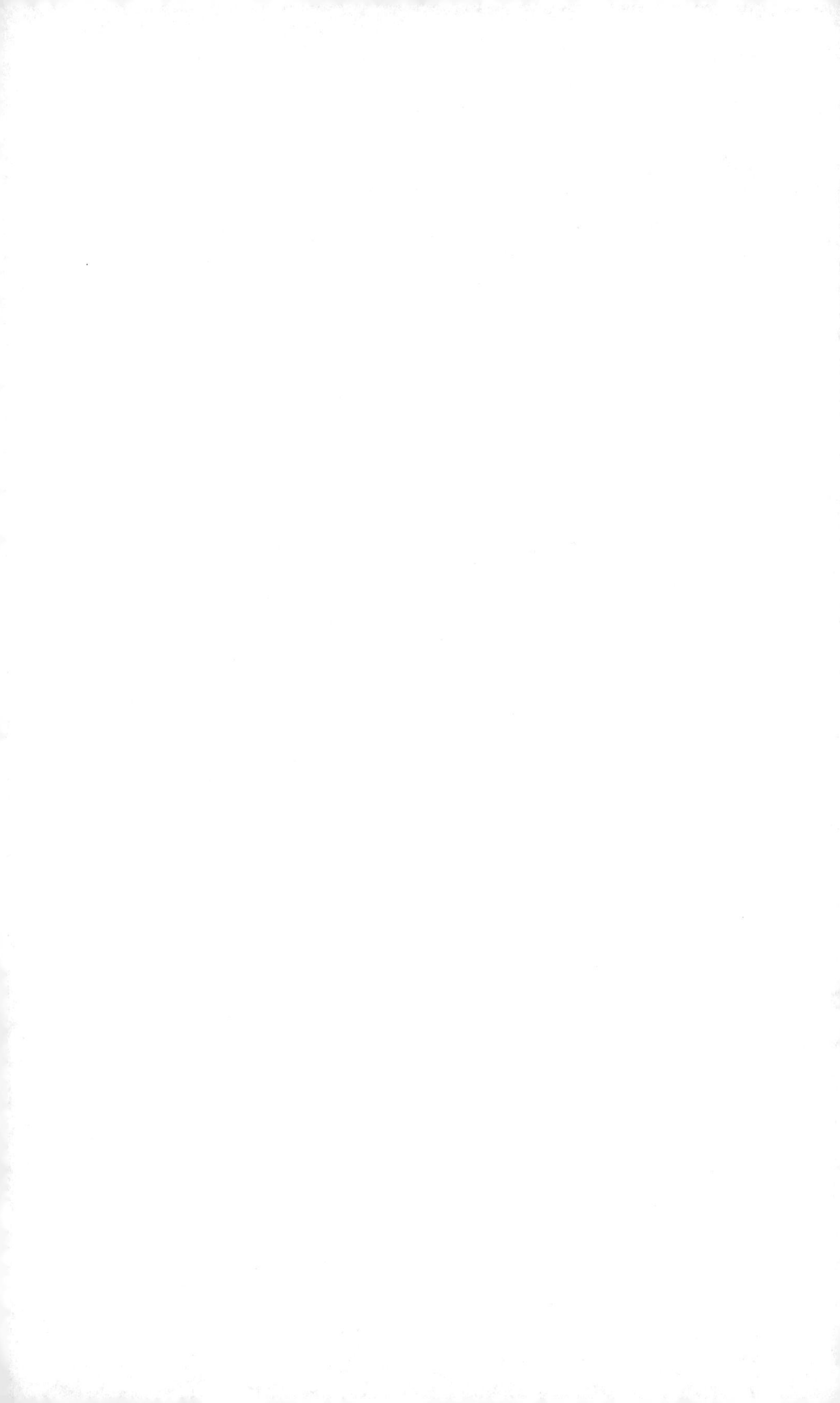

31

Bupropion

Anne Louise Stewart, M.D.
Anita H. Clayton, M.D.

Introduction

Bupropion, also known under the brand name Wellbutrin, is an oral antidepressant medication best known for its use in the treatment of major depressive disorder (MDD). Bupropion immediate-release, which is dosed three times daily, was released in 1989 after a delay to review the risk of seizures, which found that seizure occurrence was dosage related. Bupropion sustained-release (SR; dosed twice daily) and extended-release (XL; dosed once daily) were approved for all of the immediate-release indications via measures of *bioequivalence* (comparable daily doses/levels). Bupropion is also approved by the U.S. Food and Drug Administration (FDA) for the treatment of seasonal affective disorder (SAD) and nicotine use disorder. Clinical research shows that bupropion can be effective at treating attention-deficit/hyperactivity disorder (ADHD) and sexual dysfunction and is an effective adjunctive therapy to other antidepressants for treatment-resistant depression, although it lacks FDA approval for these indications. In the treatment of MDD, bupropion can take 6–8 weeks to reach its full benefit. Bupropion differs from other antidepressants in that it is unlikely to be helpful for anxiety disorders.

How Does It Work?

Bupropion's mechanism of action is unique from other antidepressants because it increases norepinephrine and dopamine effects in certain areas of the brain. Most other antidepressants affect the serotonin and norepinephrine systems.

What Is Bupropion Used to Treat?

When discussing indications for bupropion, randomized controlled trials (RCTs), systematic reviews, and meta-analyses offer the strongest evidence. Bupropion is frequently used to treat MDD, an illness that consists of low mood, lack of interest in activities, and sometimes hopelessness. People with MDD can experience changes in their sleep, appetite, energy, and ability to focus. In some cases, thoughts of suicide or of not wanting to be alive can occur to varying degrees. Because depression is one of the largest causes of disability and decreased quality of life, helpful and tolerable treatments are needed. In a meta-analysis, bupropion performed better than placebo for the treatment of MDD. Although it was not a head-to-head trial, the landmark Sequenced Treatment Alternatives to Relieve Depression (STAR*D) study aimed to assess the effectiveness of different sequences and combinations of medications and psychotherapy for MDD. In this study, bupropion was well tolerated and led to similar rates of symptom remission as the alternative treatments. STAR*D utilized bupropion as an augmentation agent to the selective serotonin reuptake inhibitor (SSRI) citalopram (Celexa), which led to greater symptom reduction but not to greater symptom resolution than the alternative treatments. As a result of these studies, bupropion might be offered at different points in MDD treatment.

SAD, now called *major depressive disorder with seasonal pattern,* is a type of depression that occurs consistently at the same time of year, most commonly in the fall or winter when days are shorter, and resolves in the spring as daylight lengthens. For someone with this seasonal pattern of depressive episodes, bupropion might be recommended over other antidepressants. In RCTs, bupropion XL at 150–300 mg/day prevented depression symptoms from occurring if given early in the season when symptoms normally begin. The medication is then often stopped during the springtime. Depression is a heterogeneous disease, so bupropion might be an option for some but not a solution for everyone.

A large, systematic review analyzed the data behind bupropion and smoking cessation. The usual dosage for this indication is bupropion SR at 150 mg/day for 3 days, then 150 mg twice a day for up to 12 weeks. The date to quit smoking is normally planned for when the medication is at steady state, about 1 week into treatment. By modulating nicotine's effects on the brain, bupropion increases the likelihood people will quit and maintain abstinence from nicotine for longer than 6 months. It can also be used in conjunction with another medication that helps with smoking cessation, varenicline (Chantix). A randomized double-blind trial showed that smoking abstinence was greater when bupropion and varenicline were used together. Bupropion often is chosen as an antidepressant when someone has both depression and nicotine dependence.

Although it lacks an FDA indication, bupropion has been studied for treatment of ADHD in children and adults because its mechanism of action increases dopamine in certain areas of the brain, similar to stimulant medication. A meta-analysis showed bupropion to be superior to placebo when a clinician rated patients' ADHD symptoms before and after treatment, but it was not superior to placebo when adults rated themselves or when parents or teachers rated ADHD symptoms in children. More studies are needed, but bupropion might be chosen as a medication if someone has MDD and ADHD or has MDD and a history of substance/stimulant abuse. Bupropion also might be chosen for patients with MDD and sexual dysfunction related to either depression or SSRI treatment of depression. In a Cochrane review of the literature, bupropion not only remained effective at treating depression in this population but also had a positive effect on most areas of sexual satisfaction and functioning on patient-rated scales.

Standard Dosing and Treatment Regimen

The usual dosing of bupropion XL is 150–450 mg/day total, taken as a once-daily dose; bupropion SR at 200–450 mg/day total, given in two divided doses; or immediate-release bupropion at 225–450 mg/day total, given in three divided doses, with the last dose of the day taken by 5 P.M. to minimize insomnia. For MDD, once-daily dosing increases adherence to treatment (remembering to take it), which improves outcomes and is better tolerated than the immediate-release formulation. With this recommended dosing, serious side effects are rare. In overdose, this medication is rarely lethal, but seizures and sustained seizures (called *status epilepticus*) have been reported. Reports also have been made of bupropion being misused via injection or snorting for its stimulant-like effect; however, when used as recommended, it is not habit-forming, and research does not show any well-documented withdrawal phenomena if stopped abruptly.

Medication Interactions

Bupropion is metabolized in the liver by the enzyme cytochrome P450 2B6. Lower dosages or an alternative antidepressant might be chosen if a patient's liver is not functioning well. Few drugs are metabolized by this enzyme, so medication interactions are rare via this elimination pathway. Bupropion decreases the activity of the enzyme cytochrome P450 2D6 in the liver. This enzyme also is responsible for metabolizing other medications; if bupropion is used, a close medication reconciliation should be completed because this agent can raise the levels of some cardiac medications and decrease the effectiveness of codeine-based pain medications. Caution also should be used when prescribing it alongside other medications that can reduce the seizure threshold.

Side Effects

Because norepinephrine can increase blood pressure, patients' vital signs should be monitored while taking bupropion. Other common side effects due to the actions of norepinephrine and dopamine include insomnia, agitation, headache, dry mouth, constipation, nausea, sweating, and anxiety, although these effects are less bothersome with once-daily dosing (i.e., bupropion XL). Bupropion is not associated with weight gain, sexual dysfunction, or sedation and may help with cognitive dysfunction or emotional blunting due to MDD or other antidepressant medication (e.g., SSRIs). Seizures have been reported when bupropion is used at higher-than-recommended dosages and in patients with predisposing factors such as an underlying seizure disorder, an eating disorder, or a history of head injury. When bupropion is taken at recommended dosages, the risk of seizure is around 1 in 1,000 people, which is similar to that of other commonly used antidepressants. Other severe side effects that have been reported but are rare include a severe allergic (*anaphylactic*) reaction and a life-threatening rash called Stevens-Johnson syndrome.

Conclusion

Overall, bupropion is an effective and generally well-tolerated medication for depressive symptoms when it is used as prescribed and use is monitored by a physician. Because bupropion has a unique way of working, a growing body of evidence indicates that it also may be helpful for treatment ADHD and sexual dysfunction, and it is now being studied as a treatment for certain substance use disorders. Bupropion can be used in all age groups, and it is one of the most-prescribed antidepressants by outpatient psychiatrists, alone or in combination with other treatments.

Recommended Reading

Centers for Disease Control and Prevention: How to Use Bupropion SR. Atlanta, GA, Centers for Disease Control and Prevention, 2022. Available at: https://www.cdc.gov/tobacco/campaign/tips/quit-smoking/quit-smoking-medications/how-to-use-quit-smoking-medicines/how-to-use-bupropion-sr.html.

National Alliance on Mental Illness: Bupropion (Wellbutrin), in About Mental Illness: Treatments. Arlington, VA, National Alliance on Mental Illness, 2023

32

Mirtazapine

Amy Claxton, Ph.D.
Steven D. Targum, M.D.

Introduction

Mirtazapine is an atypical antidepressant originally synthesized in the Netherlands in 1987 and approved by the U.S. Food and Drug Administration (FDA) in 1996 for the treatment of individuals with major depressive disorder (MDD). Mirtazapine is also used off-label for several other conditions, including anxiety and stress disorders, insomnia, reduced appetite, and pain.

How Does It Work?

Mirtazapine impacts the brain in a slightly different way than other antidepressants and may be useful for individuals whose MDD has not responded to the more commonly prescribed antidepressants. It has a dual mode of action that *antagonizes* (blocks) the presynaptic autoreceptors that in turn block the action of noradrenergic (norepinephrine) and serotonergic (serotonin) receptors. The result of this dual action is an increase of central noradrenergic and serotonergic activity that treats depression.

The peak plasma concentration of mirtazapine is reached at 2 hours after dosing. It has a half-life of 20–40 hours, and steady state levels are achieved after

4–5 days. Mirtazapine is extensively metabolized in the liver, where cytochrome P450 isoenzymes are mainly responsible for its metabolism. In the United States, mirtazapine is called Remeron and is offered in three dosages—15 mg, 30 mg, and 45 mg—and as a disintegrating tablet that dissolves in the mouth (Remeron SolTab).

What Is Mirtazapine Used to Treat?

Major Depressive Disorder

There have been many studies of mirtazapine treatment for individuals experiencing acute symptoms of depression (MDD). In most of these studies, it was more effective than placebo and just as effective as other, commercially available antidepressants. In some studies, mirtazapine revealed a rapid onset of action for depressive symptoms. In fact, a meta-analysis of 15 controlled trials reported that depressed individuals treated with mirtazapine had 74% greater likelihood of achieving *remission* (full recovery) during the first 2 weeks of treatment than those treated with selective serotonin reuptake inhibitors (SSRIs). Another meta-analysis agreed that mirtazapine was just as effective as the more commonly prescribed SSRIs and the serotonin-norepinephrine reuptake inhibitors (SNRIs). However, a respected international guideline concluded that the benefit-risk ratio for taking mirtazapine was not as good as that of the SSRIs and SNRIs. The risk relates to the known primary side effects of mirtazapine, which are drowsiness and weight gain. Consequently, mirtazapine is usually offered as a second-line treatment for MDD and given only after the patient's depression has been unresponsive to an SSRI or SNRI or when patients also experience insomnia or are underweight.

Mirtazapine has been demonstrated to prevent relapse from depression. In one study, 156 participants who had fully remitted (recovered from acute depression) were randomly and blindly assigned to receive either mirtazapine or placebo over 40 weeks of continued double-blind therapy. (*Double-blind* means that neither the doctor nor the treated individual knows whether they are receiving mirtazapine or the placebo.) In that study, 43.8% of study participants receiving placebo treatment relapsed, compared with only 19.7% of participants receiving mirtazapine.

Off-Label Uses

Beyond depression, mirtazapine has been used for many off-label purposes. Several studies of depressed individuals revealed that it had an antianxiety effect in addition to its antidepressant effect during the first 2 weeks of treatment. Consequently, one of the most frequent off-label uses of mirtazapine has been for anxiety and stress disorders. Additional uses have included insomnia, appetite disorders, pain, and substance abuse and depression after a heart attack or stroke. We review some of these therapeutic areas in the sections that follow.

Anxiety and Stress Disorders

Some evidence indicates that mirtazapine may be an effective treatment for generalized anxiety disorder, social anxiety, obsessive-compulsive disorder (OCD), and posttraumatic stress disorder (PTSD). However, no large, controlled trials are yet available to support its benefit in any of these distinct populations. Results from small, exploratory studies are often mixed. For instance, several small, placebo-controlled trials have studied mirtazapine in participants with PTSD. In one such study, a small double-blind, placebo-controlled trial of 29 patients, researchers found that it was effective in reducing the symptoms of PTSD after 26 days of treatment. A study of 100 Korean veterans determined that mirtazapine was more effective than sertraline after 6 weeks of treatment. However, a third placebo-controlled study of PTSD in 78 U.S. veterans did not show a reduction of PTSD symptoms following 8 weeks of treatment. Hence, although provocative, the results of these small PTSD studies have been inconclusive.

Insomnia

Although it is not approved for this purpose, many elderly patients receive low doses of mirtazapine for treatment of sleep difficulties. In this case, its common side effect of somnolence offers potential benefit. One open-label study of mirtazapine 30 mg nightly for sleep difficulties in individuals older than 60 years revealed a significant improvement in the sleep fragmentation index and quality of sleep, particularly in those older than 80 years.

Appetite Problems

Mirtazapine has a well-known side effect of increasing appetite and thus potentially causing weight gain. Therefore, it has been a logical choice to treat people with poor appetite or those who have eating problems associated with a medical comorbidity, such as cancer. Mirtazapine is often prescribed in low doses for elderly individuals with poor appetite as well as for sleep difficulties.

Pain Conditions (Fibromyalgia)

Three randomized, placebo-controlled trials and one open-label trial of mirtazapine have been conducted in individuals with fibromyalgia. In these studies, the medication improved measurements of pain, sleep, and quality of life. Of course, the well-known side effects of mirtazapine were also noted (e.g., somnolence, weight gain, nasopharyngitis, dry mouth, increased appetite).

Standard Dosing and Treatment Regimen

The current recommendation for using mirtazapine in MDD is to start the initial dosage at 15 mg/day with or without food. Because it is only taken once per day, it is best to take mirtazapine in the evening prior to sleep due to its tendency to induce drowsiness. Subsequently, the dosage may be increased to 30 mg/day or 45 mg/day as needed to treat symptoms. In certain subpopulations, physicians may decide to prescribe a lower dosage, such as for patients who are older or who have liver problems, because in such cases the liver may clear less medication from the body.

Use in Special Populations

Children and Adolescents

Despite some off-label use and smaller studies, mirtazapine is not approved for use in children or adolescents, and no large, published studies are available that would serve as good indicators of safety. In fact, the data remain sparse on this topic. Although one meta-analysis suggested that mirtazapine was effective and safe in children and adolescents, there are too few data to assess its merit.

Pregnancy

Some evidence indicates that mirtazapine taken during pregnancy will not negatively impact child development. A large Danish registration study found no increased risk for stillbirth, neonatal death, major congenital malformation, or miscarriage in childbearing parents who used mirtazapine during their pregnancies. However, not enough data are available to opine about the safety of this agent during lactation.

Elderly Patients

Data about the effectiveness or safety of mirtazapine in elderly patients is limited. In a trial of 255 individuals age 65 or older with MDD, mirtazapine was found to be both safe and effective compared with paroxetine. On the other hand, a large trial conducted in the United Kingdom reported that mirtazapine was not effective for the treatment of agitation associated with Alzheimer's disease. Elderly patients may experience some confusion from the common mirtazapine side effect of sedation, and some may experience the uncommon side effect of *hyponatremia* (low sodium in the blood), particularly if their diet is poor. Given the limited data, the FDA recommends caution and suggests starting with a lower dosage to assess tolerance in older patients.

Side Effects

It is important to consider the effectiveness of mirtazapine in light of its safety profile. The most common side effects include somnolence, dizziness, increased appetite, and weight gain. In a review of side effects reported during clinical trials, 54% of study participants receiving mirtazapine reported somnolence, with 10% discontinuing early because of it. In contrast, only 18% of study participants assigned to placebo reported somnolence, and only 2% dropped out because of it. Dizziness was reported in 7% of the mirtazapine group compared with 3% of the placebo group. An increase in appetite was reported by 17% of the mirtazepine group, and 8% experienced clinically significant weight gain, 15% experienced an increase in cholesterol, and 6% experienced an increase in triglycerides.

Evidence has shown that mirtazapine may affect one's ability to drive, especially during the first 1–2 weeks of daily treatment. Patients also should avoid consuming alcohol when taking mirtazapine because it could exacerbate cognitive problems and psychomotor slowness.

Overdoses of mirtazapine have been reported, but the results have been relatively mild compared with overdose of tricyclic antidepressants (TCAs). Signs and symptoms associated with mirtazapine overdose include disorientation, drowsiness, impaired memory, and increased heart rate. No reports have been published of death due to mirtazapine ingestion alone, but at least one account exists of a death due to self-poisoning with a combination of mirtazapine and lorazepam. Unlike TCAs, mirtazapine has shown no significant adverse cardiovascular effects when taken at 7–22 times its maximum recommended dosage.

Rare reports have been made of *agranulocytosis* (a dramatic reduction in white blood cells) in people taking mirtazapine. This has been reported in only 1 of every 1,000 individuals taking the medication. Fortunately, the individuals who experienced this very rare occurrence recovered when the mirtazapine was discontinued.

The abrupt cessation of mirtazapine can cause new side effects in some individuals, called a *discontinuation syndrome*, that can include anxiousness, nausea, tremor, loss of appetite, lack of desire for food, or weight loss. Therefore, a slow and gradual reduction in dosage is recommended to minimize any potential discontinuation symptoms.

Conclusion

Mirtazapine has been approved in the United States since 1996 for the treatment of MDD. Although it is a proven antidepressant medication, many people who take mirtazapine become drowsy and sluggish, have increased appetite, and gain weight. It is thus understandable that mirtazapine is considered a second-line treatment for MDD in comparison with the SSRIs and SNRIs, which have fewer profound effects on sleep or appetite. However, these treatment-emergent side effects may make mirtazapine a more desirable medication for depressed individuals who cannot sleep or have poor appetite and have led to the off-label use of the medicine for these conditions (e.g., people taking strong drugs for cancer, or elderly people who have lost weight). We consider mirtazapine to be a useful second-line antidepressant with potential utility in other conditions as well. Of course, like every powerful medication, its use must be carefully monitored, and its abrupt cessation may cause discontinuation side effects.

Recommended Reading

Alam A, Voronovich Z, Carley JA: A review of therapeutic uses of mirtazapine in psychiatric and medical conditions. Prim Care Companion CNS Disord 15(5):PCC.13r01525, 2013 24511451

Thase ME, Nierenberg AA, Keller MB, et al: Efficacy of mirtazapine for prevention of depressive relapse: a placebo-controlled double-blind trial of recently remitted high-risk patients. J Clin Psychiatry 62(10):782–788, 2001 11816867

33

Nefazodone and Trazodone

Elizabeth Deckler, M.D.
Martin B. Keller, M.D.

Introduction

Nefazodone and trazodone are both invaluable tools for psychiatrists. Nefazodone, a less-utilized but powerful antidepressant, can be prescribed to patients whose depression has failed to remit with other treatments. Trazodone, an effective antidepressant, can be used in conjunction with other psychiatric medications to improve sleep and has demonstrated efficacy in treating aggressive behavior among patients with dementia. In this chapter, we review aspects of both medications that are important for patients and their families to understand prior to starting treatment.

Nefazodone

Nefazodone, which was previously sold under the brand name Serzone, was approved by the U.S. Food and Drug Administration (FDA) in 1988 for the treatment of depression. It is a unique antidepressant that is structurally dissimilar to other antidepressant classes such as the tricyclic antidepressants (TCAs), selective serotonin reuptake inhibitors (SSRIs), and monoamine oxidase inhibitors (MAOIs). Furthermore, appreciable sexual side effects and weight gain have not been reported in patients taking nefazodone.

How Does It Work?

Nefazodone blocks the neuronal uptake of serotonin (5-hydroxytryptamine, or 5-HT) and norepinephrine, meaning it increases the amount of neurotransmitters available for the patient's brain to use. Nefazodone antagonizes the 5-HT_2 and α-adrenergic receptors, likely resulting in some of its antidepressant effect. Nefazodone is unique in that it has no significant impact on dopamine, benzodiazepine, cholinergic, beta-adrenergic, 5-HT_{1A}, or histaminic receptors, meaning it causes fewer side effects in patients than other antidepressant medications.

The half-life of nefazodone is about 8 hours, requiring patients to take it twice a day to maintain effectiveness. It takes about 1–2 weeks to reach a therapeutic blood level, and some patients have experienced initial improvement in that time. Others may need to take the medication for up to 6 weeks before noticing an improvement in depressive symptoms.

What Is Nefazodone Used to Treat?

A clinical trial that included 552 chronically depressed participants found that 55% of those treated with nefazodone alone experienced significant improvement in their symptoms, 52% of those treated with psychotherapy alone experienced significant improvement in their symptoms, and 85% of those treated with a combination of nefazodone and psychotherapy experienced significant improvement in their symptoms. This trial lasted 12 weeks and also found that participants treated with nefazodone alone improved more quickly than those receiving psychotherapy alone.

Standard Dosing and Treatment Regimen

Nefazodone is taken twice per day, once in the morning and once at night. The starting dosage of nefazodone is typically 100 mg twice per day. Physicians can increase the dosage by 100 mg/day every 7 days, aiming for a target dosage of 300–600 mg/day. The dosage should be increased until patients reach a dosage at which their depressive symptoms improve without intolerable side effects.

Side Effects

The most common side effects of nefazodone, experienced by 20% or more of patients studied in the FDA trials, include headache, dry mouth, nausea, and somnolence. These side effects generally improve over time in most patients. Nefazodone is valuable in that clinical trial data showed a relatively low incidence of sexual side effects and weight gain associated with its use. Only 1% of patients experienced a decrease in libido, and only 5% experienced an increase in appetite. These statistics are strikingly lower than the rates seen with use of other antidepressant medications.

The safety of nefazodone was established in trials published by the FDA. Safety studies included both open and double-blinded trials with more than 250 patients over the course of a year. In the *open* trials, the patients and providers knew which medication they were taking. In the *double-blinded* trials, neither the patient nor the provider knew whether the patient was given nefazodone or a placebo.

Additional Information

In 2003, Serzone, the brand version of nefazodone, was taken off the market because it was found to cause liver injury and failure in a small number of patients. The data collected estimated that it caused 1 instance of liver failure for every 250,000 patient-years of use. Despite this low incidence, it was pulled from the market for general use in depression. The generic form, nefazodone, remained on the market to be used as a later-line agent in patients whose major depressive disorder (MDD) failed to respond to first- and second-line medications. For example, a physician may opt to try nefazodone in a patient with MDD who does not experience improvement in symptoms with one or more SSRIs, such as fluoxetine or sertraline, and possibly another class of antidepressants, such as the TCAs desipramine or amitriptyline or the serotonin-norepinephrine reuptake inhibitors (SNRIs) venlafaxine or duloxetine.

Nefazodone has been taken off the market entirely in other countries but remains available in the United States with a "black-box warning" for liver injury. Of note, in the few patients who have experienced liver injuries secondary to nefazodone use, the injuries mostly occurred within the first 4 months of starting the medication. To help mitigate the risk of liver injury in patients taking nefazodone, physicians can monitor patients' liver enzymes in the blood.

Trazodone

Desyrel, the brand-name form of generic trazodone, was developed in the 1960s and approved in the United States in 1981. At that time, it ushered in a new era of antidepressant medications. Like nefazodone, it is structurally dissimilar to TCAs and MAOIs, two older classes of antidepressants that have largely been replaced by modern antidepressants such as SSRIs and SNRIs. The TCAs and MAOIs are known for causing more unwanted side effects in patients than the newer medications. Interestingly, trazodone was the first non-TCA or -MAOI medication to obtain FDA approval for treatment of depression in the United States, and it was a founding member of the class of *atypical antidepressants*. Despite trazodone's widespread use as a sleep aid, it is only FDA-approved for treatment of depression.

How Does It Work?

Trazodone inhibits serotonin reuptake. Uniquely, it stimulates the sensitivity of adrenoreceptors. It also acts as a serotonin 5-HT_{2A} receptor antagonist, blocks the α_1-adrenergic receptors, and blocks histamine (H_1) receptors. This translates to increased drowsiness and sedation with use. The half-life of trazodone is 5–9 hours, requiring twice-daily dosing for depression, and its peak plasma concentration is achieved 1–2 hours after administration.

What Is Trazodone Used to Treat?

Clinical trials published by the FDA have established trazodone as an efficacious treatment for MDD. Additional clinical trials have proven its efficacy as a sleep aid and as an agent for decreasing agitated behavior in patients with dementia, but it is used off-label for these indications.

Standard Dosing and Treatment Regimen

The necessary dosage of trazodone depends on what it is being used to treat. For depression, trazodone must be taken at a dosage of at least 150 mg/day. Patients should be started on 150 mg/ day in two divided doses of 75 mg. The dosage can be increased up to 400 mg/day in two divided doses of 200 mg. In severely depressed patients, there is evidence of successful use of up to 600 mg/day in two divided doses of 300 mg. For MDD, trazodone must be given twice per day to achieve a consistent therapeutic blood level. For treatment of insomnia, it can be dosed once per day at bedtime.

In the treatment of insomnia, trazodone can be dosed as low as 25 mg at bedtime and can be increased to 100 mg. Its hypnotic effect is seen at the lower 25-mg dose. The short half-life of trazodone can be used to its advantage in patients with insomnia. It has been shown to improve sleep initiation and maintenance without causing residual drowsiness the next day.

Medication Interactions

Trazodone has been used safely as an adjunct to other psychotropic medications. Its use is contraindicated with MAOIs, but it has been found to be generally safe in combination with other antidepressant classes. It is used off-label as a sleep aid, to improve the efficacy of other antidepressants, and to mitigate the side effects of psychotropic medications. Despite widespread use of trazodone in combination with other serotonergic agents, patients should be cognizant of the possibility of developing serotonin syndrome when using it in combination with other serotonergic agents. *Serotonin syndrome* is a condition caused by the simultaneous use of multiple medications that increase or augment serotonin. Symptoms to watch out for include insomnia, high blood pressure, sweating, increased heart rate, diarrhea, dilated pupils, confusion, and restlessness.

Side Effects

The most common side effects with trazodone, seen in 20% or more of patients included in the trials published by the FDA, were dry mouth, dizziness, drowsiness, and headache. Its common side effect of drowsiness has been used independently as a treatment for insomnia.

Conclusion

Clinical trials have established the safety of trazodone when used for treatment of depression. Importantly, unlike other agents used to treat insomnia, there is no evidence of abuse potential with trazodone.

Recommended Reading

Keller MB, McCullough JP, Klein DN, et al: A comparison of nefazodone, the cognitive behavioral-analysis system of psychotherapy, and their combination for the treatment of chronic depression. N Engl J Med 342(20):1462–1470, 2000 10816183 (Published correction appears in N Engl J Med 345[3]:232, 2001)

U.S. Food and Drug Administration: Nefazodone (https://www.accessdata.fda.gov/drugsatfda_docs/nda/2003/020152_S031_SERZONE_PRNTLBL.pdf) and trazodone (https://www.accessdata.fda.gov/drugsatfda_docs/label/2015/071196s062lbl.pdf)

34

Tricyclic Antidepressants

Robert M. A. Hirschfeld, M.D., M.Sc.*
Mark Sullivan, M.D.

Introduction

The tricyclic antidepressants (TCAs) are a class of medications used to treat depression, anxiety, and a variety of other medical and psychiatric problems. The name *tricyclic antidepressant* is derived from its chemical structure, which has three rings in it. The TCAs were first discovered serendipitously in the 1950s, and this discovery was a major breakthrough in the field of psychiatry because the TCAs were some of the first medications that were effective in treating clinical depression. They remained the primary medications prescribed for clinical depression for more than 30 years after their discovery, until newer classes of antidepressants (e.g., fluoxetine [Prozac], sertraline [Zoloft]) were developed.

How Do They Work?

A prevailing hypothesis for how TCAs impact mood is that they have an effect on the levels of chemicals called *neurotransmitters* in the brain. Neurotransmit-

*Dr. Hirschfeld was the quintessential clinician-scholar. His contributions to the field of psychiatry were great, and his mentorship and friendship will be missed by many.

ters send signals between cells. When someone experiences a depressive episode, the concentration of these neurotransmitters is believed to decrease. The TCAs increase the concentration of these neurotransmitters to help the brain improve its ability to send signals and information between cells, and this can lead to improvement in the symptoms of depression. By increasing the levels of specific neurotransmitters, including serotonin and norepinephrine, in the brain, TCAs help the brain return to its baseline functioning level.

What Are Tricyclic Antidepressants Used to Treat?

The TCAs have U.S. Food and Drug Administration (FDA) approval to treat major depressive disorder (MDD). When using TCAs to treat depression, it is important to understand that these medications take time to work. They must be taken consistently every day, although the benefits may not be apparent until 2–4 weeks after reaching an effective dosage.

Clomipramine is unique for two reasons: it is the only TCA that has FDA approval for treatment of obsessive-compulsive disorder (OCD) and the only TCA that is *not* FDA-approved to treat MDD. Although it is effective in MDD, the company that manufactured clomipramine never submitted their MDD data to the FDA for approval.

We discuss side effects later in the chapter, but one of the common side effects with TCAs can be sedation, and thus TCAs also can be used to help with sleep problems. Specifically, doxepin, used at low, non-antidepressant dosages, has FDA approval for treatment of insomnia.

Although the TCAs are not FDA-approved to treat panic disorder, they were the first medications used for this condition, and considerable evidence indicates that they can be an effective option.

Interestingly, the TCAs are effective for treating nonpsychiatric medical issues as well. Although they are not FDA-approved to treat pain disorders, including headaches, a number of studies have shown that they can be effective. Imipramine is FDA-approved to treat childhood bedwetting and is commonly used for this issue, and doxepin has FDA approval for the treatment of itching that occurs with specific skin conditions.

Standard Dosing and Treatment Regimen

Each of the TCAs has different dosage ranges (Table 34–1). The goal of treating with medications is to achieve improvement in symptoms while avoiding or

Table 34–1. Usual dosage ranges for tricyclic antidepressant medications

Medication	Usual dosage range, *mg*
Amitriptyline	150–300
Amoxapine	200–300
Clomipramine	100–250
Desipramine	150–300
Doxepin	100–300
Imipramine	150–300
Maprotiline	100–225
Nortriptyline	50–150
Protriptyline	15–60
Trimipramine	150–300

minimizing any side effects. In general, when most people use TCAs, they can tolerate the medications without significant or problematic side effects. One advantage of these medications is the fact that their blood levels can be used to optimize the dosage.

One difficulty with TCAs is waiting for them to work, and this is also an issue with newer antidepressants such as the selective serotonin reuptake inhibitors (SSRIs) and serotonin-norepinephrine reuptake inhibitors (SNRIs). It is not uncommon for people starting TCAs to experience side effects while waiting for the medications to help them. Another issue is that the symptoms of depression overlap somewhat with known side effects of the TCAs, and this can make it difficult to know whether someone is experiencing side effects.

Medication Interactions

TCAs can interact with other medications. Combining them with other agents that increase the concentration of serotonin in the body can lead to the *serotonin syndrome,* characterized by agitation, insomnia, confusion, increased heart rate and blood pressure, sweating, and headaches. Therefore, such medications—including monoamine oxidase inhibitors (MAOIs), other antidepressants (SSRIs, SNRIs), drugs of abuse (3,4-methylenedioxymethamphetamine [MDMA], cocaine), tryptophan, and other agents—should be avoided by people taking TCAs. Some medications can affect TCA levels in the body and impact patients' ability to function. People should discuss their current medicines with their providers before taking any new medication, including TCAs.

Side Effects

Some of the more common, known adverse effects of TCAs that are typically not life-threatening include blurry vision, constipation, dry mouth, urinary retention, sedation, and increased appetite. Although these medications are generally well tolerated, they have some serious risks. Desipramine is contraindicated for children younger than 12 years of age, following the tragic deaths of several children taking the medication. Patients taking TCAs are at increased risk of seizures, and people with narrow-angle glaucoma can have emergency issues related to their eyes, known as *ocular crisis*.

TCAs also can have negative effects on the heart; patients taking TCAs can experience increased heart rate and positional low blood pressure. Most notably, the TCAs can cause abnormal heart rhythms, and this effect makes these agents dangerous and potentially fatal in overdose. They should not be abruptly discontinued because patients can experience withdrawal symptoms if the dosage is not slowly lowered (*tapered*) over weeks and under clinician supervision. Symptoms of withdrawal include flu-like symptoms, headache, and anxiety, among others. When the TCAs are used during pregnancy, there is a risk of the newborn experiencing withdrawal symptoms after birth.

Conclusion

In our current era of psychiatry, TCAs are used relatively infrequently due to the development of newer antidepressant and antianxiety medications that have improved side effect profiles. One of the primary reasons for this is the risk for death in overdose. The TCAs are no longer the first-line treatment for depression and are only considered for use when patients' illness does not improve with other medications.

Recommended Reading

Hirsch M, Birnbaum RJ: Tricyclic and tetracyclic drugs: pharmacology, administration, and side effects. UpToDate, 2022. Available at: https://www.uptodate.com/contents/tricyclic-and-tetracyclic-drugs-pharmacology-administration-and-side-effects.

Nelson JC: Tricyclic and tetracyclic drugs, in The American Psychiatric Association Publishing Textbook of Psychopharmacology, 5th Edition. Washington, DC, American Psychiatric Association Publishing, 2017, pp 305–334

35

Monoamine Oxidase Inhibitors

William Coryell, M.D.

Introduction

Monoamine oxidase inhibitors (MAOIs) were the first antidepressants shown in placebo-controlled studies to be effective for treatment of depressive disorders. Their discovery, as has been the case for most medicines in use for psychiatric disorders, was a product of serendipity. Intense efforts were under way following World War II to find medications that were effective against tuberculosis. Derivatives of hydrazine were being extensively tested, in part because large amounts of this chemical were available due to its use as a component of rocket fuel during the war. One of these derivatives, iproniazid, was found to be effective against tuberculosis and, moreover, often produced a noticeable elevation in mood, sociability, and energy among the patients being treated. Further use of iproniazid was curtailed due to liver toxicity, but the finding in 1952 that this agent was an inhibitor of monoamine oxidase led to further screening of drugs with this attribute as possible antidepressants. In this way, the MAOIs isocarboxazid, phenelzine, and tranylcypromine were identified in the late 1950s as effective antidepressants.

How Do They Work?

Neurons transmit messages by releasing specific chemicals, called *neurotransmitters,* into a gap between the neurons, called *synapses.* Extensive research has indicated that relative deficiencies of certain neurotransmitters in the central nervous system play a role in the genesis of depressive disorders. The most important of these neurotransmitters appear to be serotonin, norepinephrine, and dopamine. When any of these are released into the synapse to convey a signal, they are then either inactivated by the enzyme monoamine oxidase or are reabsorbed by the nerve ending that released it. MAOIs and the more commonly used antidepressants act to increase neurotransmitter concentrations in the synapse but do so in different ways. MAOIs inhibit the enzymes, monoamine oxidases, that inactivate the neurotransmitters within the synapse, whereas other antidepressants inhibit the reuptake of these neurotransmitters. In further contrast, antidepressants in wide use affect the intrasynaptic concentration of one or two of the three neurotransmitters important to depression, whereas MAOIs affect all three.

What Are Monoamine Oxidase Inhibitors Used to Treat?

Four MAOIs have been approved for antidepressant use in the United States (Table 35–1). Although they all work by inhibiting monoamines, they do have some important differences. There are two types, A and B, and inhibition of both is necessary for antidepressant effect. Isocarboxazid (Marplan), phenelzine (Nardil), tranylcypromine (Parnate), and higher doses of oral selegiline (Eldepryl) do this. Lower doses of oral selegiline inhibit only Type B, and this is useful for early Parkinson's disease. Inhibition of Type A necessitates dietary restrictions (see "Side Effects"), and this, along with numerous medication interactions, has relegated the use of MAOIs to treatment-resistant psychiatric conditions. However, selegiline is also available in a transdermal patch that markedly lessens its effects on monoamine oxidases in the gut and thus, at recommended dosages, avoids the need for dietary restrictions.

Placebo-controlled studies have shown benefits of phenelzine for social anxiety disorder (social phobia), panic disorder, and posttraumatic stress disorder (PTSD) and of both phenelzine and isocarboxazid for treatment of bulimia nervosa. However, most of the research on treatment with the MAOIs has focused on depressive disorders. Early work showed that phenelzine was more effective for "atypical depression" than imipramine. Imipramine is a tricyclic antidepres-

Table 35–1. Monoamine oxidase inhibitors with U.S. Food and Drug Administration approval for use as antidepressants

Generic name	Brand name	Usual dosage range, *mg/day*
Tranylcypromine	Parnate	30–60
Phenelzine	Nardil	60–90
Isocarboxazid	Marplan	40–60
Selegiline	Emsam	6–12

sant (TCA), a class of medicines that was widely utilized before the advent of selective serotonin reuptake inhibitors (SSRIs; e.g., fluoxetine [Prozac]). *Atypical depression* was characterized by features of rejection sensitivity and by reverse vegetative depressive symptoms of increased sleep and appetite instead of insomnia and anorexia. Subsequent work, however, indicated that phenelzine was not more effective than SSRIs for treating patients with atypical depression. Some studies also have shown phenelzine to be superior to imipramine for *dysthymia*, a chronic form of depressive disorder.

Individuals with bipolar depression often fail to respond adequately to most classes of antidepressants, and according to a number of studies, tranylcypromine may be particularly effective for these patients. This seems to be especially true for those who have depressive states with prominent *anergia*, a severe lack of drive or energy. Case series have also reported good outcomes with dosages of tranylcypromine that are much higher than the usual upper limits, without attendant increases in side effects.

Medication Interactions

Treatment with the MAOIs also calls for important restrictions on concomitant medications. These include most other antidepressants, and a washout period of 2 weeks (6 weeks for Prozac) is usually necessary when switching from most antidepressants to an MAOI or vice versa. Any agent that stimulates the sympathetic nervous system, such as decongestants and amphetamines, are also to be avoided when MAOIs are being used. Likewise contraindicated are triptans for migraine headaches and certain opiates, such as meperidine. Patients who are prescribed MAOIs are generally advised to consult their prescriber before taking any new medication. Among the medicines that fall into these classes are those often utilized in anesthesia, and anesthesiologists may require an MAOI washout of 1–2 weeks before surgery.

Table 35–2. Monoamine oxidase inhibitor dietary restrictions

Meat	**Beverages**
Spoiled or improperly stored	Tap or non-pasteurized beer
Air dried, aged, or fermented	Red wine, sherry, liqueurs
Pickled herring	**Other**
Meat tenderizers	Concentrated yeast extract
Beef and chicken livers	Sauerkraut, kimchi
Fruits and vegetables	Supplement containing tyramine
Fava beans	Soy products
Dried fruits	
Dairy	
Aged cheese	

Side Effects

Despite broad evidence for their effectiveness in depressive disorders, most treatment algorithms relegate MAOIs to a third or fourth tier of interventions to be used in cases of poor response to more conventional antidepressants. This is due in large part to dietary restrictions that are required for all MAOIs except for selegiline at lower dosages. Nonselective MAOIs inactivate monoamine oxidases not only in the central nervous system but also in the gastrointestinal tract, where they normally break down the amino acid tyramine from dietary sources. When tyramine is not broken down in the gastrointestinal tract, and foods with high tyramine concentrations are ingested, large amounts of tyramine enter the general circulation, where it can cause excessive stimulation of the sympathetic nervous system and lead to a dangerous spike in blood pressure. Table 35–2 lists those foods most likely to contain problematically high amounts of tyramine. Many believe that the risk of hypertensive crisis with MAOIs has been overemphasized and that deaths due to hypertensive episodes are exceedingly rare. Nevertheless, MAOIs are the only psychiatric medication class that requires dietary restrictions.

Side effects with sufficient severity to interrupt treatment are more likely to occur with the MAOIs than with other antidepressants. Prominent among these are blood pressure changes and sleep disturbances. MAOIs can cause significant *postural hypotension,* a drop in blood pressure that causes faintness or dizziness when standing from a sitting or lying position. Patients may also experience difficulties falling asleep and/or afternoon drowsiness. Tranylcypromine in particular may cause early insomnia and therefore is usually not dosed in the late afternoon or evening.

Other side effects may include dry mouth, constipation, diarrhea, nausea, and sexual dysfunction, most likely in the form of delayed or absent orgasms. Low dosages of as-needed cyproheptadine may be helpful for the latter of these problems. Phenelzine may cause edema or weight gain, but tranylcypromine, isocarboxazid, and selegiline (Emsam) are generally weight neutral. Selegiline in its patch form carries a lower overall side effect burden than other MAOIs, but out-of-pocket costs for this medication can be considerably higher.

Conclusion

Dietary and medication restrictions, along with relatively high risks for a range of side effects, preclude use of MAOIs before other antidepressants have been tried and have proved unsuccessful. Nevertheless, some patients with treatment-refractory depressive illness find MAOI treatment to be much more beneficial than any other that they have been prescribed and, for such patients, treatment with an MAOI can be life changing.

Recommended Reading

Kim T, Xu C, Amsterdam JD: Relative effectiveness of tricyclic antidepressant versus monoamine oxidase inhibitor monotherapy for treatment-resistant depression. J Affect Disord 250:199–203, 2019

Krishnan KR: Revisiting monoamine oxidase inhibitors. J Clin Psychiatry 68(Suppl 8):35–41, 2007

36

Lithium

Jessica Batten, PA-C, CAQ-Psych
Stephen M. Strakowski, M.D.
Jorge R.C. Almeida, M.D., Ph.D.

Introduction

Lithium is the third element of the periodic table. It is a naturally occurring salt that has been recognized as a mental health supplement for centuries. In 1949, Dr. John Cade was the first to successfully use lithium to treat mania after a serendipitous discovery of its potential "calming" properties in unrelated rodent experiments. The U.S. Food and Drug Administration (FDA) approved lithium for the treatment of acute mania in 1970 and for maintenance treatment of bipolar disorder 4 years later.

How Does It Work?

Its affordability, efficacy, and unique neuroprotective properties have given lithium unrivaled longevity in psychiatry. The specific actions of lithium that create clinical improvement are not yet known. Substitution of or competition with other positively charged ions in the brain may contribute to its effects. Lithium has been shown to diminish excitatory signals such as glutamate and inositol, which may explain its antimanic effects. It also enhances norepinephrine and serotonin function in the brain, which may explain its antidepressant effects. Another hypothesis posits that lithium's mechanism of action may be related to neuroprotection, because it appears to stimulate several neuronal growth factor pathways.

What Is Lithium Used to Treat?

Lithium is FDA-approved for the treatment of acute mania and for bipolar disorder maintenance therapy. Based on evidence from several placebo-controlled trials, contemporary treatment guidelines consider it to be a first-line treatment for acute bipolar depression. Lithium is effective in both psychotic and nonpsychotic bipolar episodes and in rapid cycling. However, the presence of mixed states may predict a poorer response.

In addition, studies have found significant improvement in unipolar depression when lithium is used to augment a partial antidepressant response. In the large Sequenced Treatment Alternatives to Relieve Depression (STAR*D) trial, 16% of participants who did not attain remission of their unipolar depression with citalopram monotherapy and another medication trial did successfully achieve remission following the addition of lithium.

Meta-analyses of studies on lithium treatment in major mood disorders have found significantly lower suicide risk in patients receiving lithium treatment. One systematic review in 2020 included 16 ecological studies, 11 of which showed a significant inverse association between lithium levels in drinking water and suicide rates. This finding supports growing evidence that routine consumption of lithium in tap water also may have antisuicidal effects in the general population.

Lithium's potential role in the prevention of neurocognitive decline has also been suggested. A Danish study that followed up with more than 4,800 patients with newly diagnosed bipolar disorder for 10 years found that long-term treatment with lithium, but not with other psychopharmacological agents, was associated with a reduced risk of developing dementia. However, studies in primary dementias are less supportive of the therapeutic value of lithium.

Standard Dosing and Treatment Regimen

A typical dosage range for lithium is 600–2,400 mg/day. Dosing is guided by the patient's blood lithium levels, with a usual target of 0.6–1.2 mmol/L. Lithium levels should be measured 5 days after the most recent dosage change and then every 3–6 months thereafter. Kidney and thyroid function should also be assessed every 2–3 months during those first 6 months of lithium treatment. After the first 6 months, kidney and thyroid function, plus calcium, should be tested every 6–12 months.

Special Populations

Age Groups

Lithium is FDA-approved for the treatment of bipolar disorder in children as young as 12 years of age. Lithium is similarly effective, especially for mania, in adolescents, adults, and elderly populations, but the dosage required to achieve therapeutic serum concentrations decreases threefold from middle to old age due to the declining renal function that occurs as we age.

Pregnancy

Studies suggest that lithium exposure during pregnancy may increase the risk of miscarriage, especially first-trimester exposure. Although the overall risk of *Ebstein's anomaly*—a rare cardiac malformation with an incidence of 1 in 20,000 live births—may be higher with lithium use, the absolute risk associated with lithium exposure in the first trimester is thought to be less than 0.1%. In newborns, lithium exposure has been associated with hypoglycemia, nephrogenic diabetes insipidus, thyroid dysfunction, and lithium toxicity. Lithium is secreted in breast milk and passed on to the infant in clinically significant levels, with the potential to cause transient changes in infant kidney and thyroid function.

Medication Interactions

Lithium is commonly used in combination with other mood stabilizers and antipsychotics. Although such combinations can be synergistic, polypharmacy may increase the risk of adverse reactions. Lithium is almost entirely metabolized renally, so direct medication interactions are limited to other renally metabolized substances. For example, nonsteroidal anti-inflammatory drugs (NSAIDs), certain blood pressure medications, alcohol, and caffeine can alter lithium levels. Indirect interactions occur when compounds share common adverse events; for example, when lithium is used with serotonergic antidepressants, serotonin syndrome has been reported, albeit rarely.

Side Effects

Side effects of lithium may include feeling mentally slow, postural tremor, hypothyroidism, hyperthyroidism, hypercalcemia, hyperparathyroidism, and weight gain. In one double-blind trial, the average weight change over 1 year among participants was 4 kg. Lithium can induce nephrogenic diabetes insipidus, which results in the production of large-volume dilute urine, along with excessive thirst; this is usually reversible with discontinuation of the lithium. Chronic kidney disease may occur following 10–20 years of lithium treatment, although the risk of progressing to end-stage renal disease is very low (0.5%–1%). Lithium is associated with cardiac effects ranging from harmless electrocardiographic changes to fatal arrhythmias that are fortunately quite uncommon. Lithium is also associated with acne, psoriasis, eczema, hair loss, hidradenitis suppurativa, nail changes, and mucosal lesions. At toxic levels, it may cause coarse tremor, gait disturbance, delirium, memory deficits, coma, and death. Abrupt discontinuation of lithium is associated with relapse into mood episodes and suicidal behavior.

Conclusion

Lithium is a naturally occurring element and a first-line treatment for bipolar mania, depression, and maintenance. Its affordability, efficacy, and unique neuroprotective properties have given it unrivaled longevity in psychiatry.

Recommended Reading

Almeida J, Spelber D, Smith T: Lithium, in The American Psychiatric Association Publishing Textbook of Psychopharmacology, 6th Edition. Edited by Schatzberg AF, Nemeroff CB. Washington, DC, American Psychiatric Association Publishing, 2024, pp. 977–1010

Bauer M, Gitlin M: The Essential Guide to Lithium Treatment. New York, Springer, 2016

37

Lamotrigine

Erin C. Richardson, M.S.N., R.N., APRN, PMHNP-BC
D. Jeffrey Newport, M.D., M.S., M.Div.

Introduction

Lamotrigine was initially developed as an antiepileptic drug. Since its approval by the U.S. Food and Drug Administration (FDA) for seizure disorders in 1994, it has gained traction as a treatment for psychiatric disorders, most notably being FDA-approved as a maintenance treatment for bipolar disorder.

How Does It Work?

Lamotrigine blocks sodium and calcium channels on the surface of nerve cells, which in turn regulate the release of neurotransmitters such as glutamate and aspartate. It also has weak effects on serotonin and γ-aminobutyric acid (GABA) activity. However, it is unclear which, if any, of these effects within the synapse explain lamotrigine's beneficial effects on mood or seizure control.

What Is Lamotrigine Used to Treat?

Lamotrigine's only FDA approval for a psychiatric illness is as a maintenance treatment of bipolar I disorder in adults. Understanding lamotrigine's role in bipolar disorder requires careful consideration. As a maintenance treatment, lamotrigine helps adults with bipolar disorder who are currently well—that is, not depressed, manic, or hypomanic—to remain well longer. Indeed, multiple studies found maintenance therapy with lamotrigine, used alone or in combination with other mood stabilizers, was effective in prolonging time to a subsequent relapse into a bipolar depressive episode. However, lamotrigine is not effective for the treatment of manic, hypomanic, or mixed episodes. In addition, results for acute depressive episodes of bipolar disorder are inconsistent, with many studies finding lamotrigine treatment helpful but others showing no benefit. Finally, most studies indicate that lamotrigine is not helpful for rapid-cycling bipolar disorder, although one study did suggest it may improve stability.

Lamotrigine has been used off-label by psychiatrists for other psychiatric illnesses, including posttraumatic stress disorder (PTSD), obsessive-compulsive disorder (OCD), and borderline personality disorder; unfortunately, however, the data supporting its use for other psychiatric disorders are scant. For example, lamotrigine's "mood stabilizing" properties for bipolar disorder have led some to use it off-label for borderline personality disorder; however, few data support this practice. Although some studies found lamotrigine decreases impulsivity and affective instability in patients with borderline personality disorder, most show it to be no more effective than placebo. Studies of its use for autism spectrum disorder and depersonalization disorder also have shown no benefit, and most studies in treatment-resistant depression indicate that it is likewise ineffective.

A single preliminary study has suggested lamotrigine may relieve the avoidance and reexperiencing symptoms of PTSD. Another study indicated that lamotrigine augmentation of a selective serotonin reuptake inhibitor (SSRI) may improve OCD, although lamotrigine alone offers no benefit for OCD. Two preliminary studies have reported mixed results for lamotrigine in treating binge-eating disorder.

Research for the use of lamotrigine in psychotic disorders is also equivocal. Some studies suggest that adding lamotrigine to typical and atypical antipsychotics, including clozapine, helps relieve the positive symptoms and general psychopathology of psychotic disorders, but other studies have found no benefit.

Finally, lamotrigine has also been studied in the treatment of chronic pain; however, most studies have demonstrated no benefit. Preliminary evidence indicates that it may afford relief from HIV-related neuropathic pain and central poststroke pain.

Standard Dosing and Treatment Regimen

Lamotrigine's target dosage for treatment of bipolar disorder is 200 mg/day. Due to the risk of medication interactions, the target dosage for patients also taking valproate is only 100 mg/day, and the target dosage for those also taking carbamazepine (Tegretol) is 400 mg/day. Lamotrigine must be started much lower than the target dosage and increased upward in a slow, stepwise manner, in accordance with a detailed schedule, to decrease the risk of developing a serious rash. Patients begin by taking 25 mg/day for the first 2 weeks, 50 mg/day for the next 2 weeks, and then 100 mg/day beginning in the fifth week. Again, due to the risk of interactions, patients who are taking valproate start lamotrigine at half the 25-mg/day dosage, and those who are taking carbamazepine begin at twice the 25-mg/day dosage.

Patients who have been taking a stable lamotrigine dosage but miss doses for as few as 3–4 days should not immediately resume taking the previous dosage. Instead, to minimize the risk of rash, they must restart at the 25-mg/day entry dosage and again gradually increase to the target dosage.

Use in Special Populations

Children and Adolescents

Lamotrigine is not approved for the treatment of any psychiatric condition in youth; however, it is approved for the treatment of epilepsy in children as young as 2 years. When children are treated with lamotrigine, dosing is determined by the child's weight. Although some clinicians may use lamotrigine as an off-label treatment for mood disorders in adolescents, there are limited data to support this practice.

Pregnancy

Because of lamotrigine's favorable reproductive safety profile, especially compared with many other antiepileptics and mood stabilizers, it is commonly used during pregnancy. Doing so, however, requires careful dosage management. Lamotrigine is metabolized in a unique way by a single enzyme that is induced by estrogen. Thus, as estrogen levels steadily climb during pregnancy, lamotrigine levels fall, and the dosage may need to be repeatedly increased in order to offset this more rapid estrogen-induced metabolism. The dosage is then reduced after delivery as the patient's estrogen levels quickly return to pre-pregnancy levels.

Elderly Patients

There are no dosage adjustments required for use of lamotrigine in the geriatric population.

Medication Interactions

Valproate

Valproate slows the metabolism and clearance of lamotrigine, increasing lamotrigine levels by as much as 50%–60%. Those taking valproate together with lamotrigine require half the usual dosage of lamotrigine and should use a slower titration schedule when starting lamotrigine.

Carbamazepine

Carbamazepine has the opposite effect of valproate in that it increases the metabolism and clearance of lamotrigine, thus lowering its levels by 30%–50%. As a result, patients taking carbamazepine together with lamotrigine need higher lamotrigine dosages and use a more rapid titration schedule. Oxcarbazepine (Trileptal), an antiepileptic medication related to carbamazepine, does not impact lamotrigine clearance; therefore, lamotrigine dosage adjustment is not necessary when the two medications are used together.

Estrogen

Estrogen-containing agents, including contraceptives and hormone replacement treatments, increase the body's metabolism and clearance of lamotrigine in the same way as naturally occurring estrogen, decreasing lamotrigine levels by as much as 50%. Patients taking estrogen-containing medications may therefore need a higher dosage of lamotrigine. Progestin-only contraceptives do not impact lamotrigine levels.

Side Effects

Lamotrigine is generally well tolerated, with side effect rates comparable with those of placebo. In particular, it is not associated with weight gain or the so-called metabolic syndrome that plagues many medications used to treat bipolar disorder. Its chief safety concern, which prompted an FDA "black box warning," is a risk of rash, from benign to severe, when starting treatment. When lamotrigine is discontinued because the patient develops a mild rash, some evidence suggests it may be reintroduced later using a slower dosage titration schedule; however, this should not be attempted if the patient develops a severe rash.

Lamotrigine has been associated specifically with an increased risk of Stevens-Johnson syndrome (SJS), a serious life-threatening rash accompanied by a systemic hypersensitivity reaction. Development of SJS mandates immediate discontinuation of lamotrigine and may necessitate hospitalization. Patients who develop flu-like symptoms, runny nose, fatigue, patchy reddening of the skin, or a rash when starting lamotrigine should seek an emergency evaluation for SJS. Fortunately, SJS is rare, occurring in 0.08%–1.3% of participants in lamotrigine research studies. The greatest risk for severe rash, including SJS, occurs during the first 2 months of lamotrigine treatment. Other risk factors include age (pediatric), rapidly increasing the dosage, concurrent treatment with valproate, and a particular human leukocyte antigen phenotype (*HLA-B*15:02*) that can be determined with laboratory testing.

Lamotrigine has also been linked with an even more rare condition called *hemophagocytic lymphohistiocytosis*, in which a hyperactive immune system causes widespread inflammation and organ damage. Symptoms include high fever, rash, jaundice, upper right abdomen tenderness or swelling, swollen lymph nodes, difficulty walking, and visual disturbances. Fortunately, this condition is extremely rare, with only eight cases reported among patients taking lamotrigine since the medication was introduced in 1994.

Lamotrigine exposure is rarely associated with toxicity; however, large overdoses may lead to seizures, heart arrhythmias, altered consciousness or coma, and death. In severe cases of lamotrigine overdose, activated charcoal, gastric lavage, and dialysis may be necessary.

Conclusion

Aside from a few rare but serious side effects, lamotrigine is a well tolerated and efficacious medication indicated for maintenance treatment of bipolar disorder. Whether used alone or in combination with other mood stabilizers, it can prolong the time to a depressive relapse for patients with bipolar disorder. Scant data support lamotrigine for other psychiatric illnesses, although it is often used off-label. Lamotrigine must be started slowly at first due to the risk of a serious rash, and it should be restarted if more than 3 days' doses have been missed. Notable interactions that occur with carbamazepine, valproate, and estrogen may be managed successfully by dosage adjustments. Its favorable reproductive safety profile makes lamotrigine a reasonable option for pregnant people with bipolar disorder.

Recommended Reading

Edinoff AN, Nguyen LH, Fitz-Gerald MJ, et al. Lamotrigine and Stevens-Johnson syndrome prevention. Psychopharmacol Bull 51(2):96–114, 2021 34092825

Geddes JR, Calabrese JR, Goodwin GM. Lamotrigine for treatment of bipolar depression: independent meta-analysis and meta-regression of individual patient data from five randomised trials. Br J Psychiatry 194(1):4–9, 2009 19118318

38

Valproate

Ihsan M. Salloum, M.D., M.P.H.

Introduction

Valproate and its different formulations (valproic acid, divalproex sodium) are anticonvulsants that have multiple U.S. Food and Drug Administration (FDA)-approved indications and several off-label uses in psychiatric disorders. Valproic acid is a 2-propyl valeric acid, an eight-carbon branched short chain fatty acid derived from valeric acid of the valerian root *Valeriana officinalis*. It was first synthesized in 1881 and used as an inert solvent in medical research. The anticonvulsant effects of valproic acid were discovered serendipitously in 1963, and valproate was introduced as an antiepileptic in France in 1967. The antimanic and prophylactic activities of valproate were first reported in France, and its efficacy in bipolar disorder was then tested in Germany in the early 1980s and subsequently in the United States. Controlled studies in the United States then demonstrated the efficacy of valproate monotherapy for acute mania. The FDA approved divalproex sodium for treatment of acute mania in 1995.

Valproate has broad therapeutic potential due to its multiple pharmacological actions. It substantially increases γ-aminobutyric acid (GABA) levels, delays the activation of voltage-dependent sodium channels, and protects neurons from the toxic excitatory action of glutamate, in addition to regulating several cellular and transcription mechanisms. It has established efficacy for acute mania and has been found effective for rapid cycling moods, dysphoric mania, and maintenance treatment. Valproate is used in other psychiatric disorders to target impulsivity, aggression, and affective instability and is also useful in decreasing alcohol use in bipolar disorder. It is generally well tolerated by most patients, although rare but serious side effects may occur. Valproate has a substantial risk of producing malformation if used in pregnancy and has a complex medication interaction profile. Use of therapeutic drug monitoring along with regular clinical monitoring should enhance the safe use of valproate.

How Does It Work?

Valproate has multiple pharmacological actions that may explain its broad therapeutic potential. It substantially increases GABA levels, which is thought to occur via several mechanisms. It enhances GABA release through a presynaptic effect on $GABA_B$ receptors, activates enzymes involved in GABA synthesis, and inhibits enzymes involved in its degradation. These effects on GABA have been linked to valproate's antimanic and antiseizure properties. Valproate delays the activation of voltage-dependent sodium channels, suppressing high-frequency, repetitive neuronal firing, and appears to protect neurons from the toxic excitatory action of glutamate.

Furthermore, valproate appears to regulate several cellular mechanisms. Like lithium, it aids in cytoskeleton remodeling. Valproate treatment increases the growth cone area in cultured sensory neurons. It is reported to have differential effects on growth, proliferation, and differentiation in many types of cells and appears to inhibit mechanisms involved in programmed cell death. Valproate also controls the mechanism by which the genetic code is transcribed to make protein by inhibiting, in a dose-dependent manner, the expression of histone deacetylases. This mechanism is thought to underlie the birth defects caused by valproate.

What Is Valproate Used to Treat?

Approved Indications

The only FDA-approved indications for valproate in psychiatry are for the treatment of bipolar disorder. The divalproex sodium formulation is approved for the treatment of acute mania, and divalproex sodium extended-release is approved for the acute treatment of bipolar-associated manic or mixed episodes, with or without psychotic features. Valproate is also FDA-approved for the treatment of various seizure disorders and for migraine prophylaxis. Its efficacy in acute mania is well established by several randomized trials, and its use in acute mania is recommended by several clinical practice guidelines. Randomized trials have also reported valproate to be effective in mixed and rapid cycling variants of bipolar disorder.

Off-Label Use

Valproate was evaluated in controlled trials for the maintenance treatment of bipolar disorder and found to be more effective than placebo in preventing future bipolar episodes. Several studies have reported valproate to be as effective as lithium carbonate in the maintenance therapy of bipolar disorder, although other studies showed lithium to be more effective. The combination of lithium and valproate was found to be more effective than valproate alone in preventing future episodes. Findings are inconsistent regarding the efficacy of valproate in the treatment of bipolar depression. Bipolar disorder in individuals with a history of mixed episodes, rapid cycling, or a higher number of prior episodes appears to have responded better to valproate than to lithium.

Valproate has been used off-label in a number of other psychiatric disorders to target, in most cases, a specific symptom cluster. Valproate added to antipsychotics improved the symptoms of schizophrenia, and when added to clozapine treatment for schizophrenia, it led to a greater reduction in aggression and anxiety-like symptoms than clozapine alone. Valproate decreased anxiety symptoms in anxiety disorders, obsessive-compulsive disorder (OCD), and borderline personality disorder and, compared with placebo, decreased heavy alcohol use in bipolar disorder. It has proven helpful in the treatment of alcohol withdrawal and in preventing relapse to alcohol use in people with alcohol use disorder. Furthermore, valproate added to dextromethorphan substantially improved neurotrophic activity in bipolar disorder. Case reports and open-label trials have shown valproate to be useful for the treatment of agitation, aggression, impulsivity, and affective instability in patients with brain injury, dementia, or borderline personality disorder.

Use of valproate in youth is based on small trials, open-label studies, and case reports. It was found useful in the treatment of rapid cycling or dysphoric mania that did not respond to lithium and in the treatment of the depressive phase in bipolar II disorders. It also improved aggression in children with oppositional defiant disorder, conduct disorder, and disruptive behavior disorders and reduced impulsivity and aggression in those with autism spectrum disorders.

Standard Dosing and Treatment Regimen

Valproic acid is available in enteric-coated immediate-release, delayed-release (12-hour), and extended-release (24-hour) oral preparations, typically as divalproex sodium. The delayed-release formulation is available in 125-mg, 250-mg, and 500-mg tablets as well as 125-mg sprinkle capsules, and its initial recommended dosage for the treatment of mania is 750 mg/day, in divided doses. The extended-release form is available in 250-mg and 500-mg tablets intended for once-daily oral administration, and the initial recommended dosage for mania is 25 mg/kg/day. The maximum recommended dosage is 60 mg/kg/day for both formulations. The therapeutic daily dosages range from 500 mg to 2 g in adults or from 15 mg/kg to 60 mg/kg in children. The initial dosage is increased as rapidly as tolerated to achieve therapeutic plasma levels (trough plasma concentration between 50 μg/mL and 125 μg/mL) and treatment response.

Valproic acid is rapidly absorbed following oral administration. Peak serum levels depend on the formulation: 1–4 hours for valproic acid; 3–5 hours for divalproex sodium, which increases to 4–8 hours it is when taken with food; and 4–17 hours for extended-release divalproex sodium. Its serum half-life typically falls in the range of 9–19 hours. The medication is rapidly distributed throughout the body, and it is strongly bound (90%) to plasma protein. Valproate is primarily metabolized in the liver to the glucuronide conjugate. Valproate and its metabolites are excreted primarily in urine, with minor amounts excreted in feces and expired air.

Use in Special Populations

Children and Adolescents

Studies in children and adolescents (age range 10–17 years, or 3–10 years with seizure) have reported the safety and tolerability of valproate to be comparable with those of adults. Medication-related adverse reactions included somnolence, nausea, upper abdominal pain, gastritis, rash, and increased ammonia. Monitoring of total serum valproic acid concentrations is limited by variability in the free fraction of serum valproic acid. Factors that influence hepatic metabolism and protein binding should be considered when interpreting valproic acid concentrations in children. Pediatric patients younger than 2 years are at high risk of fatal hepatotoxicity, especially those with mental retardation or developmental disorders. The risk of fatal hepatotoxicity decreases progressively after age 2. Compared with adults, children younger than 10 years have 50% higher clearances of valproate, whereas those 10 and older have clearance similar to adults.

Pregnancy and Lactation

Valproate should not be administered to patients of childbearing potential unless no alternative treatments are available and the patients' condition warrants use after a risk-benefit analysis has been performed. A fetus that has been exposed to valproate is at high risk for decreased IQ, neurodevelopmental disorders, neuronal tube defects, and other major congenital malformations, such as craniofacial defects (e.g., oral clefts), cardiovascular malformations, hypospadias, and limb malformations. These effects usually occur early in pregnancy, and the risk is dose-dependent. The rate of malformations is four times higher among offspring exposed to valproate than among those who were not exposed to antiseizure medications. Observational studies have reported an increased risk of autism spectrum disorder and attention-deficit/hyperactivity disorder (ADHD) among valproate-exposed infants, and these infants are also at a higher risk for hypoglycemia, fatal hepatic failure, and potentially fatal hemorrhagic complications as a result of valproate-induced clotting abnormalities in the childbearing parent. Thus, clotting parameters should be routinely monitored in the parent. Abrupt valproate discontinuation in females with epilepsy may precipitate status epilepticus, with resulting parental and fetal hypoxia.

Patients of childbearing potential should use effective contraception while taking valproate and should receive regular counseling about the relative risks and benefits of valproate use during pregnancy. Alternative therapeutic options should be considered, especially for females who are at the onset of puberty and those planning a pregnancy. Folic acid supplementation, up to 5 mg/day, is suggested for patients who are taking valproate when they become pregnant and during their first trimester in order to decrease the risk for valproate-induced congenital neural tube defects and congenital and developmental abnormalities in the fetus.

Valproate is excreted in human breast milk, with an estimated concentration of 1%–10% of the parent's serum level. The effects of valproate on milk production or excretion are not known; however, children exposed to valproate during gestation and breastfeeding had lower IQs at age 6, and hepatic failure and clotting abnormalities have been reported. Breastfed infants should be monitored for jaundice or unusual bruising.

Elderly Patients

Elderly patients are more sensitive to the effects of valproate because of the decrease in their unbound clearance of the medication and their greater sensitivity to somnolence. The starting dosage of valproate should be reduced in this patient population, and the treatment dosage should be increased more slowly than in younger patients. Elderly patients should be monitored regularly for adverse reactions such as somnolence, dehydration, and reduced fluid and nutritional intake, and the dosage should be adjusted or the medication discontinued if such reactions occur.

Medication Interactions

Valproate has been reported to have undesirable interactions with many medications. According to Drugs.com, 386 agents had been reported to interact with valproate as of January 2023. Interactions occur because of the *pharmacokinetic* (i.e., absorption, distribution, metabolism, and excretion) and the *pharmacodynamic* (i.e., end-organ effects, classified as additive, synergistic, and antagonistic) effects of the medications used. Valproate interactions can be reciprocal and carry important therapeutic implications, including hepatic enzyme induction or inhibition, protein displacement, and pharmacodynamic interactions. The latter refers to the target effect of valproate, such as the brain. For example, valproate can cause sedation and somnolence, and this effect may be worsened if it is used with another medication that has the same side effect.

Valproate has hepatic enzyme inhibition effects on several medications, leading to an increased blood levels and potential effects/toxicity. These include, among others, lamotrigine, ethosuximide, phenobarbital, primidone, diazepam, phenytoin, amitriptyline/nortriptyline, and paliperidone. This interaction may result in a need for dosage adjustment of the affected medications. On the other hand, fluoxetine, fluvoxamine, and felbamate may decrease valproate clearance and increase its blood levels due to their hepatic enzyme inhibition of valproate metabolism.

Valproate acts as a mild hepatic enzyme inducer of olanzapine and aripiprazole. Conversely, valproate metabolism is highly inducible, which may result in decreased blood levels when it is taken along with some of the major anticonvulsants, such as carbamazepine and phenytoin, or with oral contraceptives.

Valproate has a protein-binding displacement activity that can result in increased bioavailability of the displaced agent, such as warfarin. Adjustment of the displaced medication (in this example, warfarin) and decreased dosage may be required. Conversely, valproate may be displaced by salicylates and free fatty acids, thus increasing its bioavailability and effects. The valproate and concomitant medication concentration levels should be monitored whenever interacting agents are introduced or withdrawn.

A number of medications administered with valproate can cause undesirable side effects by augmenting valproate's adverse effects. For example, the co-administration of valproate and topiramate increases patients' risk of hyperammonemia and encephalopathy; valproate use with the anticancer medication bexarotene increases their risk of pancreatic inflammation; and its use with the antiseizure agent eslicarbazepine may cause respiratory depression, sedation, and impaired attention, judgment, and psychomotor skills. Co-administration of valproate with olanzapine significantly increases patients' glycosylated hemoglobin (HbA1c), body mass index (BMI), weight, triglycerides, and triglyceride/high-density lipoprotein cholesterol compared with olanzapine alone. Risperidone administered with valproate produces similar but substantially smaller increases in these parameters.

Side Effects

Valproate is well tolerated by most patients; however, adverse effects may occur, including gastrointestinal symptoms such as upset stomach, loss of appetite, nausea, vomiting and diarrhea, and weight loss or gain. Less common adverse effects may include tremor, drowsiness, skin rash, temporary hair loss, muscle weakness, liver test abnormalities, and anemia. Others include decreased platelets, which may lead to susceptibility to bleeding, and increased ammonia levels, which may lead to confusion and organic brain syndrome. Serious reactions have been reported, such as pancreatitis and liver failure, although these are rare. Fatalities have been reported, mostly due to liver failures in a very small number of patients receiving valproate; these reports mostly involved patients younger than 2 years. Liver failure is believed to be due to an idiosyncratic reaction, not due to dosage, because it occurred in patients taking a wide range of dosages and with a variety of blood levels. Other rare and potentially serious side effects include hyponatremia; syndrome of inappropriate antidiuretic hormone secretion (SIADH) with water retention; hallucinations; psychosis; suicidality; severe skin conditions, such as toxic epidermal necrolysis, erythema multiforme, and Stevens-Johnson syndrome; problems with producing blood components due to bone marrow suppression; polycystic ovarian syndrome; hyperammonemia; hypothermia; cerebral pseudoatrophy; encephalopathy; and coma.

When valproate is to be discontinued, the dosage should be tapered down because sudden stoppage can cause withdrawal seizure in patients with seizure disorders. Contraindications to valproate include significant hepatic impairment, hypersensitivity to the medication, urea cycle disorders, mitochondrial disorders, or suspected disorders in patients younger than 2 years and patients who are pregnant (as in prophylactic use of valproic acid for migraine headache).

Valproate Poisoning

The most common manifestation of valproic acid poisoning is central nervous system dysfunction. Although most patients experience mild to moderate lethargy and recover, valproate toxicity can progress in severity to cerebral edema and fatal outcome. Symptom progression is rapid, although it could be slowed with the ingestion of delayed-release preparations. Symptoms of valproate toxicity and overdose include respiratory depression, tachycardia, hypertension, hyperthermia, hyperammonemia, hypernatremia, hyperosmolality, hypocalcemia, and metabolic acidosis. Gastrointestinal symptoms include vomiting, diarrhea, and hepatitis. Other neurological symptoms such as meiosis (pinpoint pupils), agitation, tremor, and myoclonus or muscle fasciculation can occur. Valproate serum levels should be monitored closely. Valproate is 90% protein-bound at serum therapeutic levels (trough) (85–125 μg/mL); toxic levels are those higher than 175 μg/mL (trough), and unbound, active free valproate increases with rising levels. Levels higher than 450 mg/L have been determined to cause severe life-threatening clinical manifestations. Treatment of valproate poisoning may include general supportive measures; gastrointestinal decontamination, such as the use of activated charcoal; naloxone for patients with depressed mental status; L-carnitine therapy for those with hyperammonemia, lethargy, coma, or hepatic dysfunction; and hemodialysis when indicated.

Conclusion

Discovery of the therapeutic action of valproate in bipolar disorder was an important addition to the treatment of this condition. Valproate is generally well tolerated and lacks many long-term side effects such as the movement disorders or severe metabolic syndrome related to first- and second-generations antipsychotics. However, valproate may have severe side effects, such as fetal malformation. It is safe when caution is observed in terms of the patient's general health condition and concomitant medications.

Recommended Reading

Crapanzano C, Casolaro I, Amendola C, et al: Lithium and valproate in bipolar disorder: from international evidence-based guidelines to clinical predictors. Clin Psychopharmacol Neurosci 20(3):403–414, 2022 35879025

Nayak R, Rosh I, Kustanovich I, Stern S: Mood stabilizers in psychiatric disorders and mechanisms learnt from in vitro model systems. Int J Mol Sci 22(17):9315, 2021 34502224

39

Carbamazepine

Robert M. Post, M.D.

Introduction

Carbamazepine is a major anticonvulsant for the treatment of temporal lobe epilepsy and trigeminal neuralgia that is also approved by the U.S. Food and Drug Administration (FDA) for the treatment of acute mania in patients with bipolar disorder. It works rapidly in patients with acute mania and can be started at doses of 200 mg two or three times a day, slowly increasing to a target dosage of 1,200 mg/day or a maximum of 1,600 mg/day.

How Does It Work?

The mechanism of action of carbamazepine in the treatment of epilepsy and trigeminal neuralgia is thought to be related to its acute effects in blocking sodium channels. However, because its maximal effects in depression occur only after several weeks, more chronic effects of carbamazepine could be implicated. The medication's antidepressant effects may be mediated by those atypical of many other antidepressant modalities; for example, most antidepressant medications decrease β-adrenergic receptors in the prefrontal cortex, but carbamazepine upregulates them. Most antidepressants upregulate mineralocorticoid and glucocorticoid receptors and therefore decrease cortisol, whereas carbamazepine increases plasma and urinary free cortisol. This unusual profile may explain why carbamazepine is effective for some depressed patients who have affective syndromes that are resistant to more traditional antidepressant modalities. However, like other mood-stabilizing and antidepressant modalities, carbamazepine increases levels of brain-derived neurotropic factor, which is often reduced in depression.

What Is Carbamazepine Used to Treat?

Carbamazepine is the most potent anticonvulsant, stopping seizures generated by repeated amygdala stimulation. This could be of importance in the treatment of depression and posttraumatic stress disorder (PTSD), in which there is evidence of amygdalar hyperactivity. Among depressed patients who were studied using positron emission tomography (PET) scans, those whose depression responded to carbamazepine were uniformly in the group demonstrating cortical and limbic hypermetabolism, in contrast to the typical association of depression with reduced cortical metabolism.

Carbamazepine is also effective but not FDA-approved for long-term prophylaxis of manic and depressive episodes. It works alone or as an adjunct to lithium in many patients whose condition responds inadequately to lithium. In fact, carbamazepine works well in patients who demonstrate all of the predictors of a poor response to lithium, including those with mixed or dysphoric mania; a bipolar II disorder rather than bipolar I disorder diagnosis; a history of anxiety disorders and substance abuse comorbidities; schizoaffective illness with mood-incongruent delusions; rapid or continuous cycling episodes; and a negative family history of bipolar disorder.

Carbamazepine is also effective in acute depression and prevention of depression, but it is not FDA-approved for these indications. One small series documented the antidepressant effects of carbamazepine utilizing a double-blind, placebo-controlled, off-on-off-on study design. When carbamazepine was substituted for placebo, participants' depression improved; when placebo was given instead of carbamazepine, their mood deteriorated but improved again when carbamazepine was added back.

In long-term treatment, loss of efficacy with carbamazepine (i.e., tolerance to its therapeutic effects) has been reported in a small percentage of patients, sometimes after many years of good response. This kind of tolerance is not a result of low blood levels of carbamazepine. Tolerance can be managed by adding other prophylactic medications that have different mechanisms of action or by implementing a period of time off carbamazepine and then restarting the medication later.

Standard Dosing and Treatment Regimen

Carbamazepine should be started at low dosages, especially for depression treatment, and titrated upward according to clinical effectiveness or the emergence of side effects. Routine monitoring of blood levels is not needed or indicated because there is no relationship of blood levels to clinical response. Moreover, the dosages and blood levels associated with the development of side effects vary widely; some people will experience side effects at a low blood level (4 μg/mL) and others at 6–8 μg/mL, whereas others may experience few or no side effects at dosages as high as 1,600 mg/day that achieve blood levels of 12 μg/mL or higher.

Carbamazepine in available in an immediate-release preparation, Tegretol, and extended-release preparations called Equetro and Carbitrol. If immediate-release carbamazepine is titrated upward too quickly, it can lead to breakthrough side effects about 2 hours after a given dose. Equetro has a smoother course of blood levels and the entire dose can be given at night, which can help with sleep. The lower blood levels thus achieved during the day are associated with fewer side effects. The half-life of one acute dose of carbamazepine is about 26 hours but with chronic administration decreases to about 12 hours.

Carbamazepine is converted to a 10,11 epoxide metabolite that also has anticonvulsant effects. With enzyme induction, after several weeks the amount of carbamazepine converted to the 10,11 epoxide is increased. Because this is not measured in conventional carbamazepine assays, its contribution to efficacy or side effects may be missed.

Medication Interactions

Carbamazepine induces liver enzymes of the cytochrome P450 3A4 (CYP3A4) subtype. This enzyme induction leads to lower blood levels of carbamazepine (*auto-induction*) after 2–3 weeks and to lower blood levels of many other medications metabolized by CYP3A4, including many of the atypical antipsychotics (e.g., quetiapine, aripiprazole, lurasidone, brexpiprazole, lumateperone, cariprazine). The dosages of these medications thus may need to be increased several weeks after starting carbamazepine. Some agents, such as erythromycin (and related antibiotics) and some calcium channel blockers (e.g., verapamil and diltiazem), are strong inhibitors of the action of CYP3A4 and can result in increased carbamazepine blood levels and the emergence of side effects. It is best to inform your pharmacist that you are taking carbamazepine so that they, as well as your physician, can watch out for the common interactions associated with the medication.

Carbamazepine will increase the metabolism of estrogen in birth control formulations, resulting in occasional unwanted pregnancies. Therefore, a higher-dosage form of the estrogen component or other contraceptive devices should be used. Carbamazepine is a category D substance and should be avoided during pregnancy. There is a several-percentage higher risk of spina bifida with the use of carbamazepine, and this appears to increase with anticonvulsant combination treatment.

An analogue of carbamazepine called oxcarbazepine is not a strong inducer of CYP3A4 enzymes and thus has fewer medication interactions. Its clinical profile is somewhat similar to that of carbamazepine, but it is not FDA-approved for treatment of mania. Studies suggest it may be less effective in patients with more severe or psychotic mania for whom carbamazepine is more effective.

Side Effects

Typical side effects emerging when the carbamazepine dosage is too high are dizziness, ataxia, or double vision. If these occur with initial dosing, the dosage can be reduced; later, when enzyme induction has occurred, the higher dosage may be well tolerated.

Carbamazepine can induce a mild lowering of the white blood cell (WBC) count because it blocks the effects of colony stimulating factor. Lithium stimulates colony stimulating factor and increases WBC counts; therefore, it can normalize the low counts caused by carbamazepine. However, mild lowering of the WBCs should be distinguished from more serious but rare hematological side effects, including the loss of WBCs (*agranulocytosis*) or the complete suppression of blood cell formation (WBCs, red blood cells, and platelets), called *aplastic anemia*. Because these unpredictable occurrences can manifest rapidly from a relatively normal baseline, most epileptologists do not recommend regular monitoring. Instead, they warn that if patients develop a fever or sore throat (due to the loss of WBCs) or red spots on the skin (*petechiae*, due to the loss of platelets), their physician should order an immediate complete blood count to rule out these two serious side effects. The incidence of agranulocytosis is about five to eight times higher in patients taking carbamazepine than in the general population (which is 6 per 1,000,000 of the population per year), and the incidence of aplastic anemia with carbamazepine is between 1 per 50,000 and 1 per 200,000 exposed patients, which is higher than that in the general population (for whom the incidence is about 2 per 1,000,000 of the population per year).

A serious rash progressing to sloughing of the skin, either Stevens-Johnson syndrome or toxic epidermal necrolysis, can occur with carbamazepine. It is difficult to distinguish a benign rash from these more serious forms, so the medication should be discontinued with the emergence of any rash. Considerable progress has been made in studying the pharmacogenomics of serious rash with carbamazepine. The human lymphocyte antigen *HLA-B*1502* has been associated with this syndrome in patients of Asian descent, and genetic screening may be useful in these individuals. In contrast, the risk of serious rash is lower among individuals of northern European descent, on the order of 1–6 per 10,000, and is associated with *HLA-A*3101* (which occurs in 2%–5% of Europeans), so the utility of genetic screening in these individuals is less certain.

Carbamazepine can raise cholesterol by about 20 points, but it also increases low-density lipoproteins (which are favorable), so its cardiovascular effects are uncertain. The cardiac effects are generally not prominent, although the medication does decrease atrioventricular conduction, and it is relatively contraindicated in patients with heart block. Homocysteine increases and folate decreases have been reported, so treatment with folate may also be helpful. Vitamin D levels may also be lowered by carbamazepine, with or without associated increases in osteoporosis. Whereas lithium is a blocker of vasopressin secretion through its inhibition of the second messenger cyclic adenosine monophosphate, carbamazepine appears to exert indirect facilitatory effects at the vasopressin receptor. It can also induce low levels of serum sodium (hyponatremia), particularly at high dosages and in females, which can be reversed or prevented by lithium.

Conclusion

Although carbamazepine is not as popular as a treatment for bipolar disorder now as it was several decades ago, because of its unusual properties, clinical efficacy, and mechanisms of action it may still have an important role in the treatment of patients with bipolar disorder, particularly those whose condition does not respond well enough to lithium and other mood stabilizers.

Recommended Reading

Post RM: Carbamazepine, in Comprehensive Textbook on Psychiatry. Edited by Sadock BJ, Sadock VA, Ruiz P. New York, Lippincott Williams and Williams, 2017

Post RM, Ketter TA, Uhde T, et al: Thirty years of clinical experience with carbamazepine in the treatment of bipolar illness: principles and practice. CNS Drugs 21(1):47–71, 2007 17190529

40

Other Anticonvulsants

Pregabalin, Gabapentin, and Topiramate

Mark A. Frye, M.D.
Balwinder Singh, M.D., M.S.

Introduction

Anticonvulsants were initially developed to treat convulsions in patients with epilepsy or other seizure disorders. Early clinical observations of enhanced general well-being among epileptic patients treated with anticonvulsants, as well as various early animal models of affective illness progression, have promoted controlled investigations of anticonvulsants as potential mood-stabilizing agents for bipolar disorder, other select anxiety disorders (social anxiety, panic disorder), and pain conditions. As reviewed elsewhere, a strong clinical evidence base and U.S. Food and Drug Administration (FDA) approval exists for the anticonvulsants lamotrigine, divalproex sodium, and carbamazepine in the treatment of bipolar disorder. This FDA approval identifies these anticonvulsants as mood stabilizers. Although gabapentin and topiramate were investigated substantially as potential mood stabilizers for bipolar disorder, these studies were negative. However, the anticonvulsants pregabalin, gabapentin, and topiramate are used in several select anxiety, addiction, and pain conditions.

How Do They Work?

The exact mechanism of anticonvulsant action in epilepsy or mood stabilization in bipolar disorder is not fully understood. Seizures are conceptualized as excessive stimulation of brain cells or neurons; broadly, anticonvulsants are thought to reduce excess neuronal stimulation either by decreasing excitatory stimulation or increasing inhibitory stimulation. Mechanistically, excitatory stimulation is decreased using medications that decrease glutamate (an excitatory amino acid), such as topiramate, whereas inhibitory stimulation is increased using medications that increase γ-aminobutyric acid (GABA, an inhibitory amino acid), such as gabapentin or pregabalin.

What Are These Other Anticonvulsants Used to Treat?

Gabapentin

Gabapentin is FDA-approved for the adjunctive (add-on) treatment of complex partial epilepsy and for pain management of postherpetic neuralgia in adults. It has no FDA approval for treatment of primary mental health conditions. For patients who need help safely withdrawing from alcohol use (with normal kidney function), gabapentin has demonstrated benefit with a standard dosing protocol (starting dosage 900 mg three times daily for 4 days, with the dosage tapered over the course of 5 days) in reducing the severity of alcohol withdrawal symptoms. The strongest clinical evidence base for gabapentin is for the treatment of alcohol use disorder, specifically for patients who have safely withdrawn from alcohol with the goal of maintaining sobriety. In a review of seven clinical trials (dosage range 300–3,600 mg/day, trial duration 3–26 weeks), gabapentin, compared with placebo, significantly decreased the percentage of heavy drinking days in the clinical trial; this outcome measure in general refers to 4/3 standard drinks on any day or 14/7 drinks per week for males/females, respectively. It should be noted the main outcome measure for these studies was complete sobriety or abstinence, and no difference in this outcome was detected between gabapentin and placebo. One controlled study showed benefit of gabapentin for social anxiety disorder (900–3,600 mg/day) in a 14-week trial. Gabapentin has a modest clinical evidence base for several pain conditions that commonly co-occur with mood and anxiety disorders or are often associated with secondary symptoms of depression and anxiety. Beyond its FDA approval for postherpetic neuralgia in adults, gabapentin has additional clinical data for treatment of pain conditions associated with trigeminal neuralgia, diabetic neuropathy, and fibromyalgia, in trials typically lasting 6–12 weeks in which gabapentin was given at 1,200–3,600 mg/day.

Pregabalin

Pregabalin is FDA-approved for the adjunctive treatment of adults with complex partial epilepsy, pain management of postherpetic neuralgia, diabetic neuropathy, neuropathic pain associated with spinal cord injury, or fibromyalgia; it is also the first anticonvulsant to be FDA-approved for fibromyalgia. Pregabalin has no FDA approvals for treatment of primary mental health conditions. Most of the pain management and fibromyalgia studies used dosages up to 300 mg/day. For fibromyalgia, which is often comorbid with depression and anxiety disorders, acute trials (typically 8–13 weeks in duration) consistently showed results of reduced pain, fatigue, and anxiety and improvement in sleep at dosages higher than 300 mg/day. Beyond its FDA approvals, clinical evidence has indicated that pregabalin may improve the symptoms of generalized anxiety disorder; meta-analyses of multiple studies lasting 6–8 weeks and using dosages of 300–600 mg/day reported greater anxiety symptom reduction with pregabalin than with placebo. Additional 6-month data suggest longer-term benefit for maintenance of treatment response.

Topiramate

Topiramate is FDA-approved for the treatment of complex partial epilepsy, primary generalized seizures, a severe epilepsy of childhood onset called Lennox-Gastaut syndrome, and migraine prophylaxis. It has indications in younger patients for both Lennox-Gastaut syndrome (age 6 and older) and migraine prophylaxis (age 12 and older). Like many anticonvulsants, the dosage range for topiramate for migraine (100 mg/day) is lower than that for seizure disorders (200–400 mg/day). Topiramate has no FDA approvals for the treatment of primary mental health conditions. Extended-release topiramate used in combination with phentermine (known as Qysmia) is FDA-approved as an adjunct to a reduced-calorie diet and increased physical activity for chronic weight management in obese (body mass index [BMI] ≥30) or overweight (BMI ≥27) adults who have at least one medical condition related to their weight (e.g., hypertension, diabetes, increased lipids). It has a similar adjunct indication for youth ages 12 years and older whose initial BMI is in the 95th percentile or higher. Initial daily dosing of the combination is phentermine 3.75 mg/topiramate 23 mg for the first 2 weeks, with a maintenance daily dosage range of 7.5 mg/46 mg–15 mg/92 mg; if the patient does not lose at least 5% of their baseline weight, the medication should be tapered and discontinued. A clinical evidence base—but not FDA approval—exists for topiramate monotherapy of obesity (16–384 mg/day) and type 2 diabetes (96–192 mg). Like gabapentin (but with stronger clinical evidence), topiramate has been helpful for maintenance of sobriety in patients with alcohol use disorder who have safely withdrawn from alcohol.

Over the course of 8 weeks, topiramate 300 mg/day was more effective than placebo (starting dosage 25 mg/day, final dosage 300 mg/day) on several study outcome measures (i.e., length of abstinence, drinks per day, heavy drinking days, craving for alcohol). Dropout related to side effects was higher with topiramate and was primarily related to headache, anorexia, insomnia, numbness/tingling, and taste changes.

Systematic review of three studies (8–16 weeks in duration, median dosage 300 mg/day) showed topiramate was more effective than placebo for binge eating disorder, decreasing binge frequency, weight, and BMI.

Standard Dosing and Treatment Regimen

The standard dosing regimen of gabapentin, pregabalin, and topiramate (outside of FDA indications for epilepsy), starts at a lower dosage and has slower titration.

Gabapentin

For patients with normal renal function, the starting dosage of gabapentin typically is a single dose of 300 mg on day 1, two doses of 300 mg on day 2, and three doses of 300 mg on day 3. The target dosage ranges from 1,200 mg/day (maintenance of sobriety), to 1,800 mg (fibromyalgia), and 1,800–3,600 mg/day (neuropathy). Dosage adjustments are required when there is evidence of impaired renal function, typically seen with chronic kidney disease. Given the potential risk of sedation and respiratory depression, dosing for geriatric patients should be at the lowest dosage possible.

Pregabalin

For patients with normal renal function, pregabalin is typically started at 75 mg twice daily, increased within 1 week to 150 mg twice daily. The maximum maintenance dosage is 225 mg twice daily. In the off-label use for generalized anxiety disorder, it has been prescribed up to 600 mg/day in three divided doses. Again, adjustments are required when there is evidence of impaired renal function, and given the potential risk of sedation and respiratory depression, dosing for geriatric patients should be at the lowest dosage possible.

Topiramate

For patients with normal renal function, topiramate is started at 25 mg/day, with a 25-mg dosage increase typically at weekly intervals. The target dosage is typically up to 300 mg/day. Adjustments are required when there is evidence of impaired renal function, and given the potential risk of sedation and respiratory depression, dosing for geriatric patients should be 50% that for younger adults.

Use in Special Populations

Children and Adolescents, Adults, and the Elderly

Most studies of gabapentin and pregabalin have been conducted in adults. Their use in children is based on their FDA indication for seizures. Topiramate use in children is based on FDA approval for a range of seizures, including Lennox-Gastaut syndrome, and prevention of migraine. The combination of extended-release topiramate and phentermine is FDA-approved as an adjunct for youth ages 12 years and older whose initial BMI is in the 95th percentile or higher.

Medication Interactions

Neither gabapentin nor pregabalin is metabolized by the liver, and they are excreted unchanged in the kidneys. Thus, there are no concerns regarding their use with other medications metabolized by the liver. However, patients' lithium levels should be monitored when they are taking gabapentin or pregabalin because all three medications are excreted renally. Topiramate may reduce hormonal contraception levels. It also may magnify central nervous system (CNS) depression (spectrum from sedation and lack of arousal to marked confusion and coma) when used with other agents that increase CNS depression. Concurrent use of topiramate with other anticonvulsants can result in decreased levels of topiramate (when used with carbamazepine) or increased levels of ammonia (when used with valproate).

Side Effects

Gabapentin

Gabapentin has a highly favorable side effect profile. Sedation, drowsiness, dizziness, gait unsteadiness, dry mouth, and weight gain are the most common side effects noted in controlled studies; it is not common for patients to stop the medication because of side effects. Serious side effects are uncommon but can have serious psychiatric implications, including induction of mania and aggression. Gabapentin has a broad therapeutic index and appears to be safe in overdose. It has been clinically observed to have the potential for misuse and abuse, most commonly in individuals with a history of addiction.

Pregabalin

Similarly, the pregabalin side effect profile is mild. Common side effects have included dizziness, sedation, dry mouth, edema, blurred vision, weight gain, and concentration difficulties. Rare side effects have included an allergic hypersensitivity (*angioedema*). Pregabalin has been clinically observed to have the potential for misuse and abuse, most commonly in individuals with a history of addiction.

Topiramate

Side effects with topiramate can include weight loss, confusion, dizziness, impaired cognition, numbness/tingling, metabolic changes in blood referred to as *acidosis*, and kidney stones. Rare serious side effects include severe rash, liver failure, glaucoma, and increased ammonia.

Conclusion

Although gabapentin, pregabalin, and topiramate have not received regulatory approval for their use in the treatment of major depression or bipolar disorder, careful investigation of these non-mood-stabilizing compounds has provided clinical evidence suggesting therapeutic benefit for the target symptoms of anxiety and pain. This is, on balance, an overall benefit because patients with mood disorders commonly have comorbid anxiety disorder, migraine headache disorder, and a number of neuropathic conditions.

Recommended Reading

Coplan JD, Aaronson CJ, Panthangi V, et al: Treating comorbid anxiety and depression: psychosocial and pharmacological approaches. World J Psychiatry 5(4):366–378, 2015 26740928

Garakani A, Murrough JW, Freire RC, et al Pharmacotherapy of anxiety disorders: current and emerging treatment options. Front Psychiatry 11:595584, 2020 33424664

41

Typical Antipsychotics

Fabiano G. Nery, M.D., Ph.D.
Henry A. Nasrallah, M.D.

Introduction

The first typical antipsychotic, chlorpromazine, was synthesized during the early 1950s as an anesthetic agent for tranquilization and sedation before surgery. It was observed in 1952 that patients would become calmer and more indifferent to the environment following surgery, beyond the period of sedation. Chlorpromazine was then tested in psychiatric patients, especially hospitalized patients with psychosis, and it was found to improve delusions and hallucinations in those patients. The introduction of chlorpromazine was soon followed by that of many other antipsychotics with a similar structure and, in 1965, by haloperidol. These are known as *first-generation antipsychotics* or *typical antipsychotics*. This class of medications played a key role in enabling the discharge of patients from long-term institutions in the second half of the twentieth century. Many patients who had been chronically hospitalized were able to return to the community and receive outpatient medication treatments and psychosocial rehabilitation. However, these medications have intolerable neurological side effects and now have been largely replaced by the *second-generation antipsychotics*, also known as the *atypical antipsychotics*, which have a different side effect profile.

How Do They Work?

Typical antipsychotics work by blocking the dopamine receptor function (especially the subtype 2, or D_2, receptor). When they bind to the dopamine receptor, they limit the ability of dopamine to bind to that same receptor and thus decrease dopamine activity. It is believed that psychotic symptoms (delusions and hallucinations) are caused, in part, by an excess of dopaminergic activity in certain brain areas, which explains why typical antipsychotics work against delusions and hallucinations. These agents differ in their ability to block dopamine receptors, but their exact mechanism of action remains unknown.

What Are Typical Antipsychotics Used to Treat?

Schizophrenia is the primary psychiatric condition that typical antipsychotics are approved to treat. Almost all typical antipsychotics are U.S. Food and Drug Administration (FDA)-approved to treat this condition. Early clinical trials have confirmed their efficacy in treating delusions and hallucinations in schizophrenia; for example, 75% of hospitalized patients treated with chlorpromazine, thioridazine, or fluphenazine markedly improved versus 23% of those treated with placebo. These three typical antipsychotics were also efficacious in treating psychotic symptoms of depression. Several long-term clinical trials in schizophrenia showed that typical antipsychotics are also helpful in reducing relapse rates and hospitalizations, preventing relapse, and preventing treatment discontinuation for any cause (e.g., due to side effects). Long-acting injectable antipsychotic formulations of typical antipsychotics have been shown to be more effective than oral tablets in preventing relapses and rehospitalizations because adherence to oral pills can be inconsistent.

Although not FDA-approved for this indication, typical antipsychotics are also effective for the treatment of other psychotic disorders (e.g., brief psychotic disorder) and are often prescribed for treatment of psychotic symptoms associated with other conditions (e.g., acute confusional states such as delirium, dementia, drug intoxication). Chlorpromazine is FDA-approved to treat manic episodes in bipolar disorder. Haloperidol is also considered efficacious to treat acute mania, a condition in which it might have some advantages over other options (e.g., lithium) because it provides rapid sedation and control for patients with psychotic symptoms. Some typical antipsychotics are FDA-approved to treat hyperactivity, agitation, and severe childhood behavioral problems, but these now have been largely substituted by the newer atypical antipsychotics. Some of the typical antipsychotics also have FDA approval to treat severe generalized anxiety disorder due to their tranquilizing effect, which is unrelated to their antipsychotic efficacy. Finally, two typical antipsychotics, pimozide and haloperidol, are FDA-approved to treat Tourette's disorder, which is postulated to be caused by a hypothetical hyperdopaminergic state in the nigrostriatal pathway. Table 41–1 provides a summary of the typical antipsychotics, with indications for age group and dosage range.

Standard Dosing and Treatment Regimen

The appropriate dosing of typical antipsychotics is important because higher-than-necessary dosages are more likely to cause undesirable side effects. Some studies have shown that psychosis can be controlled by blocking about 65% of dopamine D_2 receptors, but once the blockade exceeds 80%, patients experience abnormal movement and endocrinological side effects. In clinical trials, the dosage found to produce clinical response is listed in Table 41–1. However, individual responses may account for some variability. For instance, some patients may need a lower or a higher dosage of the antipsychotic than others, but it is wise to start at a low dosage and increase it gradually to avoid side effects.

Use in Special Populations

Children and Adolescents

Most clinical studies have been done in adults ages 18–65 years. However, typical antipsychotics have been used in children and adolescents for pediatric bipolar disorder or for agitation or hyperactivity not associated with psychosis. The main issue with using typical antipsychotics in youth is the agents' long-term effects on hormonal development, weight gain, and brain development. These effects are not well understood, but some evidence indicates that typical antipsychotics are associated with brain tissue loss (thinning of cerebral cortex) and shrinkage, in addition to the brain atrophic changes related to psychosis itself.

Elderly Patients

The elderly patient population is more prone to motor side effects of antipsychotics and also may be taking various medications for other health conditions, increasing the risk of medication interactions (discussed in the following section). Elderly people metabolize medications slower than do younger adults, which results in higher levels; this may explain their propensity to develop side effects. Therefore, daily dosages for elderly patients are usually one-half to one-third the dosages typically used in younger adults.

Table 41–1. U.S. Food and Drug Administration–approved first-generation antipsychotics

Generic drug name	Indications	Age group	Dosage range
Chlorpromazine	Schizophrenia	Adults	200–800 mg/day
	Acute manic episodes in bipolar disorder	Adults	400–800 mg/day
	Agitation/aggression associated with psychiatric disorders (IM)	Adults	25–200 mg/day
	Severe behavioral problems (acute agitation)	Children	0.55 mg/kg/dose every 4–6 hours, maximum 100 mg/day
Droperidol	Agitation (IM or IV)	Adults	2.5–10 mg/dose, maximum 20 mg per episode
Fluphenazine	Psychotic disorders	Adults	1–5 mg/day
Haloperidol	Schizophrenia	Adults	2–20 mg/day (PO); 50–150 mg/month (LAI)
	Tourette's disorder	Adults, children age 3+ years	0.05–0.075 mg/kg/day
	Acute agitation (IM)	Adults	2–20 mg/day
Loxapine	Schizophrenia	Adults, children age 12+ years	60–100 mg/day
Perphenazine	Schizophrenia	Adults, children age 12+ years	12–64 mg/day
Pimozide	Tourette's disorder	Adults, children age 12+ years	1–10 mg/day for adults; 0.05 mg/kg/dose/day for children
Prochlorperazine	Schizophrenia	Adults, children age 2+ years weighing >20 lb	15–150 mg/day
	Generalized nonpsychotic anxiety disorder	Adults	15–20 mg/day
Thiothixene	Schizophrenia	Adults, children age 12+ years	6–60 mg/day

Table 41–1. U.S. Food and Drug Administration–approved first-generation antipsychotics *(continued)*

Generic drug name	Indications	Age group	Dosage range
Thioridazine	Schizophrenia	Adults, children	150–800 mg/day
Trifluoperazine	Schizophrenia	Adults, children age 6+ years	4–40 mg/day
	Nonpsychotic anxiety	Adults	2–4 mg/day

Note. IM=intramuscular; IV=intravenous; LAI=long-acting injection; PO=oral (by mouth).

Source. www.fda.gov/drugs.

Medication Interactions

"Drug-drug interactions," or medication interactions, are what we call events that happen when the effect of one medication is affected by the coadministration of another. Patients with psychotic disorders, particularly schizophrenia, often have multiple medical conditions and may be taking other medications besides antipsychotics. These agents may affect each other during the absorption process, metabolism process, or when binding to the targeted region (e.g., the brain). Smoking increases the activity of some liver cytochrome P450 enzymes, which affects the absorption, distribution, metabolism, and elimination of some antipsychotics, such as haloperidol, fluphenazine, and thiothixene, and thus may decrease their clinical efficacy. Thisis not caused by nicotine but by the aromatic polycarbons in tobacco. Therefore, nicotine replacement therapies (e.g., gums, patches, lozenges) are safe to prescribe for patients taking typical antipsychotics. If a patient stops smoking and starts using nicotine replacement therapy, their antipsychotic blood levels may increase, and they may require a reduction in the antipsychotic dosage. Some antidepressants (e.g., fluoxetine, paroxetine, bupropion) may increase the blood levels of some antipsychotics, such as haloperidol and fluphenazine, by inhibiting a liver enzyme that metabolizes those medications. This may cause QTc prolongation, which increases the risk of cardiac arrhythmias, or it may reduce the seizure threshold and thus increase the risk of seizures. Serotonergic medications (e.g., fluoxetine) may also increase dopamine blockade, increasing the chance of neuroleptic malignant syndrome; conversely, antipsychotics may increase the serotonergic effects of serotonergic agents, increasing the chance of serotonin syndrome. In addition, many antipsychotics are sedating, and when used together with other sedating agents, such as antihistamines for anxiety or allergies or benzodiazepines for anxiety or agitation, they may cause extra-sedation.

Side Effects

The amount of dopamine blockade in the mesolimbic brain areas required to improve psychotic symptoms can also cause the undesirable side effects of typical antipsychotics, because this blockade happens throughout the brain. Therefore, although dopamine blockade in the mesolimbic brain areas will improve psychotic symptoms, in the mesocortical areas it may cause emotional blunting and indifference, cognitive slowing, and apathy; in the nigrostriatal areas it may cause motor abnormalities, such as tremors, rigidity, shuffling gait, akathisia, and tardive dyskinesia; and in the tuberoinfundibular areas, it may cause endocrine abnormalities, such as engorged breasts, milk excretion from the nipples, and lack of menstruation (all attributed to an increase in prolactin).

Typical antipsychotics also differ in the way they block other types of brain neurotransmitters. For example, some typical antipsychotic medicines also block cholinergic receptors (in the brain and other parts of the body, such as the gut), giving rise to side effects such as dry mouth, constipation, blurred vision, and cognitive slowing; histaminic receptors, causing increased appetite, weight gain, and drowsiness; or adrenergic receptors, causing tachycardia, orthostatic hypotension, and drowsiness. In overdose, typical antipsychotics can cause cardiac arrhythmias, severe hypotension, severe sedation, coma, and mental confusion. Such severe reactions are related to the medications' massive effects on adrenergic, histaminic, or cholinergic receptors.

On the other hand, typical antipsychotics that block cholinergic receptors, if stopped abruptly, may cause *cholinergic rebound* (e.g., sleep disturbance, vivid dreams, nightmares, anxiety, nausea, diarrhea, sweating, confusion, delirium), supposedly due to the sudden acute increase in cholinergic activity. Likewise, typical antipsychotics that block dopamine receptors may lead to increased dopaminergic activity if stopped abruptly, leading to *rebound psychosis* (fast reemergence of psychotic symptoms). Therefore, typical antipsychotics should be slowly tapered down in dosage before being discontinued.

Although rare, typical antipsychotics may also be associated with a condition called *neuroleptic malignant syndrome.* The clinical manifestations of this syndrome include fever, muscle rigidity, abnormal mental status, irregular pulse or blood pressure, tachycardia or cardiac arrhythmias, hypotension or hypertension, and diaphoresis. Neuroleptic malignant syndrome is a medical emergency. Patients taking typical antipsychotics who present these symptoms should be evaluated in an emergency room, where other diagnoses can be ruled out, the antipsychotic agent may be safely discontinued, and supportive treatment may be provided.

Conclusion

Typical antipsychotics started the pharmacological revolution in the treatment of severe psychiatric disorders such as schizophrenia and bipolar disorders; however, with the advent of the atypical antipsychotics in the 1990s (e.g., risperidone, olanzapine, and quetiapine, agents with lower risk of neurological movement disorders), the use of the typical, first-generation antipsychotics declined substantially. This was good for psychiatric patients, who often discontinued their typical antipsychotics and subsequently experienced psychotic relapses leading to rehospitalizations, brain damage, imprisonment, and suicide.

Recommended Reading

Guiroy I, Wright T, Wu BW, et al: Role of antipsychotics in mood disorder treatment, in The American Psychiatric Association Publishing Textbook of Mood Disorders, 2nd Edition. Edited by Nemeroff CB, Schatzberg AF, Rasgon N, et al. Washington, DC, American Psychiatric Association Publishing, 2021, pp 285–296

Nasrallah HA, Tandon R: Classic antipsychotic medications, in The American Psychiatric Association Publishing Textbook of Clinical Psychopharmacology, 5th Edition. Edited by Schatzberg AF, Nemeroff CB. Washington, DC, American Psychiatric Association Publishing, 2017, pp 603–622

42

Atypical Antipsychotics

Philip D. Harvey, Ph.D.

Introduction

Atypical antipsychotic medications are characterized as "atypical" because they have additional mechanisms of action compared with older medications. The new neuroscience-based nomenclature aims to realign psychotropics in terms of their pharmacological properties. For antipsychotics, instead of their previous classifications as *first-generation* and *second-generation* (i.e., typical vs. atypical), the nomenclature now emphasizes the medications' underlying mechanism. For antipsychotics, the terms *dopamine-receptor antagonists* and *serotonin-dopamine antagonists* (SDAs) are now used. This allows for a mechanism-based rather than disease-based classification.

This chapter describes the SDAs, including their actions and side effects. In addition, the medications approved by the U.S. Food and Drug Administration (FDA) are described and compared with medications that are used "off-label." Off-label usage is not inappropriate; it is fully allowed by standards of medical practice. However, standards of evidence are consistent for approved medications and may be different for unapproved uses. Obtaining FDA approval also requires a series of studies for which older, generic medications do not have financial support to develop.

How Do They Work?

SDA medications have several shared features. They block the dopamine D_2 receptor and serotonin-2A (5-hydroxytryptamine $[5\text{-HT}]_{2A}$) receptor. Although the oldest SDA, clozapine, was not intentionally developed for this purpose, the later medications were developed with these joint mechanisms in mind. Risperidone was the first agent developed to intentionally block both receptor systems, and its development was, in fact, the result of the intentional mechanistic combination of two older medications—haloperidol, a dopamine antagonist, and ritanserin, a 5-HT_{2A} antagonist.

The extent to which SDAs block dopamine and serotonin receptors varies across the medications. Although initially developed to treat psychotic conditions, most of these medications also have wider use in mood and anxiety disorders. Several have FDA approval for the treatment of depression that responds poorly to antidepressant treatment (known as *refractory depression*), depression associated with bipolar disorder (*bipolar depression*), and maintenance treatment of bipolar disorder aimed at preventing relapse of both mania and depression symptoms.

These medications are also commonly utilized for anxiety disorders that respond poorly to other treatment efforts. No SDAs are FDA-approved for these uses, but some clinical evidence has shown them to be effective in certain cases. This information is reviewed later (see "Anxiety Disorders").

What Are Atypical Antipsychotics Used to Treat?

Conditions With Depression

Refractory depression and bipolar depression are challenging conditions and involve high levels of disability and morbidity. Patients with bipolar depression also have the highest risk of suicide attempts and death from suicide of all psychiatric conditions. Treatment efforts targeting symptom reduction are thus critical. Data indicate that treatment with SDAs for these conditions has a response rate that justifies their use. The adverse events that may arise with the SDAs are not substantial enough to raise safety concerns in general, although these agents have quite a bit of variability in their tolerability. As a general rule, when treating refractory or bipolar depression, the medication with the lowest side effect burden is best, given the lack of data suggesting substantial differences in efficacy among the various options. Augmentation with or transition to an SDA would be optimal clinical practice at present for patients with either of these conditions who experience inadequate response or are unable to tolerate other treatments.

FDA approvals for the SDA medications are still in flux. For instance, long-acting injectible (LAI) paliperidone (9-hydroxyrisperidone) palmitate (Invega) is not approved for bipolar disorder maintenance, but risperidone (Risperdal Consta) is. One variant of LAI aripiprazole (Maintena) has been approved for maintenance therapy in bipolar disorder, but a version manufactured by another company (Aristada) is not, despite being the same medication.

Refractory Depression

Refractory depression is defined as a depression without any lifetime history of manic features that does not respond adequately to treatment with suitable dosages of antidepressants. To truly be classified as refractory depression, adequate trials—in terms of dosage and duration—of antidepressants with more than one mechanism of action (i.e., selective serotonin reuptake inhibitors [SSRIs], serotonin-norepinephrine reuptake inhibitors [SNRIs], dual reuptake inhibitors) must have been completed. Depression is not truly refractory if the patient simply cannot tolerate antidepressants or does not adhere adequately to treatment, the dosage tried was too low, or the trial was too short. The severity level of depression that remains despite treatment is not rigidly defined, but *remission* is defined as the near-total absence of depression, so any residual depression that is causing distress is a potential treatment target.

Bipolar Depression

Bipolar depression is complex because it can occur both in the presence and absence of the concurrent euphoric/irritable symptoms of bipolar disorder. The severity of bipolar depression can vary markedly, but even residual sad moods or minor depression symptoms are known to be associated with reduced quality of life and disability. The more time someone with bipolar disorder spends in a sad or depressed mood, regardless of severity, the poorer their quality of life. Thus, even low-level depression is a treatment target.

Bipolar depression is rendered more challenging because the antidepressant medications used to treat unipolar depression are ineffective for many patients. Older medications, known as tricyclic antidepressants (TCAs), are known to potentiate mood switches into mania, although the medications most commonly prescribed for major depression (i.e., SSRIs) have a notably lower risk.

Maintenance Treatment of Bipolar Disorder

Some medications are approved for maintenance therapy (i.e., relapse prevention) of bipolar disorder, although not specifically for bipolar depression. Because relapses can have either polarity (although they are much more common for bipolar depression), approved maintenance treatments are also essentially

Table 42–1. Approved uses of serotonin-dopamine agonists in mood and anxiety disorders

Medication	Depression	Refractory depression	Bipolar depression	Bipolar maintenance
Oral medications				
Aripiprazole[a]		X	X	
Asenapine[b]	X			
Brexpiprazole		X		
Cariprazine			X	
Iloperidone[b]	X			
Lumateperone			X	
Lurasidone[a]			X	
Olanzapine-fluoxetine[a]		X	X	
Paliperidone[c]			X	
Quetiapine[a]	X	X	X	
Long-acting injectables				
Abilify Maintena				X
Paliperidone[d]				
Risperdal Consta				X

[a]Generically available in the United States.
[b]Rarely used, may not be available.
[c]Approved for mania.
[d]Approved for schizoaffective disorder.

treatments for bipolar depression. Table 42–1 presents all of these current medications and their approved uses. As can be seen in the table, multiple medications have been approved for treatment of the conditions just discussed. A few are LAIs, only some of which are approved for maintenance treatment, whereas others are orally administered. Thus, various options are available, and some of the orally administered medications are available in generic form in the United States. Most health insurances cover the cost of at least one of the LAIs and some, if not all, of the brand name medications.

The advantage of having multiple approved medications is that in the event of side effects or inadequate benefits, alternatives are available. Furthermore, considerable evidence from randomized trials indicates that essentially all SDA medications have efficacy for refractory depression, and their lack of FDA approval in some cases is simply because the manufacturer did not pursue approval before the medication became generic. That said, insurance companies can deny claims for non-approved medications, even if they are low-cost generics.

Anxiety Disorders

Many medications have FDA approval for the treatment of anxiety disorders, including both generalized anxiety disorder (GAD) and panic disorder (PD). As noted earlier, none of the SDA medications has FDA approval for any anxiety disorder. Are there cases in which an SDA might be helpful? Is the risk/benefit profile suitable? We examine these issues in the discussion that follows.

Some of the medications used for anxiety disorders are among those with the highest risk for addiction, although it can be difficult to differentiate patients with anxiety disorders from those with a history of benzodiazepine addiction. The commonly used and approved non-addictive medications for anxiety disorders are the SSRIs, SNRIs, and buspirone. SDA medications have no addiction potential, so there is an inherent motivation to test them for efficacy.

Many studies of the SDAs, predominantly quetiapine, have been conducted in the treatment of GAD and PD, but the results have not been adequately positive for FDA approval. Studies of the rates of response and side effects have indicated that the former are not as high as the rates seen in mood disorders, and discontinuations due to the latter are common. That said, many cases of GAD and PD involve significant symptoms and poor treatment response. Experimenting with quetiapine as an off-label strategy seems worthy of consideration, because case series reports have shown that some patients respond to that medication. Although quetiapine can cause daytime sedation, this may not be a significant adverse effect in people who have excessive arousal and anxiety.

Agitation

Both major depression and bipolar disorder can be associated with agitated behavior. Historically, one treatment used for agitation was dopamine antagonists, such as haloperidol, but these have largely been replaced by the SDAs. Using SDAs for agitation avoids the addiction potential associated with benzodiazepines and may effectively treat the underlying mood disturbance. Short-term risks with SDAs are quite low for occasional use for agitation, although a new treatment specifically targeting agitation in bipolar disorder, rapidly dissolving dexmedetomidine, has recently been approved and may be a viable alternative to either SDAs or benzodiazepines for the rapid reduction of agitated behavior. For now, it is only available in emergency department or inpatient settings, but trials are under way to obtain approval for at-home use, either self-administered or administered under the guidance of a caregiver.

Standard Dosing and Treatment Regimen

Like all current psychotropic medications for mood disorders, the SDA medications are not curative. Because they are commonly started only after previous treatment. The dosages used as augmentation therapy can be reduced to manage side effects once mood symptoms improve, but no evidence has shown improved long-term outcomes after discontinuing a single effective course of treatment.

Furthermore, there is no evidence that these treatments have effects other than on clinical symptoms and related subjective reports of quality of life. Disability is common with mood disorders, and symptomatic treatments have not been shown to eliminate disability. In fact, people with bipolar disorder who do not have any current symptoms of depression do not necessarily show improvement in functioning consistent with functional recovery. Other interventions, including psychosocial interventions and computerized cognitive training, have been demonstrated to improve everyday functioning and symptom stability and are clearly a first step in that direction.

In bipolar disorder, some of the approved treatments have been found to be effective as monotherapy for acute and maintenance treatments. Because lithium requires considerable monitoring and has some risks, the fact that Risperdal Consta, lurasidone, and lumateperone have been approved as monotherapy expands treatment options.

Only a few of the currently available LAI medications have been approved for use in bipolar disorder. Although the approved and unapproved medications are chemically interchangeable, the latter may not be approved by insurance and carry considerable cost as a result. LAIs have several advantages, including more stable blood levels of the medication, which is associated with reduced side effects and improved adherence because receiving the medication on a biweekly (Risperdal Consta) or monthly (Sustena) basis or every 3 months (Trinza) eliminates day-to-day challenges with self-administration and obtaining prescription refills. LAIs also allow early detection of nonadherence because missing an injection is a clear sign that the patient is not receiving medication, something that can be challenging to confirm with patients taking oral medications.

SDA *polypharmacy* (i.e., use of multiple medications) is common in people with schizophrenia. However, evidence supporting this strategy in schizophrenia is very limited compared with the considerably greater evidence supporting careful dosage titration and selection of the single best possible medication. For mood disorders, there is essentially no evidence on the use of more than one SDA. Thus, switching medications, rather than adding another agent from the same class, is a preferable strategy when treatment with a given SDA fails to produce a response.

Use in Special Populations

Elderly Patients

All of the SDA medications have a class warning regarding risk of stroke in patients age 65 and older. Thus, extreme caution is required when elderly patients are receiving treatment with these medications.

Side Effects

All of the SDA medications occupy the dopamine D_2 receptor, and the higher the dopamine receptor blockade, the more likely parkinsonian-like symptoms will occur. Most of these medications are also associated with weight gain, with this effect varying considerably across the different agents. Some of these medications also are associated with significant sedation. When patients experience euphoric or irritable manic symptoms, this sedation may be beneficial; however, it can lead to cognitive challenges and daytime somnolence, which can be hazardous when they are driving or performing certain work-related activities.

Conclusion

SDAs are a viable treatment option when mood disorders fail to respond optimally to other approaches, and they also may have use in the treatment of certain anxiety disorders. Although these medications have well-understood risks, the risks associated with poorly treated depression, both unipolar and bipolar, are probably greater. The only long-term danger with SDAs is tardive dyskinesia (TD), which is a long-term neurological side effect. The risk of developing TD is much lower with SDAs than with dopamine antagonists, but any emergence of parkinsonian side effects during SDA treatment requires careful evaluation because such effects can signal greater individual risk. Studies have suggested that TD has an incidence of less than 1% annually with SDAs and that prediction of TD risk is feasible. In fact, a long-term surveillance study of the use of aripiprazole in major depression determined that new-onset cases of TD arose in just 37 participants out of the 6 million treated to that point. The estimated risk with quetiapine is even lower. Thus, on an individual basis, the risk of development of TD, particularly with careful management, is very small.

Recommended Reading

Stahl SM: Prescriber's Guide: Stahl's Essential Psychopharmacology. Cambridge, UK, Cambridge University Press, 2020

Zargorski N: Antipsychotics increasingly prescribed for bipolar disorder. Psychiatric News, June 25, 2020. Available at: https://psychnews.psychiatryonline.org/doi/10.1176/appi.pn.2020.6a35.

43

Sedative-Hypnotics

Andrew D. Krystal, M.D., M.S.

Introduction

This chapter provides information about a group of medications referred to as *sedative-hypnotics.* These medications are generally used to help people fall or stay asleep. As a result, their primary use is to treat *insomnia,* which is defined as sustained difficulty falling or staying asleep that is associated with impairment in function or quality of life. Although nearly everyone has problems with sleep from time to time, persistent difficulty accompanied by impairment occurs in 10%–20% of the population. Notably, insomnia occurs in roughly three-quarters of individuals with major depression and in an even higher percentage of those with anxiety disorders. Although sometimes considered nothing more than a nuisance, a large body of research has established that untreated insomnia has important health consequences. It is associated with a substantial increase in risk for major depression, substance use disorders, and cardiovascular disorders. It is also a leading cause of automobile and work accidents and is one of the strongest predictors of having suicidal thoughts and suicide attempts. As such, it is critical that anyone affected by insomnia discuss their sleep difficulty with their health care provider so appropriate treatment can be administered.

When a decision is made to pursue treatment for insomnia, one option to consider is cognitive-behavioral therapy for insomnia (CBT-I). CBT-I is a multimodal psychotherapy that has been solidly established to be helpful for many patients and is recommended as a first-line treatment for insomnia in several clinical guidelines because of its effectiveness and safety profile. When CBT-I is either ineffective or unavailable, the mainstay of treatment is sedative-hypnotic medications. A variety of sedative-hypnotics are available for treating insomnia. These include some approved by the U.S. Food and Drug Administration (FDA) for this purpose, including benzodiazepines, nonbenzodiazepines, selective antihistamines, orexin antagonists, and melatonin agonists. Others sometimes used include agents originally developed, FDA-approved, and marketed for the treatment of other conditions that are being used "off-label" for insomnia. This includes some antidepressants and antipsychotics. In addition, people sometimes take nonprescription treatments obtained "over-the-counter" (OTC) from their pharmacy to treat insomnia, nearly all of which are nonselective antihistamines.

Different types of medications have different effects that impact how well-suited they are for use in a given individual with insomnia. Their relevant characteristics are described in the following discussion. The treatment of insomnia in clinical practice has, by and large, been a one-size-fits-all endeavor without any appreciation for the differences between medications. However, these differences matter, and awareness of them makes it possible to tailor the choice of treatment for each patient to achieve better results.

Benzodiazepines

The benzodiazepines have been available for many years for treatment of insomnia. They include some that may be familiar, such as triazolam (Halcion), temazepam (Restoril), and flurazepam (Dalmane), and are highly effective for helping people fall asleep. Temazepam has established benefit for helping people to stay asleep. Flurazepam, however, is rarely used due to its excessive duration of effect.

The most important adverse effects of these medications are an increased risk of falls and memory difficulty during active treatment at night and sedation/impairment the next day in the subset of individuals for whom the duration of effect is too long. They also have the potential to be abused by those with a predisposition to substance use problems. Because of these risks, benzodiazepines are generally reserved for use in patients whose insomnia fails to respond to treatment with other medications, particularly those with trouble falling asleep, as well as those with significant amounts of anxiety, because these medications have potent anxiety-reducing effects.

Nonbenzodiazepines

A group of medications with the same types of effects as the benzodiazepines but unrelated to them in their chemical structure are those often referred to as nonbenzodiazepines. These include well-known agents such as zolpidem (Ambien), zolpidem controlled-release (Ambien CR), zaleplon (Sonata), and eszopiclone (Lunesta). Although the therapeutic and adverse effects of these medications are similar to those of the benzodiazepines, they are used more often because their duration of effect is generally shorter, decreasing the risk of daytime adverse effects. In fact, zolpidem and zaleplon are FDA-approved only for helping people fall asleep because they have very limited ability to help people stay asleep. Notably, zaleplon has an ultra-short duration of effect, such that levels in the blood are negligible within 4 hours of taking it.

Zolpidem controlled-release and eszopiclone are both FDA-approved for helping people fall asleep and stay asleep and can be very effective treatments in those without liability for abusing substances. Eszopiclone has been found to be especially effective in those with depression and anxiety disorders. Several research studies have suggested that, when given along with an antidepressant or anxiety-reducing medication, eszopiclone not only improves sleep in people with depression and anxiety disorders but also has an augmenting effect, increasing the improvement in depression or anxiety beyond the effects of the antidepressant or anxiety-reducing medication.

Generally, these medications are used for individuals who have severe difficulty falling asleep or problems falling or staying asleep that fails to respond to other medications. Eszopiclone is reasonable to consider for use along with a medication such as a selective serotonin reuptake inhibitor (SSRI; e.g., fluoxetine [Prozac], sertraline [Zoloft], escitalopram [Lexapro]) in patients with insomnia accompanying depression or anxiety.

Selective Antihistamines

Another type of sedative-hypnotic medication is the selective antihistamines. One such medication, doxepin (Silenor), has been approved by the FDA for insomnia therapy, but it is approved only for helping people *stay* asleep because it has only modest benefit for sleep-onset problems. Doxepin was originally FDA-approved for the treatment of depression in doses of 75–150 mg. However, its FDA approval for insomnia is in doses of just 3–6 mg because its antihistamine effects are so potent that it remains clinically effective for insomnia even when given at less than 10% of the antidepressant dose but at this smaller dose it impacts only sleep and essentially nothing else. The benefit of this selectivity is a favorable side effect profile. If the doxepin dosage is too high, patients may experience side effects such as dry mouth, blurred vision, constipation, memory difficulty, or daytime sedation. A notable feature of doxepin in the 3–6 mg range is that it still has potent effects in the last third of the night without increasing the risk for daytime impairment. This is not possible with benzodiazepines or nonbenzodiazepines, making this medication ideally suited for those with early morning awakening but no difficulty falling asleep. Doxepin also is not associated with a risk of abuse, so it is an ideal medication for individuals with difficulty staying asleep who are prone to abusing medications.

It is important to be aware of the distinction between doxepin and the medications that are available OTC to treat insomnia, which are also antihistamines (i.e., diphenhydramine and doxylamine). Doxepin 3–6 mg is substantially more selective in its antihistaminergic effect than the OTC agents and thus is associated with significantly lower risks of the side effects described earlier. Furthermore, doxepin has been determined in a rigorous set of research studies to have robust benefit for treatment of insomnia as well as a good safety profile. In contrast, the OTC agents have not been rigorously studied, so it remains unclear how effective they are and whether their risk/benefit ratio favors their use.

Selective Melatonin Agonists

Another type of medication that is FDA-approved for insomnia therapy are the selective melatonin agonists. One such agent is ramelteon (Rozerem), which is approved only for helping people fall asleep due to its very short duration of effect. Ramelteon has an excellent safety profile, including lack of risk of abuse; however, its therapeutic effects are relatively inconsistent, which limits its utility. Nonetheless, it is a valuable option for individuals with difficulty falling asleep who are prone to abuse medications or any individual with difficulty falling asleep for whom it is important to avoid side effects.

Orexin Receptor Antagonists

The last group of medications with FDA approval for insomnia are the orexin receptor antagonists. These agents block the wake-promoting effect of orexin, the chemical our body uses to keep us awake during the day. Orexin also plays a role in keeping people awake at night, which is the basis for the therapeutic effect of these medications. Three types are currently available: suvorexant (Belsomra), lemborexant (Dayvigo), and daridorexant (QUVIVIQ). They are approved by the FDA for use in people who have difficulty falling or staying asleep. Like low-dosage doxepin, they have therapeutic effects during the last third of the night without increasing daytime sleepiness. The main risks of these medications are daytime dizziness/sedation and abuse liability. They are generally well tolerated and thus can be effective for people with trouble falling or staying asleep who are not prone to medication abuse. However, they are particularly good for people who have problems with both falling asleep and early morning awakening.

Off-Label Medications

A number of medications that are FDA-approved for the treatment of depression (e.g., trazodone [Desyrel], amitriptyline [Elavil]) and the treatment of psychosis (hallucinations/delusions; e.g., quetiapine [Seroquel], olanzapine [Zyprexa], risperidone [Risperdal]) but not for insomnia are often used off-label for this purpose. Although these agents do not have a robust body of research establishing their therapeutic effects and risks in individuals with insomnia, some are widely prescribed; in fact, trazodone is the most-prescribed treatment for insomnia. One large study of trazodone did not show it to have therapeutic effects for insomnia, but several small studies have suggested it might be helpful. However, the dosage of trazodone must be tailored for each person, and no sufficiently large studies have yet demonstrated it to be therapeutic for insomnia when flexible dosing is employed.

The risks of these off-label uses vary with the medication and dosage. All are associated with a risk of dizziness and daytime sedation, but none is associated with significant risk of abuse. Antidepressants other than trazodone are often associated with dry mouth, blurred vision, constipation, and memory difficulty. Antipsychotic medications are associated with risks of weight gain, insulin resistance, muscle stiffness, and, rarely, the development of involuntary movements referred to as *tardive dyskinesia*. Owing to the lack of established therapeutic effects and safety profiles, off-label medications cannot be recommended for first-line insomnia treatment. However, they are among the options for those whose insomnia fails to respond to other available therapies.

Conclusion

A variety of medications are available for the treatment of insomnia, but they differ in their profiles of risks and benefits. Optimal treatment requires finding the agent with the risk/benefit profile that best matches each patient's particular type of insomnia (e.g., difficulty falling or staying asleep, early morning awakening) and their vulnerability to adverse effects.

Recommended Reading

Krystal AD, Ashbrook LH, Prather AA: What is insomnia? JAMA 326(23):2444, 2021 34932076

Sateia MJ, Buysse DJ, Krystal AD, et al: Clinical practice guideline for the pharmacologic treatment of chronic insomnia in adults: an American Academy of Sleep Medicine clinical practice guideline. J Clin Sleep Med 13(2):307–349, 2017 27998379

44

Ketamine and Esketamine

Chris A. Kelly, Ph.D.
James W. Murrough, M.D., Ph.D.

Introduction

Ketamine was first approved by the U.S. Food and Drug Administration (FDA) for use as an anesthetic, and among such medications, it is known to be safe and reliable. Ketamine also has other clinically useful properties, including sedation, pain relief, and anti-inflammation effects. When taken at dosages lower than those needed to induce anesthesia, it can cause mind-altering and out-of-body experiences; these properties led to its illicit use as a "party drug," and it would eventually be designated in 1999 as a Schedule III controlled substance in the United States.

In the late 1990s, researchers began investigating ketamine's antidepressant effects. Continuing research into the 2000s suggested that, unlike other antidepressants approved for use in depression at the time, ketamine showed strong and rapid (within 72 hours of a single dose) antidepressant effects, even in patients with chronic and severe forms of depression. Ketamine typically occurs as a mixture of two mirror forms, called *R* and *S*. In more recent years, the S form of ketamine (also known as *esketamine*) has been developed as an antidepressant and, in 2019, received FDA approval for use in treatment-resistant depression (TRD). In general, *treatment-resistant depression* refers to depression that fails to benefit from two or more standard antidepressant medications. Of note, esketamine did not appear to be as effective in older adults as in younger adults, and there was some debate in the field regarding the strength of the clinical evidence on which its FDA approval was based. Following its approval for adults with TRD, esketamine subsequently gained FDA approval for the treatment of depressive symptoms in adults with major depressive disorder (MDD) with suicidal thinking, the first approval of its kind in the United States. Because ketamine and esketamine work differently in the brain than other antidepressants, such as selective serotonin reuptake inhibitors (SSRIs), they have also significantly shifted the direction of antidepressant research. It should be noted that although hundreds or even thousands of ketamine or esketamine clinics across the United States currently offer in-person or telehealth care, not all of these follow the guidelines for appropriate care recommended by the American Psychiatric Association task force's consensus report.

How Do They Work?

One way ketamine is thought to work as an antidepressant is by stimulating the growth and rapid regrowth of brain connections that may have been lost during periods of high stress and depression. Ketamine exerts its primary effects via the brain's glutamatergic system, most importantly at the glutamate *N*-methyl-D-aspartate (NMDA) receptor but also at other receptors in the brain, including opioid receptors. *Glutamate* is an important neurotransmitter (i.e., brain chemical) that is a necessary component in the communication between nerve cells, and ketamine may help to improve communication between the nerve cells, especially in areas of the brain involved in mood. It is not yet known precisely how ketamine affects brain function to relieve depression; for example, although one small study showed that the opioid system was involved in response to ketamine, another study did not support the role of this system.

What Are Ketamine and Esketamine Used to Treat?

Intranasal esketamine (brand name Spravato), when used together with an oral antidepressant, is FDA-approved for use in adults with TRD and in adults with MDD who have suicidal thinking or behaviors. Intravenous ketamine is not currently FDA-approved for treatment of any psychiatric disorder; however, many controlled clinical trials support its efficacy for TRD and suicidal thinking in depression. Additional—albeit more limited—research suggests that ketamine may be helpful for treatment of bipolar disorder, obsessive-compulsive disorder (OCD), and posttraumatic stress disorder (PTSD).

Standard Dosing and Treatment Regimen

Dosing for both ketamine and esketamine is given at the *subanesthetic* level, meaning that the individual may be less aware of their surroundings but is not fully knocked out. They can be given in an outpatient setting, and dosing plus recovery time lasts up to 3 or 4 hours before the patient is allowed to be taken home by a designated friend or family member (patients should not drive or operate heavy machinery until they have had a restful night's sleep following treatment).

For adults with TRD, dosing with intranasal esketamine occurs in two phases: an *induction* phase and a *maintenance* phase. The induction phase lasts 4 weeks, during which it is sprayed into the nostrils twice weekly. Administration of the spray itself is very quick, but the most significant side effects last about 45 minutes to 1 hour. Patients are monitored for 1–2 hours after administration as the side effects continue to wear off. Dosing starts at 56 mg on day 1 and either remains at 56 mg or is increased to 84 mg on subsequent dosing days, depending on whether the physician and patient think it is helping the depression enough. The maintenance phase lasts another 4 weeks, during which esketamine is given once weekly at either 56 mg or 84 mg. Beyond this, dosing may occur weekly or every 2 weeks at either 56 mg or 84 mg, with the frequency and dosing strength determined by the lowest needed to keep the patient feeling better.

For adult MDD with suicidal thinking or behaviors, intranasal esketamine dosage typically starts and stays at 84 mg twice weekly for 4 weeks. If the depression does not respond by the end of week 4, treatment is discontinued and alternative options may be suggested.

Currently, there is no standard dosing regimen for intravenous ketamine. Community-based regimens typically follow a schedule of four to six intravenous ketamine infusions, with dosing typically starting at 0.5 mg/kg infused over a period of 40 minutes. Limited data support increased dosing up to 1.0 mg/kg, although studies to date do not show a clear dose-response relationship for ketamine. Patients are monitored for the next 1–2 hours as the side effects of the medicine wear off. An assessment is made at the end of the infusion cycle to determine whether the medicine is working and the treatment should continue.

Use in Special Populations

Most of the research into the antidepressant and antisuicidal effects of ketamine and esketamine are in the adult population, ranging in age from 18 to 65 years. Research data from patients in community settings show that approximately half of those treated with intravenous ketamine had some response to treatment and just under one-third were no longer depressed by 1-month follow-up. A small percentage of patients (less than 10%) worsen. Although data are sparse in populations outside this age range, some research indicates ketamine may be safe and effective for treating adolescents (13–17 years of age) with TRD and suicidal thinking or behaviors. Esketamine also shows promise for TRD in later life, with the one research trial to date of intranasal esketamine suggesting that it may be helpful for TRD specifically in older adults (ages 55–74 years). Depression symptoms in adults age 75 and older did not improve with esketamine. Data on the use of ketamine as an antidepressant in children are limited to anecdotal reports unrelated to TRD and limited by the different presentation of clinical depression in children younger than 13.

Medication Interactions

Most people who are prescribed ketamine or esketamine take it in combination with their existing psychiatric medications. Available data suggest that combination treatment with nonselective monoamine oxidase inhibitors (MAOIs) and reversible inhibitors of monoamine oxidase-A can be done safely but requires monitoring. Examples of commonly prescribed MAOIs include isocarboxazid (Marplan), phenelzine (Nardil), selegiline (Emsam), and tranylcypromine (Parnate). Because ketamine and esketamine can temporarily raise a person's blood pressure and heart rate, they should be used with caution when taken with psychostimulants or with medications that cause blood vessels to constrict or narrow. Examples of some commonly prescribed psychostimulants include mixed amphetamine salts (e.g., Adderall, Vyvanse), methylphenidate (e.g., Concerta, Ritalin), and modafinil (e.g., Provigil). The list of medications that constrict or narrow blood vessels is long but includes any agent that raises blood pressure. Medications processed by the cytochrome P450 enzymes CYP3A4 and CYP2B6 may affect how well the body processes ketamine or esketamine; however, no significant interactions with most antidepressants, second-generation antipsychotics, lithium, or anticonvulsants that are FDA-approved for the treatment of bipolar disorder have been reported.

Side Effects

The side effects of ketamine and esketamine are similar, although they may be more pronounced depending on which agent is given, whether it is given intravenously or intranasally, and whether it is given in high or low doses. The most common side effect that occurs during acute dosing is *dissociation*, which is a feeling of being disconnected from one's thoughts, feelings, surroundings, or even one's sense of self. This effect is experienced by most individuals given intravenous ketamine, but fewer than half of those given intranasal esketamine. There is a small risk that taking ketamine could spark psychosis in people who have a family history of psychosis or a psychotic disorder. Other side effects include sensory distortions, abnormal sensations, a feeling of unreality, unusual thoughts or beliefs, and intense blissful feelings. These side effects tend to peak around 40 minutes after receiving the medicine and to subside within 1–2 hours. Drowsiness, dizziness, and lightheadedness are also common side effects, along with temporary increases in heart rate and blood pressure. Some may experience heart palpitations, arrhythmias, chest pain, and low blood pressure while receiving the medication. Changes in blood pressure tend to peak within 20–50 minutes of administration and return to normal within 2–4 hours. Patients may also have some trouble with attention and making decisions, and they are recommended to avoid making major life decisions on the same day they receive ketamine or esketamine. There does not appear to be an issue with withdrawal syndromes if the medicine is abruptly stopped during infusion or after a full course of ketamine or esketamine is given.

Recreational use of ketamine has been associated with unconsciousness and dangerously slowed breathing. Long-term recreational use could cause bladder and kidney problems, stomach issues such as ulcers, poor memory, and depression. Ketamine and esketamine should not be mixed with alcohol because this could be fatal. However, medically supervised use of ketamine and esketamine as a treatment for depression has typically not been associated with the same kinds of negative outcomes identified in long-term recreational use. Taking ketamine, even under medical supervision, may increase patients' risk of misusing it in recreational settings, although this risk appears to be small.

Conclusion

The use of ketamine and esketamine has marked a significant shift in depression treatment, particularly for TRD and MDD with suicidal thoughts. Approved by the FDA for these indications, a single dose of ketamine or esketamine can offer rapid relief, acting through unique mechanisms in the brain's glutamatergic and reward systems. However, their antidepressant effects following a single administration are not long-lasting, and multiple administrations are typically needed. Use requires careful monitoring due to the short-term medication effects, such as increases in blood pressure, reduced heart rate and respiratory function, and potential mental effects such as dissociation and sensory distortions. Although the data are promising, further research on the safety of long-term use of these medications and on their use in special populations is needed. The risk of misuse highlights the need for controlled medical supervision.

Recommended Reading

Mathew SJ, Zarate CA Jr: Ketamine for Treatment-Resistant Depression: The First Decade of Progress. New York, Springer, 2016

McInnes LA, Qian JJ, Gargeya RS, et al: A retrospective analysis of ketamine intravenous therapy for depression in real-world care settings. J Affect Disord 301:486–495, 2022 35027209

45

Benzodiazepines

Rebecca C. Kass, M.D.
David V. Sheehan, M.D., M.B.A.

Introduction

Benzodiazepines are controversial. Patients, family members, and providers fall into two camps when it comes to these medications: all for or all against. Our aim in this chapter is to provide a balanced presentation of the facts on these medications to enable patients to make an informed choice.

The first benzodiazepine was discovered in 1959, and it was not until the late 1980s that the first agent in this class received U.S. Food and Drug Administration (FDA) approval for treatment of panic disorder (PD). By 2013, the short-acting benzodiazepine alprazolam was the most widely prescribed psychiatric medication in the United States. Benzodiazepines continue to be broadly prescribed for treatment of both generalized anxiety disorder (GAD) and PD. Since the 1990s, the serotonin-modulating selective serotonin reuptake inhibitors (SSRIs) and serotonin-norepinephrine reuptake inhibitors (SNRIs) have become physicians' first choice for treatment of anxiety disorders, but the benzodiazepines are often used in conjunction with these medications or even as monotherapy for patients whose symptoms do not fully respond to SSRI or SNRI treatment.

How Do They Work?

Benzodiazepines work in conjunction with a specific neurotransmitter in the brain called γ-aminobutyric acid (GABA). This neurotransmitter has a number of functions, including reducing anxiety, promoting sleep, preventing seizures, and relaxing muscles. Benzodiazepines help GABA exert a stronger interaction on its receptor and thereby enhance its effects. For this reason, they are helpful in the treatment of insomnia, anxiety, muscle spasms, agitation, and acute withdrawal from alcohol (which also acts at the GABA receptor) and with inducing anesthesia.

Different benzodiazepines have different speeds of onset and durations of effect. These are related not only to the properties of each drug but also to individual patient factors, such as body weight and metabolism, its absorption in the gastrointestinal tract, the degree to which it is stored in fat tissue, and the rate at which it is eliminated from the body. Longer-acting benzodiazepines provide more extended periods of symptom relief, but with the trade-off that side effects also may last longer.

Most benzodiazepines are broken down in the liver, with three exceptions: lorazepam, oxazepam, and temazepam. For this reason, patients with impaired liver function, increased age, or those who are already taking medications that affect the breakdown of other drugs in the liver are usually prescribed one of these medications to avoid potentially harmful accumulation of the medication in the body.

To reduce the side effects associated with benzodiazepines, other sedative-hypnotics were developed for the treatment of insomnia, including zopiclone, eszopiclone, and zaleplon, which act at a similar site in the brain, but more selectively. More recently, suvorexant and lemborexant, which act upon different sites in the brain (at orexin A and B receptors), were developed to further reduce the side effects and disadvantages of the older benzodiazepines and sedative-hypnotics while providing similar benefit in the treatment of insomnia.

What Are Benzodiazepines Used to Treat?

Benzodiazepines are FDA-approved for treatment of GAD, PD, insomnia, and seizures. Alprazolam, clonazepam, and lorazepam are FDA-approved for treatment of PD (Table 45–1). Rapid symptom improvement is observed within the first week in the form of decreased panic attacks, phobic fears and avoidance, anticipatory anxiety, and disability, but they are not effective in the treatment of depressed mood or major depressive disorder. The concomitant initial use of a benzodiazepine with an antidepressant may hasten recovery from anxiety and

Table 45–1. Benzodiazepine dosage by indication

Generic name	Trade name	GAD, *mg*	PD, *mg*	Insomnia, *mg*
Alprazolam	Xanax	0.75–4	1–10	
Clonazepam	Klonopin	1–4	0.5–4	
Lorazepam	Ativan	2–8	2–8	
Oxazepam	Serax	30–120		
Diazepam	Valium	5–20	5–15	
Chlordiazepoxide	Librium	10–100		
Temazepam	Restoril			7.5–30
Flurazepam	Dalmane			15–30
Triazolam	Halcion			0.125–0.25
Zolpidem	Ambien			5–10
Sonata	Zaleplon			5–10
Eszopiclone	Lunesta			1–3
Suvorexant	Belsomra			5–20
Lemborexant	Dayvigo			5–10

Note. GAD=generalized anxiety disorder; PD=panic disorder.

panic symptoms and is a reasonable approach for rapid relief of symptoms in patients who are in acute anxiety crisis. In such cases, the benzodiazepine can be slowly tapered after several weeks. For insomnia, the short-acting benzodiazepine temazepam has received FDA approval for short-term use (7–10 days) to precipitate sleep.

No benzodiazepines are FDA-approved for the treatment of social anxiety disorder (social phobia), although they continue to be prescribed off-label for this condition. Benzodiazepines are thought to be ineffective in the treatment of obsessive-compulsive disorder (OCD), and although they may improve sleep and agitation initially in posttraumatic stress disorder (PTSD), they are not particularly effective for the core symptoms of this disorder in the longer term. An added complication is that patients with PTSD have higher rates of abuse and dependence than the general population. For these reasons, benzodiazepines are not recommended for PTSD treatment.

Benzodiazepines can play a role in the acute management of anxiety and agitation in psychotic disorders, permitting more moderate dosages of antipsychotic medications to be used effectively in such cases. However, benzodiazepines are not effective against psychotic symptoms.

Standard Dosing and Treatment Regimen

The most reliable place to locate the standard FDA-approved daily dosing regimen of various benzodiazepines for GAD, PD, and insomnia is on the FDA website at www.accessdata.fda.gov/scripts/cder/daf. The total daily dosages are usually divided up and given across multiple doses throughout the day. Most benzodiazepines only have a duration of action against anxiety of 4–7 hours, and doses may need to be spaced accordingly for optimal effect. The half-life of each benzodiazepine is not a good guide to its duration of therapeutic action. Always follow the recommendations of your prescriber when taking benzodiazepines.

Use in Special Populations

Young and elderly patients typically require lower dosages to achieve the same effect. Other special considerations in specific patient populations are described in the sections that follow.

Children and Adolescents

Benzodiazepines may be required in children and adolescents for psychiatric or medical reasons. They are used in pediatric epilepsy to prevent seizures. In this population, extended- and sustained-release formulations with longer duration of action may be used so that less frequent dosing is required. For young patients who need the medication in emergencies or are unable to tolerate pill swallowing, some benzodiazepines also come as suppositories or inhalants.

Pregnancy and Lactation

There is mixed evidence surrounding the use of benzodiazepines during the first two trimesters of pregnancy, with some literature pointing to a risk of fetal malformations and other research disputing this risk. High-dosage or long-term use of benzodiazepines by a pregnant female has been linked with neonatal withdrawal, which presents as irritability and hyperactivity at birth. Third-trimester use may lead to "floppy baby" syndrome, which presents as lethargy, and even to respiratory depression. Short-term use of benzodiazepines during labor does not appear to be harmful to the fetus.

Benzodiazepines are transmitted through breast milk and should ideally be avoided by breastfeeding females.

Elderly Patients

Current guidelines recommend short-term, as-needed use of benzodiazepines in adults older than 65 years. Medication tapering should always be done slowly in this age group, especially if the patient has been taking a high dosage for a long time.

Medication Interactions

Benzodiazepines are broken down by enzymes in the liver. Patients with liver disease, those who are elderly, or those who are already taking medications that affect this breakdown process may require lower dosages. Three benzodiazepines (i.e., lorazepam, oxazepam, and temazepam) are broken down by a different liver enzyme process, which makes them less likely to need adjustments because of liver disease or medication interactions. Ask your physician for a list of medications that can interfere with the breakdown of the benzodiazepine you are prescribed, because such interactions could either increase the side effects or reduce the benefit of the medications.

Side Effects

A common side effect of benzodiazepines, particularly at higher dosages and when first starting treatment, is impairment in motor skills. This can lead to an increased risk of falls and motor vehicle accidents. All patients should be cautioned about the use of benzodiazepines when operating machinery. The effects of benzodiazepines may be potentiated when they are combined with alcohol or illicit substances. The FDA has issued a "black box warning" for increased risk of death when combining benzodiazepines and opiate medications. Benzodiazepines can also cause somnolence, slurred speech, and, in very high doses, respiratory depression. In the event of a benzodiazepine overdose, dangerous alterations in vital functioning can occur, and emergency medical care should be sought. Flumazenil can be used as an "antidote" to benzodiazepine overdose; however, because it can precipitate withdrawal symptoms and occasionally seizures, it should only be administered by a trained medical provider.

Rapid or abrupt discontinuation of benzodiazepines can lead to withdrawal symptoms such as irritability, hyperactivity, insomnia, and, in very severe cases, psychosis, delirium, and seizures. A very slow taper is the best approach to avoid withdrawal symptoms when discontinuing benzodiazepines and increases the success of getting patients off the medication.

Substance use disorder is associated with ongoing, compulsive consumption of a substance despite negative consequences, leading to impairment in functioning in multiple domains. If a patient is prescribed a benzodiazepine appropriately by a medical professional, their symptoms should not meet criteria for a substance use disorder at any time during treatment. However, patients with a history of substance use disorder are more likely to abuse benzodiazepines and to seek out these medications from nonmedical sources to self-treat withdrawal symptoms or to augment the effects of other substances. Benzodiazepine abuse among adolescents is also a growing concern. Prescribers should check for evidence of abuse and exercise caution when prescribing benzodiazepines to adolescents or adults.

Conclusion

Benzodiazepines remain a mainstay of treatment for a number of psychiatric conditions, including PD, GAD, and insomnia. Although caution must be exercised when taking benzodiazepines due to their effects on motor function and potential for abuse, they are generally a safe and effective choice when prescribed and managed by a trained professional.

Recommended Reading

Salzman C: The APA Task Force report on benzodiazepine dependence, toxicity, and abuse. Am J Psychiatry 148(2):151–152, 1991

Sheehan DV: Benzodiazepines, in The American Psychiatric Association Publishing Textbook of Psychopharmacology, 5th Edition. Edited by Schatzberg AF, Nemeroff CB. Washington, DC, American Psychiatric Association Publishing, 2022, pp 563–584

46

Buspirone

Laura J. Miller, M.D.
Charles F. Gillespie, M.D., Ph.D.

Introduction

Buspirone, also known by the trade name Buspar, received marketing approval for the treatment of generalized anxiety disorder (GAD) from the U.S. Food and Drug Administration (FDA) in 1986. Originally developed for treatment of psychosis, buspirone was found in clinical trials to have very limited effects on the core symptoms of psychosis, which include hallucinations, delusional thoughts, and disorganized behavior. Subsequent clinical studies investigating alternative uses for buspirone found that it possessed significant antianxiety, also known as *anxiolytic*, properties and was generally well tolerated in terms of side effects. These clinical findings led to the present use of buspirone as a treatment for anxiety. Buspirone went off-patent in 2001 and is widely available in generic form.

How Does It Work?

Pharmacological

Buspirone is a partial agonist of the serotonin-1A (5-hydroxytryptamine [5-HT]$_{1A}$) receptor. These receptors are located in regions of the brain that contribute to the regulation of emotion, motivation, and memory. Disturbances in the function of these regions, which include the cerebral cortex, hippocampus, amygdala, and midbrain raphe nuclei—the primary source of serotonin in the brain—are strongly associated with the presence of clinically significant depression, anxiety, and panic. As a partial agonist, buspirone is able to "mimic" the effects of serotonin on 5-HT_{1A} receptors to a limited degree. Specifically, it activates 5-HT_{1A} receptors in some regions of the brain and blocks the effects of serotonin on 5-HT_{1A} receptors in others. This pharmacological mimicry allows it to alter the flow of neural information conveyed by serotonin and is thought to be responsible for its positive clinical effects on the symptoms of anxiety.

Metabolism

Buspirone is metabolized primarily in the liver, and its metabolites are excreted by the kidneys. In healthy human volunteers, it has a short half-life of approximately 2.5 hours, necessitating dosing two or three times daily to obtain consistent levels in the body. Taking buspirone with food reduces the impact of liver metabolism on buspirone absorption and may facilitate earlier and more consistent attainment of therapeutic blood levels of the medication. Patients who have impaired liver or kidney function will need a lower dosage of buspirone and close monitoring by their physician to avoid side effects caused by the reduced metabolism and excretion of its metabolites. In the liver, buspirone is metabolized into several pharmacologically active metabolites that have clinically relevant effects. In particular, the metabolite 1-pyriminidinylpiperazine (1-PP), which stimulates activity of norepinephrine-releasing neurons in a part of the brain known as the *locus coeruleus*, may worsen symptoms of anxiety and panic in patients with co-occurring panic disorder or in patients who are undergoing withdrawal from benzodiazepines. As a result, buspirone should be avoided in such patients so as not to worsen these conditions, unless the patient is being treated with a separate medication specifically for panic disorder or benzodiazepine withdrawal.

What Is Buspirone Used to Treat?

Generalized Anxiety Disorder

Buspirone is FDA-approved for the treatment of GAD in adults. This approval was granted based on the results of several randomized clinical trials demonstrating that buspirone was as effective as the benzodiazepine diazepam and superior to placebo in the treatment of anxiety. Subsequent studies comparing other benzodiazepines with buspirone confirmed these findings. Although buspirone and benzodiazepines have comparable efficacy in the treatment of anxiety, there are some important differences in the clinical response to these agents. The onset of anxiolytic effects on the physical symptoms of anxiety such as muscle tension and insomnia is much faster with benzodiazepines than with buspirone. This delay in relief from physical anxiety symptoms often leads patients and physicians to "give up" on buspirone before it has reached its full effect. This is most frequently observed in patients switching their current treatment from benzodiazepines to buspirone or in those recently treated with benzodiazepines who have had a relapse of anxiety and are initiating treatment with buspirone. On the other hand, buspirone does not share the risks for progressive physical dependence that are characteristic of benzodiazepines. Buspirone also may be rapidly stopped without the risk of clinically significant physical withdrawal symptoms or relapse of anxiety, which is not the case with benzodiazepines.

Mixed Anxiety-Depression, Antidepressant Augmentation, and Sexual Dysfunction

Other recognized uses of buspirone include treatment of anxiety that co-occurs with limited depressive symptoms, known as *mixed anxiety-depression*, and as an augmentation agent to enhance the effects of conventional antidepressants in the treatment of major depressive disorder. Initial clinical trials found buspirone to be helpful in the treatment of mixed anxiety-depression, with improvement of both depressive and anxiety symptoms. These findings were replicated and led to the use of buspirone to treat mixed anxiety-depression. Subsequent studies identified and confirmed a role for buspirone to augment the effects of conventional antidepressants in the treatment of major depressive disorder with co-occurring GAD and to further improve depressive symptoms in patients whose symptoms have partially, but not fully, responded to antidepressants. Finally, coadministration of buspirone is often helpful in reducing the intensity of sexual side effects, such as delayed or inhibited orgasm, sometimes experienced by patients during treatment with certain antidepressant medications.

Anxiety With Smoking Cessation and Alcohol Use Disorder

A number of randomized and placebo-controlled studies have documented the utility of buspirone in the treatment of anxiety in patients undergoing smoking cessation treatment and in patients with ongoing alcohol use disorder. The lack of abuse liability and absence of mental or physical impairment with buspirone position it well for treatment of anxiety in these two groups of patients when they are actively using and not yet sober.

Standard Dosing and Treatment Regimen

The starting dosage for buspirone is 10–20 mg/day divided into two or three doses. Based on clinical response in terms of tolerability and impact on symptoms of anxiety, the dosage of buspirone may then be gradually increased to a total dosage of 30–60 mg/day.

Use in Special Populations

Most of the clinical research studies investigating the use of buspirone to treat anxiety and anxiety with depression have been conducted with adults. However, clinical studies with buspirone have also been conducted with children, adolescents, and elderly patients. Although the results of these studies are more variable with respect to the efficacy of buspirone on treatment of anxiety in these patient groups, no safety concerns with use of buspirone in these populations have been identified, and buspirone is considered safe for use in children, adolescents, and elderly patients.

Medication Interactions

Although medication interactions with buspirone are relatively limited, there are several important ones to note. Medications such as verapamil, diltiazem, erythromycin, itraconazole, and nefazodone, along with grapefruit juice, inhibit the activity of the primary enzyme, cytochrome P450 3A4, that metabolizes buspirone. As a consequence, blood levels of buspirone and its metabolites are increased, and side effects may emerge. Conversely, co-administration of rifampin with buspirone leads to reduced blood levels of buspirone and its metabolites, and therapeutic effects may be lost. Buspirone may increase the blood levels of haloperidol and cyclosporin-A, and coadministration of buspirone with these medications should be done with careful clinical oversight. The combination of buspirone with monoamine oxidase inhibitors (MAOIs) should be avoided due to the risk of serotonin syndrome.

Side Effects

Data summarized from a series of 17 clinical trials indicate that the most common side effects of buspirone observed in adult patients are dizziness (12%), sleepiness (10%), nausea (8%), headache (6%), increased anxiety (5%), fatigue (4%), insomnia (3%), lightheadedness (3%), dry mouth (3%), and excitement

(2%). Sedation, in addition to the side effects seen in adults, may be observed in children and adolescent patients. It is important to note that most patients do not experience these side effects, and, when they do occur, they are generally mild to moderate and resolve over a few weeks at a steady medication dosage. Studies examining psychomotor function (e.g., memory, concentration, complex driving skills) in patients treated with buspirone have found no evidence of impairment in these areas of mental and behavioral function. Finally, there are no documented cases of death in overdose with buspirone alone.

Recommended Reading

Barnett SR: Anxiolytics and sedative/hypnotics: benzodiazepines, buspirone, and others, in Pediatric Psychopharmacology, 2nd Edition. Edited by Martin A, Scahill L, Kratochvil C. New York, Oxford University Press, 2011, pp 338–349

Robinson DS: Buspirone, in The American Psychiatric Publishing Textbook of Psychopharmacology, 5th Edition. Edited by Schatzberg AF, Nemeroff CD. Washington, DC, American Psychiatric Association Publishing, 2017, pp 585–600

47

Pharmacological Treatments in Development

Grace S. Pham, D.O., Ph.D.
Sanjay J. Mathew, M.D.

Introduction

Although conventional antidepressants (e.g., selective serotonin reuptake inhibitors [SSRIs]) and psychotherapy continue to be the first-line treatments for anxiety and depression, if they should fail, numerous investigational agents have emerged as potential alternatives. In addition, the therapeutic potential of naturally occurring and synthetic psychedelic compounds in treatment of anxiety and depression has recently been studied more closely, despite decades of stringent federal regulation surrounding their use. The medications discussed in this chapter are novel and behave differently than standard antidepressants, and many are still being evaluated and tested on a large scale for safety and efficacy. Just as no two people are alike, neither are their brains nor the way their anxiety and depression manifest. Novel agents and therapeutics, acting through different pathways and mechanisms, and either solo or in tandem with conventional antidepressants and psychotherapy, may help patients who have more treatment-resistant forms of depression and anxiety.

The new agents discussed here target brain receptors and systems other than serotonin, dopamine, and norepinephrine, which are the classic targets of existing medications. These agents are in clinical development for treatment of depression and related conditions, but as of late 2023, only one is approved by the U.S. Food and Drug Administration (FDA), as discussed in the following section.

N-Methyl-D-Aspartate Receptor Modulators

N-methyl-D-aspartate (NMDA) receptors regulate excitatory glutamate neurotransmission, meaning they activate *neurons* (brain cells) and cause messages to be passed further in the brain. While NMDA receptor dysregulation is classically associated with psychosis, it may also be implicated in depression and conditions associated with negative emotions. NMDA receptors also play a role in *neuroplasticity*, or the brain's ability to adapt to new conditions. Agents that antagonize, or oppose, NMDA receptors (e.g., ketamine and esketamine nasal spray) may rapidly decrease depressive symptoms in people with depression. Sigma-1 receptors have also been found to be potential targets in depression and anxiety and are affected by the conventional antidepressants bupropion and venlafaxine.

AXS-05

The novel agent AXS-05 (dextromethorphan-bupropion, brand name Auvelity) received FDA approval for treatment of major depressive disorder (MDD) in 2022. This medication acts as a hybrid of two existing agents: dextromethorphan, a substance commonly used as a cough suppressant, and bupropion, an antidepressant that prevents the reuptake of norepinephrine and dopamine. The dextromethorphan component opposes NMDA receptor activity while promoting sigma-1 receptor activity. The bupropion component increases the brain availability of dextromethorphan while also preventing reuptake of norepinephrine and dopamine. Across a number of clinical trials involving several hundred patients, AXS-05 was more effective at treating depressive symptoms compared with bupropion alone and, in a separate trial, compared with placebo. AXS-05 was well tolerated, with side effects similar to those of existing antidepressants (e.g., dizziness, nausea, dry mouth).

REL-1017

Psychiatrists frequently "augment" an antidepressant by adding a second medicine with a different mechanism of action. Combinations that have this built-in augmentation simultaneously and synergistically affect multiple pharmaceutical targets and are specially formulated to have an optimal ratio of their components. REL-1017, also known as esmethadone, is an NMDA receptor blocker that is currently undergoing phase-III clinical trials for MDD. Esmethadone is a specific chemical variant of methadone, a medication used for moderate to severe pain as well as opioid addiction, that at low dosages does not act as an opioid. It is believed to specifically block hyperactive subtypes of NMDA receptors rather than affecting the activity of normally functioning ones.

Gamma-Aminobutyric Acid-A Receptor–Positive Allosteric Modulators

γ-Aminobutyric acid (GABA) receptor dysfunction has been linked to depression and anxiety through its role in the areas of the brain that mediate stress. GABA is the major inhibitory neurotransmitter in the brain, meaning that it blocks messages between neurons, which helps counter and balance excitatory glutamate transmission in the brain. GABA transmission also plays a principal role in neural maturation and in areas of the brain that pertain to memory, which are both processes promoted by antidepressants. Benzodiazepines, including commonly known medications such as alprazolam and clonazepam, rapidly dissipate anxiety by acting at GABA receptors but are more likely to be misused and may cause cognitive deficits later in life.

New agents targeting GABA receptors that have lower misuse potential may be helpful in anxiety and depression. Zuranolone may be effective for rapid relief of symptoms in MDD and is taken by mouth once daily for 2 weeks. A synthetic compound that acts as a neurosteroid targeting $GABA_A$ receptors, zuranolone was developed as an improved, oral version of brexanolone, an intravenously administered infusion approved in 2019 for treatment of postpartum depression. It is now being tested in clinical trials for use in MDD, postpartum depression, insomnia, and bipolar depression, among other indications. The shorter time frame for zuranolone treatment—2 weeks—is especially novel considering that existing antidepressants typically require 4–6 weeks to achieve any sort of therapeutic effect and are generally prescribed for a minimum of 6–9 months. The goal of this "episodic" treatment approach is to facilitate a quick remission and prolonged symptom-free period; if the patient relapses, another 2-week treatment course would be quickly instituted.

Medications That Impact Ion Channels

Other investigational medications target specific ion channels in the brain in order to impact the relay of messages.

BI1358894

BI1358894 is an experimental agent that targets transient receptor potential canonical (TRPC) calcium channels in the *amygdala*, an area of the brain that handles the experience of emotions, and it may thereby be therapeutic in post-traumatic stress disorder (PTSD), depression, and stress-related conditions. The amygdala is hyperactive in conditions such as PTSD, mediating excessive fear circuitry activity and leading to hypervigilance and increased startle response. This medication is also currently being studied in clinical trials to determine its efficacy in depression and borderline personality disorder, the latter of which is frequently associated with anxiety and depression.

XEN1101

XEN1101 is a new formulation of an existing medication, ezogabine, which is used to treat epilepsy by targeting a specific type of potassium channel. In a clinical trial with MDD patients, ezogabine treatment resulted in improvement of depressive symptoms and was well tolerated without serious adverse effects. Ezogabine appears to mediate these actions via the *ventral striatum*, known as the "reward center" of the brain, and may reverse *anhedonia*, or loss of the ability to experience pleasure, which is a common feature of depression. Compared with ezogabine, which needs to be taken three times daily, XEN1101 only needs to be taken once a day. XEN1101 is currently being evaluated in clinical trials for treatment of MDD.

Brain Peptide Antagonists

Orexins are proteins formed in the brain that promote arousal, wakefulness, and appetite. Compared with other types of neurons, there are relatively fewer orexin neurons, although they play an important role in adjusting the brain's response to stress. Although the exact cause of hyperarousal in MDD is not currently known, it is associated with negative effects on circadian rhythms, which leads to sustained difficulty in falling asleep. Opposing the orexin receptors, which normally work to promote wakefulness, is a novel approach to treating insomnia and is now also being studied for MDD. Suvorexant (brand name Belsomra), is a medication that was approved by the FDA in 2014 for treatment of insomnia and works by targeting both orexin-1 and orexin-2 receptors. In recent clinical trials, suvorexant was found to be effective in treating insomnia in patients who were already taking antidepressants for MDD. Lemborexant and daridorexant are medications that also work against both orexin-1 and orexin-2 receptors and are FDA-approved for insomnia. So far, one medication that specifically targets orexin-2 receptors—seltorexant—has been found to improve sleep difficulties and depressive symptoms in patients diagnosed with both MDD and insomnia. It is being further studied in other clinical trials including elderly populations, which is significant because many existing medications for sleep (e.g., zolpidem [Ambien] and eszoplicone [Lunesta]) are not well tolerated in elderly patients.

Kappa Opioid Receptor Antagonists

Recent studies have supported the role of kappa opioid receptor antagonists in promoting stress resilience, thereby providing potential benefit in conditions such as depression and anxiety. Researchers have discovered that activating kappa opioid receptors in humans and animals may lead to anxious and dysphoric responses. By contrast, agents that oppose these receptors have antidepressant effects and lessen addictive behavior in animal models. Neumora Therapeutics is currently investigating NMRA-140, a selective kappa opioid receptor antagonist, in phase-II clinical trials for treatment of MDD. Janssen Pharmaceuticals is currently developing aticaprant, a different selective kappa opioid receptor antagonist, for MDD, with aims of submitting a regulatory application for FDA approval by 2025.

Psychedelics

Psychedelics were outlawed and classified as Schedule 1 substances by the Controlled Substances Act of 1970 but have reemerged as promising treatments for depression and anxiety. They include naturally occurring compounds such as psilocybin and N,N-dimethyltryptamine (DMT) and synthetic substances such as 3,4-methylenedioxymethamphetamine (MDMA) and lysergic acid diethylamide (LSD). At this time, these substances continue to be criminalized in most states, although impending legislation may lead to the more widespread use of psychedelics in mental health treatment. Most studies investigating their use in mental health conditions involved guided psychotherapy, a context that is likely to change previous popular notions of psychedelics as substances of abuse. Formal training for therapists and mental health practitioners to become certified in MDMA-assisted psychotherapy, for example, is currently available due to the FDA designating it as a breakthrough therapy.

Psilocybin

Psilocybin is a naturally occurring hallucinogenic compound found in more than 200 strains of psychoactive mushrooms. It is converted to the active component *psilocin* after ingestion and interacts with serotonin receptors. Serotonin helps mediate psychological states, including happiness, optimism, and satisfaction. Psilocybin is said to have a noetic quality, promoting mystical experiences and deeper meditation. A clinical trial investigating its therapeutic effects in patients with terminal cancer found that improvement of depressive symptoms correlated most with the strength of participants' mystical experiences. A recent study found that psilocybin was comparable with escitalopram, an SSRI, over a 6-week period. COMPASS Pathways has formulated standardized doses of psilocybin, COMP360, and 25-mg doses of COMP360 were found to decrease depressive symptoms in patients with treatment-resistant depression compared with 10-mg and 1-mg doses. The drug was found to be generally well tolerated and safe in the context of psychotherapy.

Lysergic Acid Diethylamide

LSD, also known as acid, impacts both serotonin and dopamine neurotransmission, causing significant psychoactive effects that tend to last longer than those produced by other psychedelics—on average, 8–12 hours. In a controlled research setting, a single dose of LSD was found to be safely tolerated without producing adverse physiological effects. MM-120, produced by the company MindMed, is an orally administered form of LSD that is currently undergoing studies for the treatment of depression and was recently cleared by the FDA to be administered in a clinical trial for patients with generalized anxiety disorder.

3,4-Methylenedioxymethamphetamine

MDMA, also known as Ecstasy, is a synthetic psychedelic drug that helps promote serotonin, norepinephrine, and dopamine release. Recent evidence suggests that MDMA also may promote oxytocin release, which would help explain how it facilitates openness and social bonding. Compared with psilocybin and LSD, which interact with serotonin-2A (5-hydroxytryptamine $[5\text{-HT}]_{2A}$) receptors, MDMA causes the release of serotonin from nerve cells. Due to its interactions with these neurotransmitters, MDMA acts as both a hallucinogen and a stimulant. The stimulant effects help explain MDMA's toxicity when taken in excess; in rare cases, overdose may lead to dangerous increases in body temperature, with subsequent muscle breakdown and kidney injury. MDMA appears to have more addictive potential than psilocybin, likely because of these stimulant properties. However, in controlled settings, its use with guided psychotherapy was found to promote fear extinction, making it highly effective in PTSD. In late-stage clinical trials for PTSD, MDMA-assisted psychotherapy was highly effective, demonstrating significant improvement after three sessions.

Although numerous psychedelics and regulated forms of psychedelic compounds are emerging in popularity, there are concerns regarding whether these promising findings from studies will necessarily lead to similar outcomes in patients with anxiety, depression, and other mental health conditions. One concern is that the studies may not be truly *double-blinded*, meaning that study organizers may be aware of who receives the psychedelic versus the placebo, and positive bias may skew data accordingly, leading to overly promising results. Many of these trials also incorporate psychotherapy interventions, sometimes having two therapists present, which may not be feasible or cost-effective for real patients. Finally, some psychedelics may have a higher abuse liability due to their hallucinogenic effects.

Psychedelics are already used recreationally, which can be dangerous because the manufacturing of psychedelics is not regulated, and it is highly likely that recreational psychedelics may be spiked with other illicit substances. Prescribed psychedelic compounds have the potential of being *diverted*, or sold to people who are not prescribed them, for recreational use. Overall, more federally funded studies are needed to investigate the use of psychedelics in mental health conditions, especially substance use disorders.

Less is known about the effects of *microdosing*, or repeatedly taking smaller, sub-hallucinogenic doses of psychedelics that do not produce overt psychoactive effects. Microdosing has become increasingly popular in the media, but scientific literature on this practice is lacking.

Nevertheless, these are all relative obstacles, and the safety and general lack of adverse effects make psychedelics appealing alternative treatments. Because many psychedelics interact with serotonin receptors, there is a theoretical risk of serotonin syndrome in patients who are already taking antidepressants. *Serotonin syndrome* is a serious condition caused by serotonergic medications in which there is excess serotonin and overactivation of serotonin receptors in the brain and the rest of the body. However, evidence of serotonin syndrome occurring in the setting of psychedelic use is scant. Overall, information about how psychedelics impact people who are already taking antidepressants is limited, and additional research is needed on this specific topic.

Conclusion

A number of investigational agents, as well as natural and synthetic psychedelic compounds, are actively being evaluated in clinical trials as promising treatments for anxiety, depression, PTSD, and other mental health conditions. Some appear promising based on their known mechanisms of action within the neural pathways implicated in anxiety and depression, but they require long periods of monitoring and observation among large groups of healthy study participants as well as those with mental health conditions. Mental illness is a complex entity that results from the intersection of biological, psychological, and social factors in the context of a society and world that are constantly in flux. It is thus not surprising that certain treatments for anxiety and depression may work for some people and not others or that certain people may experience anxiety and depression that does not respond to most approved treatments. If you or someone you know has experienced a lack of efficacy with antidepressants, you or they may be eligible to participate in one of these ongoing studies for treatment with an investigational drug or a psychedelic compound. Such clinical trials will help researchers and psychiatrists better understand the real-life applications of these substances and eventually lead to the standard practice of developing treatments for people with treatment-resistant depression or treatment-refractory anxiety.

Recommended Reading

Carhart-Harris R, Giribaldi B, Watts R, et al: Trial of psilocybin versus escitalopram for depression. N Engl J Med 384(15):1402–1411, 2021 33852780

Tabuteau H, Jones A, Anderson A, et al: Effect of AXS-05 (dextromethorphan-bupropion) in major depressive disorder: a randomized double-blind controlled trial. Am J Psychiatry 179(7):490–499, 2022 35582785

Part IV

The Treatments

Neuromodulation

48

Electroconvulsive Therapy

Nicholas Ortiz, M.D.

Introduction

Electroconvulsive therapy (ECT) is a safe and effective medical treatment used for a variety of neuropsychiatric illnesses, including major depressive disorder, bipolar disorder, schizophrenia, and catatonia. ECT has been used in the United States for more than 80 years, and annually more than 1 million people around the world receive ECT treatment.

ECT is a brief outpatient procedure performed by a psychiatrist in a hospital setting and may be conducted while patients are receiving inpatient or outpatient psychiatric treatment. During ECT, patients are given general anesthesia, and a painless modified electrical current is administered to their scalp, resulting in a brief generalized seizure in the brain. This seizure is carefully monitored using electroencephalography to ensure safety and response to stimulation. After the seizure is finished, patients regain consciousness and continue to recover from the effects of general anesthesia. Patients can often expect to be released and able to return home within 1 hour after their treatment.

Although not a curative treatment, because relapse may still occur after a treatment course, ECT can significantly and expeditiously improve severe psychiatric symptoms. Patients often receive an initial course of 6–12 treatments, usually administered multiple times per week. Such an initial treatment course is often followed by a taper of decreasing treatment frequency or, in certain circumstances, ongoing maintenance treatments. More details regarding ECT treatments are discussed in the following sections.

What Is It Used to Treat?

ECT is used when initial treatments, such as medications, are ineffective at improving symptoms or when patients are deteriorating so rapidly that their condition is considered life threatening. The American Psychiatric Association, the American Medical Association, and the U.S. Surgeon General all endorse ECT as a valuable tool for the treatment of depression, and the U.S. Food and Drug Administration (FDA) has issued statements on the safety and effectiveness of ECT in treating patients older than 18 years of age who have severe episodes of depression associated with major depressive disorder and bipolar disorder. In addition, large international reviews have shown ECT to be safe and effective for catatonia, treatment-resistant mania, and treatment-resistant schizophrenia. Its safety and effectiveness have also been demonstrated in individuals younger than 18 years who have treatment-resistant illness and in those with life-threatening neuropsychiatric conditions. ECT has also been successfully used in pregnant and postpartum patients experiencing severe psychiatric symptoms (psychosis), and it remains a valuable treatment option especially when pharmacotherapy options would pose a significant risk to the fetus.

How Is Electroconvulsive Therapy Performed, and How Many Treatments Should Be Expected?

Prior to receiving ECT, patients are evaluated by a primary care physician who performs a medical history and physical examination to determine the patient's relative risk of undergoing ECT treatments. No specific medical conditions absolutely disqualify someone from receiving ECT; however, some conditions can increase a person's relative risk of experiencing complications during the procedure. Patients with neurological problems such as strokes, brain bleeds, or *aneurysms* (outpocketing of blood vessels), as well as those with heart problems such as a recent heart attack or heart failure, can have an increased risk of complications during ECT. Similarly, patients with severe lung problems or bone fractures can also be at an increased risk for complications during treatment. Having implantable medical devices such as pacemakers or nerve stimulators does not automatically disqualify someone from receiving ECT.

During an ECT treatment, patients are placed under general anesthesia and do not "feel" the treatment being delivered. They are put on an intravenous line and first given a medication that results in unconsciousness, followed by another medication that reduces muscular contractility in order to minimize the intensity of their convulsions during the seizure. Patients may also be given medications to regulate their heart rate and blood pressure during the treatment if necessary.

Modern ECT involves delivery of a small amount of modified electric current that is briefly passed through the scalp into the brain, resulting in a seizure. Modern constant-current ECT devices use square-wave pulse trains that can be modified in frequency, pulse width, and duration. This stimulation is typically introduced on the right side of the brain to minimize the potential side effects associated with applying stimulation over the language centers of the brain, which are typically located on the left side. Bilateral treatment may be indicated in patients who do not respond to unilateral treatments or for those with life-threatening neuropsychiatric illness, such as malignant catatonia or neuroleptic malignant syndrome. A conducting gel is used to facilitate the flow of electricity and to prevent injury or irritation to the skin. A soft mouth guard is also used to prevent any dental injuries that could result from contraction of jaw muscles that may be activated during the stimulation.

The waveform of the patient's seizure, as well as other physiological parameters, including their blood pressure, blood oxygenation, and pulse rate, are carefully monitored throughout the treatment. Although seizures induced by ECT typically resolve on their own, medications can also be given to assist in ending a seizure in the event it continues beyond a desired duration.

Patients wake up in the treatment room within seconds to minutes after the seizure stops and are evaluated by staff who ensure they are not experiencing any confusion or discomfort. Mild nausea and headache sometimes occur after treatment. Patients are typically ready to be driven home 30–60 minutes after the treatment is complete.

ECT is typically administered in an initial course of between 6 and 12 treatment sessions, with such sessions occurring two or three times per week until improvement is observed. Once a patient has improved, many psychiatrists recommend gradually spacing out additional ECT sessions before completely stopping treatment. Tapering treatments while continuing psychiatric medications has been shown to reduce the risk of relapse following discontinuation of ECT.

Does It Work? How Does It Work?

ECT is one of the most effective treatments for unipolar and bipolar depression, with roughly 75% of patients responding (i.e., "getting more than half better") and 50% experiencing a total remission of depressive symptoms. More than 80% of patients with catatonia respond to ECT; among patients with schizophrenia (especially those for whom medications have had little effect), response is likely in 30%–50%, but total remission is still unlikely.

In a recent study of severely depressed patients, ECT was found to outperform intravenous ketamine. After six treatments (ECT sessions or ketamine infusions), 63% of the ECT group experienced a total remission of their depressive symptoms compared with 43% of the intravenous ketamine treatment group. A larger percentage of patients in the ketamine treatment group were unable to complete the study compared with the ECT group.

The exact mechanism underlying the therapeutic effects of ECT is not understood. Therapeutic links between seizures and mental illness have been observed in patients whose psychosis or depression resolved following seizures. Early attempts at inducing seizures with medications such as camphor oil or Metrazol were successful but had many side effects. ECT was developed as an alternative way to induce seizures that had fewer side effects and was safer than previous pharmacological methods. ECT has been demonstrated to increase patients' cerebral blood flow, neurotransmitter and neuropeptide levels, neurogenesis (new neuron growth) and gliosis (growth of glial cells that support neuron health), and brain chemicals implicated in neuron health, such as brain-derived neurotrophic factor and vascular endothelial growth factor.

Side Effects

All medical treatments have potential risks, and patients should have a comprehensive conversation with their psychiatrist to discuss whether ECT is appropriate for their condition. Overall, ECT is very safe and carries risks similar to those associated with any procedure involving general anesthesia. The risk of death associated with anesthesia is 1 in 80,000, which is considered to be very low, and there is no special added risk of death associated with ECT and anesthesia. Prior to the treatment patients may experience pain, bruising, or skin irritation associated with placement of the intravenous line. It is imperative that patients not eat or drink anything 8 hours prior to treatment to minimize the risk of aspirating stomach contents during the procedure. After awakening from treatment, they may experience temporary confusion or disorientation, which typically resolves in several minutes. They may also feel mild muscle soreness, jaw or neck pain, headache, or fatigue following treatment. *Side effects are the same for pregnant patients. Fetal heart rate can slow and uterine contractions may occur, but these most often resolve without need of intervention.*

Difficulties with memory, mainly *anterograde amnesia* (forgetting events that happen between treatments), have been reported with ECT. Although some case reports have described patients who have experienced difficulty with long-term memories after ECT treatment, large systematic reviews have found that ECT does not have a major impact on long-term memory and tends to actually improve patients' cognitive and executive functioning. Difficulties with memory have been reported to improve as the frequency of ECT sessions is reduced. Memory issues are less commonly seen in patients who receive unilateral treatments and ultra-brief pulse width stimulation (*pulse width* refers to the duration of each square-wave pulse, with ultra-brief pulses being shorter than 0.5 ms).

Additional Information

What Do Patients Think of Electroconvulsive Therapy?

Most patients tolerate treatments well, and many experience a significant reduction in symptoms and an improved quality of life. In a recent study performed by the Mayo Clinic, 91% of participants who received ECT indicated that they were "glad I received treatment," and more than 50% would choose to receive ECT again.

Acknowledging the History and Stigma of Electroconvulsive Therapy

Despite the compelling evidence for its safety and effectiveness, ECT has been a target of negative social publicity and controversy due to its historical association with frontal lobotomies and depictions of early unmodified ECT without the use of anesthesia. Many cite an image of Jack Nicholson in the film *One Flew Over the Cuckoo's Nest* as their main familiarity with ECT and see the treatment as a form of punishment, coercion, or torture. These associations and depictions bear no resemblance to modern ECT, which is conducted only after obtaining informed consent from the patient or their guardian and is administered in a manner to preserve the utmost safety, care, and respect for the patient.

Conclusion

ECT is a safe and effective treatment option for specific neuropsychiatric conditions, but it is often underutilized due to logistical limitations and stigma. We hope the information presented here helps patients and their families to make informed decisions regarding their care and improves public awareness of the safety and efficacy of ECT.

Recommended Reading

Dukakis K, Tye L: Shock: The Healing Power of Electroconvulsive Therapy. New York, Avery, 2007

Manning M: Undercurrents: A Therapist's Reckoning With Her Own Depression. San Francisco, CA, HarperSanFrancisco, 1994

49

Transcranial Magnetic Stimulation

Susan K. Conroy, M.D., Ph.D.
Paul E. Holtzheimer, M.D., M.S.

Introduction

History of Device Development

Transcranial magnetic stimulation (TMS) is a noninvasive, in-office treatment in which a stimulator is placed over a particular area of the patient's scalp and delivers a series of magnetic pulses to a specific region of the brain. These magnetic pulses, in turn, create an electrical current in the brain that stimulates the nerve cells in that region. TMS treatment is delivered while patients sit in a chair similar to a recliner. No anesthesia is needed during TMS, and patients remain awake during the session, which can take about 3–40 minutes depending on the type of TMS delivered.

TMS technology was first developed in the 1980s, when Dr. Anthony Barker, an English neurosurgeon, showed that delivering a single magnetic pulse over the part of the brain that controls movement could produce movements in the corresponding part of the person's body. The early clinical uses of TMS involved "mapping" brain function in this way in neurological disorders. As technology advanced in the early 1990s, repetitive TMS (rTMS) became possible, such that many pulses in a row could be quickly delivered, creating longer-lasting changes in brain function. This led to the potential for therapeutic uses of TMS in the treatment of psychiatric disorders. The first and still most common clinical use of TMS is for treatment of major depressive disorder (MDD); after multiple clinical trials, the first rTMS device was cleared by the U.S. Food and Drug Administration (FDA) in 2008 for this indication. Today, several FDA-cleared devices are used in clinical practice.

What Is It Used to Treat?

For TMS, FDA clearance is acquired by the manufacturer of each TMS device, and this involves a review of clinical studies of TMS treatment for each different indication (condition) specific to the brain region being targeted and the number and pattern of magnetic pulses being delivered at each session. TMS to the left dorsolateral prefrontal cortex (DLPFC) was FDA-cleared in 2008 for treating unipolar MDD in adults whose symptoms had not responded to one or more medications. A number of other psychiatric indications have also received FDA clearance, including obsessive-compulsive disorder (OCD) in 2018 and smoking cessation in 2020; TMS for each of these indications includes a component of symptom provocation as part of each session because the state of the brain during treatment may be important for maximum effect (e.g., a patient with OCD would be instructed to think about their fear of germs before and during treatments).

TMS is not currently FDA-cleared for other psychiatric disorders but has been studied in a number of conditions. Reasonably good evidence indicates that TMS is safe and effective for treatment of major depressive episodes in patients with bipolar disorder; as with any antidepressant treatment, there is concern about causing a "manic switch" in such patients, but this does not appear common. TMS has also shown preliminary benefit for treating posttraumatic stress disorder (PTSD), but the best method for delivering TMS in PTSD remains unclear. There are some limited data for use of TMS in generalized anxiety disorder. Substance use disorder treatment with TMS (beyond smoking cessation) is an active area of research as well.

In addition, some evidence has revealed that TMS treats depression when it is delivered to brain regions other than the left DLPFC or in different stimulation patterns than the current FDA-cleared protocols. Examples include the right DLPFC at low frequency, the dorsomedial prefrontal cortex, and "bilateral" treatment protocols in which regions on both sides of the brain are stimulated during the treatment session.

How Is Transcranial Magnetic Stimulation Treatment Performed, and How Many Treatments Should Be Expected?

The strength of the magnetic pulses is customized to each individual by determining their *motor threshold*, which is the amount of energy required to produce movement in hand muscles about half the time, for example, in 5 out of 10 stimuli. Dosing of TMS is then relative to the patient's motor threshold. In clinical practice, TMS is usually delivered at 100%–120% motor threshold. The area of the scalp overlying the DLPFC, where the stimulator is placed when treating MDD, is typically identified by moving a certain distance forward from the area that stimulates the muscles of the thumb or index finger or by measuring distances between various "landmarks" on a person's head (e.g., bridge of nose, center of ears) and calculating where the DLPFC is likely to be. Multiple types of stimulator coils are available; both regular figure-of-eight shaped and "deep" TMS coils target the DLPFC in all cleared treatment protocols. Both coil types show similar efficacy in depression; for OCD and smoking cessation, only deep TMS has been FDA-cleared. For some devices, a swimming cap–like hat worn during treatment is used to mark the treatment spot so it can be quickly found at subsequent treatment sessions.

All effective TMS treatment protocols involve multiple sessions, and most FDA-cleared protocols consist of once-daily sessions, 5 days per week, for multiple weeks (4–6 weeks for MDD and 6 weeks for OCD). "Accelerated" TMS protocols, with multiple sessions per day, are an active area of research but are not yet in widespread clinical use. The number of magnetic pulses delivered per session in FDA-cleared protocols varies between 1,800 and 3,000; depending on the protocol's timing/pattern of pulse delivery, a session can take between 3 minutes and 30 minutes. The very short, 3-minute sessions employ a stimulation pattern called *theta burst stimulation* that seems to be at least as effective as other forms of TMS for depression.

Does It Work? How Does It Work?

The electrical current that is generated during TMS alters the way brain cells in the targeted region operate, making the region either more or less active. When multiple treatments are delivered over time, this can increase or decrease activity in certain brain regions and change the way regions interact with each other, which is believed to underlie the improvement in psychiatric conditions seen with TMS. TMS treatment for depression is typically delivered to the DLPFC, an area connected to many parts of the brain that are important in mood regulation. Although its exact mechanism of action is not fully known, brain imaging studies have confirmed that TMS delivered to the DLPFC can change functioning in brain regions connected to that region. TMS is also associated with changes in neurotransmitter systems thought to be involved in the etiology of depression, such as serotonin, norepinephrine, and dopamine.

Multiple studies have confirmed that TMS leads to greater reductions in depression severity compared with placebo, or *sham*, treatment. For MDD, rates of TMS response (typically defined as a 50% decrease in depression symptoms from before treatment begins) are about 50% overall, meaning that about half of patients find that a course of TMS makes their symptoms significantly better. A smaller proportion, about 20% of patients in most studies, achieve *remission*, meaning they have few to no depression symptoms at the end of a course of treatment. For OCD, clinical studies show that about 40% of patients experience a significant reduction in symptoms; "real-world" data collected in the years following FDA approval show somewhat higher numbers. For smoking cessation, the number of daily cigarettes smoked, cravings, and proportion of patients who quit smoking continuously for several weeks at a time are improved somewhat with TMS.

For all indications, maintenance treatment following an initial series of TMS, either to keep a patient well or to "rescue" them when symptoms begin to recur, is an active area of research, and currently no clear consensus has been reached in the field regarding best practices.

Side Effects

TMS does not cause memory trouble or confusion and requires no recovery period following treatment. However, headaches and pain under the stimulation site are common; these typically diminish over time or can be well treated with over-the-counter pain relief medicines. Twitches of the facial muscles near the stimulator can occur during treatment sessions; these may be annoying to the patient but are not dangerous. TMS treatment is loud and could be associated with ringing in the ears and transient, mild hearing loss; patients and TMS administrators typically wear ear protection, such as earplugs, during stimulation to reduce these effects. Lightheadedness and, rarely, fainting can also occur during TMS sessions. A rare but serious side effect is seizures, but for patients with no preexisting increased risk of seizure, the risk with TMS is extremely low. However, for patients who are already at a higher risk for seizures, the risk is much greater, and TMS may not be the safest treatment option. As with most antidepressant treatments, there is a theoretical risk of inducing mania or hypomania, but very little evidence has been found of this actually occurring with TMS. The magnetic field associated with TMS can cause some metal objects to heat up, so patients with pacemakers and certain types of metal in their head or neck should not receive this treatment.

Additional Information

Use in Special Populations

A number of studies have demonstrated that TMS is safe and well tolerated in children, but very little good quality data are available showing it to be effective in this patient population. Some earlier trials of TMS for depression in adolescents suggested benefit, but the largest, most well-conducted studies do not support antidepressant effects of TMS over sham stimulation. TMS in older adults has been studied and has good evidence for efficacy, although the stimulus intensity often has to be increased because of the greater distance between scalp and brain that occurs with the natural loss of brain tissue that happens as people get older.

Case Vignette

Carol is a 58-year-old female with an episode of MDD that has been occurring for 3 years. She has tried three different medications, each for multiple weeks and at a dosage high enough to theoretically be effective. She also recently completed a course of cognitive-behavioral therapy. However, despite receiving multiple adequate treatments, her depressive symptoms have remained significantly distressing and impair her ability to function. Finally, her psychiatrist referred her for a course of TMS. Following the first treatment, Carol had a headache, but she found this was not a problem if she took acetaminophen before each subsequent treatment. After approximately 2 weeks of daily treatments, her depressive symptoms began to improve, and after 6 weeks of treatment she had minimal depressive symptoms. She continued psychotherapy and medications during and after the TMS course.

Conclusion

TMS is a safe and effective in-office treatment for depression that has few side effects. A number of approved treatment protocols are already in place, and new protocols are an active area of research. Use of TMS is expanding to treat other psychiatric conditions as well.

Recommended Reading

Brennan N: Neal Brennan: 3 Mics (Netflix Comedy Special). Netflix, 2017. Available at: https://www.netflix.com/title/80117452.

Trivedi M, Downar J: The role of transcranial magnetic stimulation in major depressive disorder. In Discussion: Major Depressive Disorder Podcast, Medscape, May 11, 2022. Available at: https://www.medscape.com/viewarticle/968557.

50

Vagus Nerve Stimulation

Charles R. Conway, M.D.
Britt M. Gott, M.S.

Introduction

Use of Vagus Nerve Stimulation in Treatment-Resistant Depression

The use of vagus nerve stimulation (VNS) for treatment-resistant depression (TRD) evolved from studies in which this therapy was being used for treatment-refractory epilepsy. For years, VNS had been successfully used in epilepsy patients, and neurology researchers noticed that patients with refractory epilepsy who were receiving VNS were also experiencing improvements in their mood, independent of the reduction in seizures. This led to formal study of mood changes in treatment-refractory epilepsy, which demonstrated significant depressive mood improvement and eventually led to the study of VNS in TRD.

Earliest Studies

The initial studies of VNS in TRD were *open-label studies*, meaning that all patients were implanted with real VNS devices and were aware that they were receiving active stimulation. These studies were very promising, with depressions responding to treatment in 30.5% of participants. Furthermore, patient follow-up showed that 44.1% sustained response 1 year after the stimulation. This is important because many TRD treatments cannot sustain antidepressant effects.

The ideal study of a new treatment is a *placebo-controlled, double-blind study*. In 2002, this type of study was conducted with VNS for TRD: all patients had VNS devices implanted, but only half of the devices were turned on, and neither the patients nor the depression raters knew who was receiving active treatment. At the time, depression researchers did not know the stimulation time required to achieve an antidepressant response. This study provided 10 weeks of stimulation (2 weeks of dose current titration and 8 weeks of stimulation). At the end of the 10 weeks, no statistically significant difference was seen between placebo (VNS device off) and active treatment (VNS device on) for the primary depression measure used in this trial (although a secondary depression measure did achieve statistical significance). Fortunately, the researchers had built an open-label extension phase into this trial in which all participants had their devices turned on in order to study the continued effects of VNS on mood. It was noted in this extension that with each passing month, the number of patients whose depression responded to treatment increased. The primary finding emerging from this trial was that *most patients who respond to VNS take many months to experience an antidepressant benefit.* Although some people may be "early responders," most require 6–12 months of treatment to experience benefit.

Large Ongoing Studies

Despite VNS receiving U.S. Food and Drug Administration (FDA) approval for TRD in 2005, the Centers for Medicare and Medicaid Services (CMS) issued a "no coverage" decision in 2007 that concluded the evidence supporting VNS for TRD was not adequate to support Medicare coverage. This decision had the unfortunate effect of making VNS inaccessible to most TRD patients. In 2019, CMS agreed to cosponsor, along with the device maker LivaNova, a "coverage with evidence" trial. This trial, entitled the RECOVER Study, is a large, multicenter (70–100 U.S. sites), double-blind trial (all patients were implanted with VNS, but only half had their devices turned on). The blinded portion lasted 1 year, after which all participants had their devices turned on, and they were to be followed for another 4 years. At this time, the RECOVER trial has completed recruitment of the unipolar TRD arm (500 participants). Results are expected in 2024.

Additional Studies

A large, open-label study of VNS in TRD, the RESTORE LIFE Trial, is now under way in Europe. In addition to that and the other studies just described, several other open-label studies of VNS in TRD have been conducted, and all have demonstrated that a significant proportion of patients experience and maintain an antidepressant response with VNS. Other questions addressed in subsequent VNS studies included those in the section headings that follow.

What Is It Used to Treat?

Currently, VNS has only one FDA-approved psychiatric indication: "chronic or recurrent depression, either unipolar or bipolar, with a history of failure of the depression to respond to at least four antidepressant interventions." Patients are not required to have failed to achieve response with electroconvulsive therapy (ECT) to be eligible for VNS. Currently, VNS is being studied for several other indications as well, including inflammatory disease.

How Is Vagus Nerve Stimulation Performed, and How Many Treatments Should Be Expected?

Several studies have addressed specific clinical issues related to VNS in TRD. One study attempted to understand which electrical "dose" of VNS was most likely to bring about the best antidepressant benefit. Patients in this trial were assigned to three different groups based on electrical parameters (i.e., low, medium, and high). After participants were randomly assigned to one of the dosing groups, the results demonstrated that all three groups had roughly equivalent response rates, although patients ino the higher dosing group had greater *long-term* response rates.

Dosing

The VNS device is programmed using a "wand" that is positioned over the skin covering the implanted device. A handheld computer tablet then allows the programmer to adjust the device settings. Four device "parameters" are used in VNS: *current, frequency, pulse width*, and *duty cycle*.

Current

Measured in milliamps (mA), the *current* represents the amount of electrical charge being administered. We now know that the current is the most important electrical setting of VNS. Work has demonstrated that greater current is associated with more sustained antidepressant benefit. For this reason, the current is titrated to the patient's highest tolerable setting. The VNS device increases the current in increments of 0.25 mA, up to a maximum of 3.5 mA, and this is typically done gradually, with the programmer increasing the current and allowing the device to cycle three or four times to assess whether that current is tolerable. Clinical experience has shown that patients best tolerate only two or three increments of current increase per session over one or two sessions per week. These slow current adjustments allow patients to better tolerate the increases and to achieve an overall higher tolerable current level.

Frequency

VNS devices are programmable to three different *frequency* settings, measured in cycles per second, or *Hertz* (Hz): 15 Hz, 20 Hz, and 30 Hz. Most patients are started at 20 Hz and held at this frequency. Clinical experience suggests that patients tend to better tolerate 20 Hz or less.

Pulse Width

The *pulse width* is the duration of each stimulatory burst measured in microseconds (μsec). Programmable pulse widths available with VNS include 130 μsec, 250 μsec, and 500 μsec. Clinical experience suggests most patients best tolerate 130 μsec and 250 μsec, with 250 μsec being the most common pulse width used.

Duty Cycle

Duty cycle is the percentage of time that the VNS device is "on," or actively stimulating. The typical starting duty cycle is 10%, which represents 30 seconds on, 5 minutes off. Typically, this initial duty cycle is not altered until the patient has had prolonged exposure to VNS (usually 6–9 months or longer). The duration of active stimulation ranges from 7 to 14, 21, 30, and 60 seconds, and the duration of inactivity ranges from 0.2 to 0.3, 0.5, 0.8, 1.1, 1.8, 3, 5, and 10 minutes. Stimulation duty cycle (time on/total time) should not exceed 50%.

Two weeks following surgical implantation (allowing 2 weeks for recovery), the patient presents to their mental health worker for programming. Typical device settings are a frequency 20 Hz, a pulse width 250 μsec, and a duty cycle of 30 seconds on, 5 minutes off (10%). At this first appointment, the patient is informed that device titration will occur over several meetings, usually one or two times per week. Starting at 0.25 mA, the device is allowed to cycle three or four times (about 20 minutes) to determine if the patient tolerates the settings. Most patients do not report discomfort while receiving VNS at very low currents. In a given titration session, the device current can be increased by two or three increments (e.g., in session one, it may be increased by 0.25 mA to 0.5 mA and

0.75 mA), as tolerated. After these first three increments, patients return for further increases until their maximal tolerated current is achieved (this is typically 1.5–2.0 mA), after which their treatment is held at those parameters for a sustained period, typically 6–9 months. During this period, patients regularly undergo clinical observations to determine whether the stimulation is effective at reducing their depression.

If Sustained Stimulation Is Not Effective

If no or very minimal response is noted at 6–9 months, adjustments can be considered for potential improved treatment. The existing literature suggests that the amount of charge delivered over time may be a primary predictor of response to VNS in TRD. With this in mind, the mental health provider may consider increasing the duty cycle (either decreasing the inactive, or "off," time [most common] or increasing the active, or "on" time). Another strategy is to increase the stimulation current or frequency. Over time, many patients have reported improved mood with VNS parameter adjustments.

Does It Work?

How Does Vagus Nerve Stimulation Compare to Existing Treatments for Treatment-Resistant Depression?

One landmark study compared groups of equivalently ill TRD patients who had received either add-on VNS or treatment as usual (TAU; i.e., any treatment available, including ECT) over the course of 5 years. For both antidepressant response (a 50% drop in depressive symptoms) and remission (essentially minimal residual depressive symptoms), add-on VNS was determined to be superior both in the speed to response/remission and in the number of patients whose depression responded/remitted during that period. This study was instrumental in demonstrating the clinical superiority of VNS using an open-label, naturalistic design that was similar to how patients are treated in clinical practice.

Can Patients Who Fail Electroconvulsive Therapy Respond to Vagus Nerve Stimulation?

Another question addressed by these researchers was how patients who had previously received ECT subsequently responded to VNS. They found that patients whose TRD had previously failed to respond to ECT were slightly less likely to achieve response to VNS than those whose TRD had responded to prior ECT *but were more likely to respond to VNS than TAU.* This is a very important finding because it indicates that VNS often will be effective in patients whose TRD has previously failed ECT.

How Does Vagus Nerve Stimulation Impact Quality of Life?

Researchers looking at VNS in TRD had found that often patients whose TRD had not responded to VNS (using the classic definition of *response* as a 50% improvement in depressive symptoms from baseline) reported that their lives had significantly improved with VNS. This prompted a group of researchers to assess how VNS impacted patients' quality of life, and, using data from a previous VNS study, they found that patients receiving add-on VNS were more likely to experience improvement in quality of life than those receiving TAU. Furthermore, VNS patients who had experienced significantly lower reductions in depression (a 34% drop of depressive symptoms from before implantation, rather than the standard 50%) had statistically significant improvement in their quality of life. This is also a critical finding because TRD is a chronic, long-lasting illness, and quality of life is likely the most important clinical outcome factor. Why VNS is associated with this improvement in quality of life independent of reduction in depression symptoms is not clear; however, evidence has shown that VNS brings about improvements in anxiety, alertness, and cognition, and perhaps these lead to the improvement in perceived quality of life.

A considerable amount of science has gone into understanding how VNS accomplishes its effects in TRD. For a full review of this topic, please refer to the Conway and Xiong paper in the "Recommended Reading" section at the end of this chapter. Here we provide a general discussion of proposed mechanisms of action of VNS in TRD.

How Does It Work?

Increased Activation and Deactivation of Regions Historically Associated With Depression

When the vagus nerve is stimulated, nerve impulses travel upstream into the brain. These fibers enter the brain through the brain stem (i.e., the lower portion of the brain, called the *medulla*), and the impulses go farther up into the cortex (the outermost "shell" portion of the brain) and the subcortex (regions below the cortex). Brain imaging studies, which can assess activity in different parts of the brain, have shown that patients receiving VNS experience increased activation in brain regions known to be associated with depression (i.e., regions that may have been deactivated naturally due to depression prior to treatment) and that these changes, as in the clinical studies noted earlier (see "Earliest Studies"), tend to be delayed, in many instances occurring after 4–6 months of stimulation. Unfortunately, we do not yet have the ability or precision to use brain imaging to determine who is likely to respond to VNS prior to surgery, but there is some suggestion that certain brain activation patterns are more likely to respond to VNS.

Activation and Increased Turnover of Brain Neurotransmitters Known to Be Critical in Depression

The upstream brain stem and brain pathway of the vagus nerve intersects with the regions of cells that contain the primary brain chemicals associated with depression, the neurotransmitters norepinephrine and serotonin. Animal studies show that chronic VNS is associated with increased firing of these serotonin and norepinephrine neurons. Furthermore, another neurotransmitter critical in depression—dopamine—also undergoes changes with VNS. One study examined cerebrospinal fluid taken before and after VNS in patients with TRD and found that those receiving active VNS had increased metabolites of dopamine in their cerebrospinal fluid, whereas those receiving *sham*, or placebo, VNS (implanted but not turned on) did not. Other researchers using positron emission tomography (PET) scans found that 12 months of VNS led to significant activation of the primary brain stem center for dopamine in patients whose symptoms responded to VNS, but not in those whose symptoms did not respond.

Other Possible Mechanisms of Action

Evidence has shown that VNS has powerful anti-inflammatory abilities, which may have a positive influence on its effectiveness in TRD. As noted earlier in the discussion of quality of life improvement, VNS also has positive effects on anxiety, alertness, and cognition in patients with TRD, which may collectively contribute to the treatment's overall clinical and biological effectiveness.

Side Effects

Potential side effects in patients who receive the implanted device for VNS are generally mild, well tolerated, and occur specifically during device stimulation. More than 22 studies have summarized the most common side effects as pain related to implantation, voice alterations and hoarseness, coughing, headache, and throat and neck pain. Possible rare (less than 3% of patients), more severe side effects include development of manic-depressive symptoms (which sometimes resolve when stimulation parameters are adjusted), worsening of depression, heart complications, infections at the implantation site, and worsening of sleep apnea. There are currently no known antidepressant medication contraindications to VNS, and ECT is allowed as long as the VNS device can be turned off prior to ECT treatment. The treating psychiatrist (and other specialists as needed) and the implanting surgeon will review these side effects and patients' personal medical histories prior to surgery to discuss any concerns.

Additional Information

Use in Special Populations

Currently, VNS is only approved for patients who are 18 years of age and older. It has not been carefully studied in children and adolescents with TRD. VNS is approved for treatment of both unipolar and bipolar TRD. Thus far, studies examining VNS treatment in different age groups (i.e., young adulthood, middle age, and geriatric) have not found any age differential in response to VNS.

Vagus Nerve Stimulation Device and Surgery

The VNS device is a small, implantable pulse generator (similar to a cardiac pacemaker) that is implanted in the chest, just below the collarbone (clavicle). Typically, this surgery is performed by a neurosurgeon or ear, nose, and throat surgeon who has undergone specific training in this procedure. The surgery is done under general anesthesia and is considered an outpatient procedure (patients go home the same day). Two incisions are made, one in the armpit (axilla) that allows the device to be positioned under the skin below the collarbone, and a second incision in the neck region. A lead from the device is tunneled beneath the skin and attached to the vagus nerve in the neck. Typically, patients recover for 2 weeks following surgery before the VNS device is activated.

Conclusion

Although VNS for TRD received FDA approval in 2005, the decision by Medicare in 2007 to not cover the treatment has limited its availability. Despite this limitation, numerous studies continue to demonstrate that VNS has sustained therapeutic antidepressant benefits in TRD. Additionally, ongoing studies offer considerable hope that VNS will become more widely available for those with very resistant TRD. Many questions remain regarding VNS for TRD, including optimizing which patients will respond and further refining how the treatment is delivered (e.g., optimizing electrical parameters).

Recommended Reading

Conway CR, Xiong W: The mechanism of action of vagus nerve stimulation in treatment-resistant depression: current conceptualizations. Psychiatr Clin North Am 41(3):395–407, 2018 30098653

Conway CR, Hristidis VC, Gott BM, et al: Vagus nerve stimulation for treatment-resistant depression: current status of this novel treatment. Psychiatr Ann 52(7):272–282, 2022

51

Deep Brain Stimulation

Patricio Riva-Posse, M.D.
Helen S. Mayberg, M.D.

Introduction

Neurosurgical treatments for psychiatric illnesses have existed since before there were effective pharmacological options such as antidepressants or antipsychotics. Observations that specific areas in the brain corresponded to particular functions were made in the nineteenth century, allowing for the initial descriptions of language or motor areas by Broca (in 1865), Jackson (in 1873), and others. Clinicians observed that people who had experienced brain lesions had changes in behavior, and they began to develop ways to surgically create such lesions as interventions for patients with various psychiatric disorders. A variety of different lesions were tried, and the many case reports available from the middle of the twentieth century describe improvement in symptoms for many patients.

From today's perspective, these interventions are clearly unsafe, but in many cases they represented physicians' last-ditch attempts to bring relief to patients for whom no other options were available. "Psychosurgical" treatments have always been considered controversial; the widespread, indiscriminate use of the transorbital lobotomy during the mid-twentieth century resulted in profound ethical ramifications that persist to this day. The first treatments with modern psychopharmacology, such as antidepressants and antipsychotics, only became available in the 1950s and 1960s, but with the advent of effective pharmacological options, neurosurgical interventions fell out of favor. However, standard treatments such as pharmacology, psychotherapy, and noninvasive neuromodulation (e.g., electroconvulsive therapy [ECT]) are not effective for all patients.

Understanding Psychiatric Disorders as Neural Circuit Disorders

A new paradigm in the way neuropsychiatric disorders are understood as dysfunctional brain networks, advances in functional stereotactic neurosurgery, and successes in treatment of neurological disorders such as Parkinson's disease made the exploration of neurosurgical interventions for severe depression possible. Invasive technologies for electrical stimulation (as opposed to the creation of brain lesions) offer the possibility of reversing side effects and allowing for a precise modulation of the targeted brain circuits.

Deep brain stimulation (DBS) involves implanting thin electrodes within certain areas of the brain that deliver electrical impulses from a pacemaker-like device implanted under the skin in the patient's upper chest. The electricity then modulates how neurons and their axons communicate with each other. In order to place the electrode in the desired brain region, neurosurgeons apply three-dimensional coordinates based on information from brain imaging (a method known as *stereotaxis*) to determine the correct location for the electrode and the trajectory of the lead. The DBS programming allows for multiple parameter settings (i.e., voltage or current, frequency, and pulse width), and each of the leads has multiple contacts (usually separated by a few millimeters), which offers physicians the ability to explore which settings lead to the most improvement and avoid side effects.

DBS became available in the late 1990s for treatment of neurological illnesses such as Parkinson's disease and essential tremor. DBS technologies have since improved and currently are approved by the U.S. Food and Drug Administration (FDA) to treat severe cases when standard medical approaches have failed. It is estimated that approximately 100,000 patients have received DBS worldwide for neurological indications.

What if, similar to how a patient's tremor improves with DBS, the delivery of precise electrical pulses could modify patients' mood symptoms?

What Is It Used to Treat?

In 2005, a case series was published describing the results of DBS treatment in a group of six patients with treatment-resistant depression (TRD). Six months after the surgery, four of the patients had improved in their depression scores by more than half. In the following years, various groups in North America and Europe began researching protocols to evaluate the efficacy of this novel treatment for patients with chronic and severe depression. More than 15 years later, many open-label series and clinical trials have had varying results, but advances in the mechanisms of antidepressant effects, newer technologies to deliver and sense stimulation, and improved imaging techniques have moved the field forward, although it is still considered experimental. Considering the prevalence of depression, the levels of treatment resistance, and the continuing high rates of suicide, the total number of patients who have received DBS for TRD remains in the low hundreds, although numbers in several orders of magnitude greater could potentially benefit from this intervention.

Does It Work? How Does It Work?

Subcallosal Cingulate White Matter

The *subcallosal cingulate gyrus* (SCC) is the portion of the cingulum that lies below the *corpus callosum* (the brain region that connects both hemispheres). This region is a critical node in mood regulation networks involved in negative mood and antidepressant treatment response. Patients who received DBS in the SCC during the original trials conducted in Canada and the United States experienced a sustained antidepressant response, with about two-thirds demonstrating response to treatment after 1 year of stimulation. Following these auspicious early results, an industry-sponsored, double-blind, randomized controlled multicenter study was initiated, with the intention of recruiting 200 participants in North America. This study was halted after 90 patients were recruited because the interim analysis predicted a low chance of the study meeting its primary outcome. After 24 weeks of stimulation, less than one-quarter of patients had improved, and no difference was observed between the active treatment group and the group receiving "sham" stimulation. However, there were some positive aspects: patients who continued the open-label phase of the study gradually improved, and after 24 months, response rates were much better, with about half of patients showing clinical response and one-third in remission of depression.

Investigation then turned to the reasons why this trial failed to replicate the results of the open-label studies, and a more in-depth understanding of the SCC anatomy was developed. Using an advanced neuroimaging technique called *tractography*, the researchers looked more closely at the location of the DBS leads in the SCC. This technique allows a visual representation of nerve tracts using data collected by magnetic resonance imaging (MRI). It became apparent that patients who responded to DBS in the SCC had received stimulation in a group of white matter fibers that communicated with other key regions of the mood network in the frontal lobes, the subcortical areas, the rest of the cingulate cortex, and other locations. With this insight, studies were conducted prospectively and showed an increase in the efficacy of the intervention; in recent case series, 70%–80% of patients responded to treatment and achieved response faster.

In addition to improving depression in a relatively shorter time frame, DBS has demonstrated long-term efficacy and sustained antidepressant results. This is important because the related surgery is certainly more invasive, risky, and costly than other treatments. Patients with TRD experience years of depression and, in many cases, only a brief response to treatment. Several publications have now highlighted the long-term duration of antidepressant effects with DBS.

Ventral Capsule/Ventral Striatum

The *ventral capsule/ventral striatum* (VC/VS), also referred to as the *ventral anterior limb of the internal capsule*, has long been recognized as another intervention target for both depression and anxiety. Even before DBS, surgical lesions to this region had been an effective approach for treatment-refractory psychiatric disorders since 1949. Early indications of DBS in this target area were for the treatment of obsessive-compulsive disorder (OCD). Tractography imaging has recently refined DBS in this region, allowing the target to be selected in a precise manner. The first open-label DBS study in the VC/VS involved 17 participants with TRD, of whom 53% demonstrated response at 1 year. Following the same trajectory as that used in the SCC, a multicenter, randomized, sham-controlled clinical trial was designed in the United States with the goal of providing a higher level of evidence supporting the VC/VS target for TRD. However, this trial did not find clinical significance in treatment response rates after 16 weeks of treatment (20% response in the treatment group, and 14% in the sham group).

A different study, designed and conducted in the Netherlands, had better results, although they were not directly comparable with the initial clinical trial. Following 1-year of open-label stimulation, 40% of patients showed response. Afterward, participants entered a blinded discontinuation phase (their stimulation was stopped), and within a couple of weeks their depression returned. DBS studies targeting the VC/VS are ongoing, and researchers hope that use of improved imaging and electrophysiological signals will ultimately improve patient outcomes.

Medial Forebrain Bundle

The *medial forebrain bundle* (MFB) is a collection of myelinated and unmyelinated fibers that connect dopaminergic areas in the brain stem to other subcortical nuclei. The MFB has long been considered an essential structure related to psychobehavioral functioning in both animals and humans. Interestingly, although other targets within the reward system (i.e., the ventral striatum and nucleus accumbens) had already been tried, the difficulties identifying the MFB using standard imaging had delayed its potential use as a target for DBS in depression. Advanced imaging is needed to pinpoint the exact region in the brain stem to insert the electrodes. An original pilot study in Germany assessed the safety and efficacy of DBS in the MFB in seven patients with TRD. Interestingly, the antidepressant effects were very rapid in their onset. Within the first week of stimulation, six of the seven patients had achieved symptom response, and four were in remission. These improvements were also reported to be sustained; about half of the patients were still in remission at 1 year, which continued until the 4-year follow-up. Other groups replicated these findings, and although they had slightly less dramatic responses, their results showed that about two-thirds of participants experienced a significant antidepressant effect. A separate group in the United States replicated these early findings. Three of six patients had a greater than 50% decrease in depression scores relative to baseline 1 week following stimulation initiation.

Due to the MFB's proximity to regions in the brain that control eye movements, possible adverse effects of DBS in this target region are blurred vision and strabismus. There are also reports of an abrupt return of depressive symptoms if treatment is discontinued.

In a clinical study that used a randomized controlled onset of stimulation, 16 participants received DBS or sham treatment in a double-blind, randomized-control condition for 8 weeks following implantation surgery, after which all patients received active stimulation. All patients reached the response criterion, and most ($n=10$) responded within 1 week; 50% were classified as remitters after 1 year of stimulation. It appeared that the double-blind phase of 2 months was not long enough, but regardless, this evidence of a sustained response with DBS is very encouraging. More clinical trials are under way in this target region.

Conclusion

After almost two decades of research in DBS for treatment of depression, this approach remains experimental, and few patients have received this potentially game-changing intervention. Fortunately, incremental advances have been made in the understanding of depression neurocircuitry, in electrophysiology, and in neuroimaging that open the possibility for better-designed clinical trials to categorically determine whether DBS is a viable option for patients with TRD. Several research groups are moving the field forward with new insights into the changes that stimulation generates in the brain; in this way, they are preparing new technologies for delivering electrical impulses to the brain in response to wave patterns that signal a "depressed" state.

Cumulative evidence from different research groups investigating different targets indicates that the antidepressant response to DBS is long lasting in most patients. Although patients must continue taking antidepressant medications, many are able to reduce the dosages and achieve more tolerable pharmacological combinations following DBS treatment. Most groups have also identified benefits of conducting psychotherapy while DBS is effective.

The hopes of many people whose depression has failed to respond to other treatments rely on the scientific community, the device manufacturers, and research funding agencies. More comprehensive knowledge of the neuroscience and clinical aspects behind TRD will also help predict which DBS targets might be indicated for unique subpopulations in the future. Patients with TRD who have experienced incapacitating symptoms for years and have withdrawn from society and from their families seek and value psychotherapeutic strategies that will help them rehabilitate to a full functional recovery.

Recommended Reading

Crowell AL, Riva-Posse P, Holtzheimer PE, et al: Long-term outcomes of subcallosal cingulate deep brain stimulation for treatment-resistant depression. Am J Psychiatry 176(11):949–956, 2019 31581800

Dandekar MP, Fenoy AJ, Carvalho AF, et al: Deep brain stimulation for treatment-resistant depression: an integrative review of preclinical and clinical findings and translational implications. Mol Psychiatry 23(5):1094–1112, 2018 29483673

52

Light Therapy and Chronotherapeutics

Michael Terman, Ph.D.
Jessica Rao, M.P.H.

Introduction

Bright light therapy is well-known for its antidepressant action in patients under clinicians' guidance, as well as in unsupervised self-treatment, for seasonal affective disorder (SAD). It was first described in the late 1970s by the National Institute of Mental Health's (NIMH) Clinical Psychobiology Branch following their discovery that bright light delivered at night would quickly terminate the release of the hormone melatonin by the pineal gland deep within the brain.

The connection to psychiatry was the insight of a patient—a scientist himself—who had logged his changing mood and energy for many years. His log revealed the reoccurrence of depression each year as day length diminished before winter. His state in spring, by contrast, was energetic, creative, and productive, although with the sleep loss characteristic of hypomania and mania. He speculated that bright artificial light, recently found to suppress melatonin, could be used to replenish the absent light in winter and reverse his depression. Under guidance from the NIMH research team, his depression remitted within days of using bright light exposure at the edges of long winter nights, thus shortening the night. The specific light level closely matched outdoor light just after the sun rises over the horizon and just before sunset, which was significantly brighter than typical indoor room light.

Does It Work? How Does It Work?

This finding sparked an international research effort with hundreds of volunteers replicating the antidepressant action of bright light. Tabletop light boxes in the best current commercial designs made it convenient for SAD patients to obtain in-home treatment (Figure 52–1). These contrast with the miniaturized (and less expensive) devices on the unregulated open market, which have not met clinical standards.

- The original treatment regimen used both morning and evening light therapy sessions at 2,500 lux for a total of 4–6 hours per day, which was too time intensive for daily use by individuals with workday schedules and family obligations. This was replaced by far brighter light exposure at 10,000 lux for 30 minutes in the morning, matching the level of outdoor skylight approximately 40 minutes after sunrise.
- Dual morning and evening sessions were dropped when morning light alone proved sufficient.
- Light boxes were designed to sit on a desk or table, allowing time for work or breakfast, and tilted downward toward the head (like sky cover) for increased visual comfort.
- Light box screens blocked ultraviolet radiation (UVR) as a safety measure for the eyes and skin. Earlier speculation that UVR participated in the antidepressant effect was disproved.
- The timing of morning light exposure was set according to the individual's personal circadian rhythm—early to late relative to the solar cycle—as determined by a Web program that is anchored to the melatonin rhythm, the Automated Morningness-Eveningness Questionnaire (available at https://chronotype-self-test.info/index.php?sid=61524&newtest=Y).

The proliferation of controlled research trials of light therapy for SAD led to the formation of the Society for Light Treatment and Biological Rhythms in 1988, the formation of the Center for Environmental Therapeutics in 1994, a confirming independent meta-analysis by an American Psychiatric Association (APA) work group in 2005, and conditional approval as a complementary or alternative treatment in APA clinical guidelines in 2019.

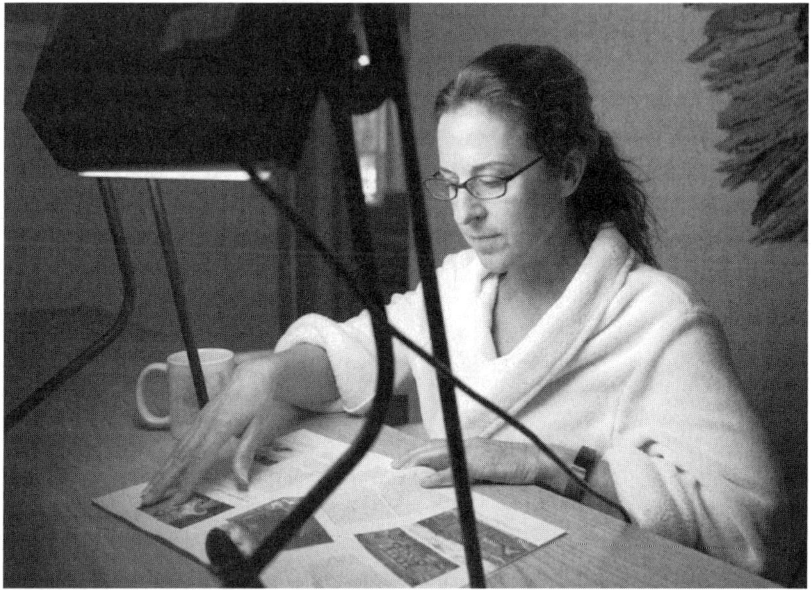

Figure 52–1. Model seated at 10,000 lux downward tilted light box (Northern Light Technologies BOXelite OS).

Source. Photo courtesy of the Center for Environmental Therapeutics.

What Is Light Therapy Used to Treat?

The scope of successful investigations of bright light therapy has extended well beyond SAD, although further independent clinical trials are still needed. Applications include light therapy for nonseasonal major depressive disorder and peripartum depression. Exploratory studies have also shown benefit for patients with attention-deficit/hyperactivity disorder (ADHD), premenstrual dysphoric disorder, binge-eating disorder, and fibromyalgia. A unique expansion of the method, "triple chronotherapy," has shown great promise for patients with bipolar disorder, leading to rapid remissions of depression within 1 week. This method combines light therapy with two sleep manipulations: nights spent totally awake, followed by recovery sleep in gradually earlier steps. The underlying concept encompassing all these light-responsive disorders is a mismatch of the person's circadian rhythm with the solar cycle and extends to nonpsychiatric sleep and medical disorders such as delayed sleep phase disorder, Parkinson's disease, and diabetes.

Bright Light Therapy Versus Antidepressant Drugs for Nonseasonal Depression

The APA's 2019 clinical guidelines suggest light therapy as an adjunct to medication (assuming an insufficient response to medication, as is often the case), which implies that bright light therapy is not on an equal treatment level with medication. A 2016 multicenter study, the largest of its kind, led by the University of British Columbia and published by the *Journal of the American Medical Association*, suggested otherwise. This study demonstrated that participants had a large positive response to light therapy that was superior to the smaller response recorded to fluoxetine alone (Figure 52–2). Although fluoxetine by itself was not significantly different from placebo, improvement was better when the medication was used in combination with light therapy.

This clinical trial clearly showed that the response to light did not depend on seasonality of depression and that it could be effective year-round. Although most psychiatrists prescribe medication before recommending light therapy, a different approach has worked for patients in open treatment at Columbia University who experienced residual symptoms after trying several antidepressants. Light therapy was added to their established medication, and if they experienced rapid major improvement, they could discontinue the medication or taper the dosage gradually to see whether light alone was sufficient.

Side Effects

Although patients should be advised of the potential mild side effects (mainly jumpiness/jitteriness, headache, and nausea) and guided in dosage manipulations to reduce them, attention also should be drawn to the greater overall benefit than risk for the same symptoms. It is also important to note that there are different challenges to using light therapy across age groups. For example, some children may have trouble sitting still in front of a light box in the morning before school, and parents may feel torn between caring for children and maintaining the light therapy schedule.

Additional Information

A New Look at Light Therapy: Dawn Simulation

With the timing of morning bright light therapy focused on a mismatch between a person's circadian rhythm and the solar cycle—discrepancies as little as

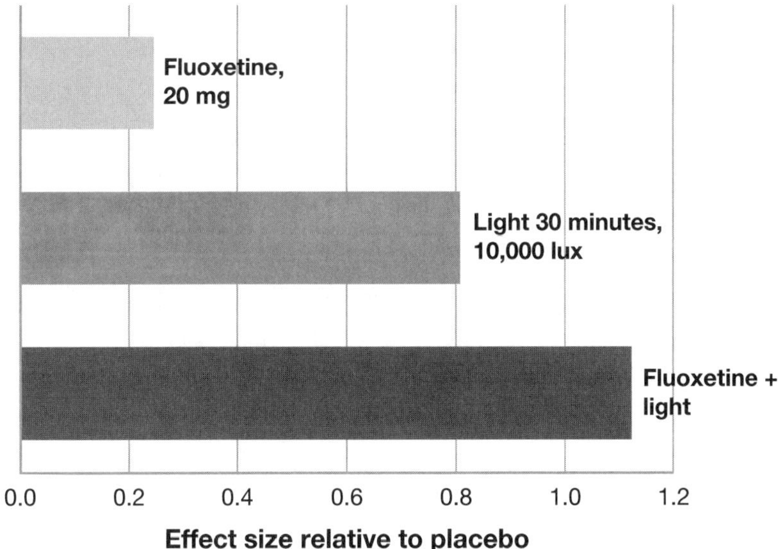

Figure 52–2. Comparison of antidepressant response to drug (n=31), light (n=32), and their combination (n=29), relative to placebo (n=30).

Source. Analysis of multicenter study and graphic by the Center for Environmental Therapeutics, from Lam RW, Levitt AJ, Levitan RD, et al: "Efficacy of Bright Light Treatment, Fluoxetine, and the Combination in Patients With Nonseasonal Major Depressive Disorder: A Randomized Clinical Trial." *JAMA Psychiatry* 73(1):56–63, 2016.

30 minutes—the therapeutic objective is to reconcile this mismatch by shifting the rhythm into concert with day and night. In most cases the rhythm is delayed; indeed, chronic circadian phase delay has been recognized as a risk factor for depressed mood. In SAD, for example, the delayed sunrise of winter can precipitate mild to severe depressions that are absent in summer. The circadian system responds selectively to light presentation in early morning, whereas it shows no major phase shifting at midday, and has an opposite effect that exacerbates the phase delay in the late evening and first part of the night.

The most sensitive time of day for phase correction of delayed rhythms is the pre-sunrise dawn interval, a period of relative darkness outdoors. The dawn gradually ends at sunrise, with winter dawns being later than those in spring or summer. Animal laboratory research has repeatedly shown exquisite sensitivity to artificial dawn illumination, even including the ability of the signal, when presented on a non-24-hour cycle, to shift the rhythm farther from 24.0 hours than the sudden-onset of bright light. This basic research inspired development

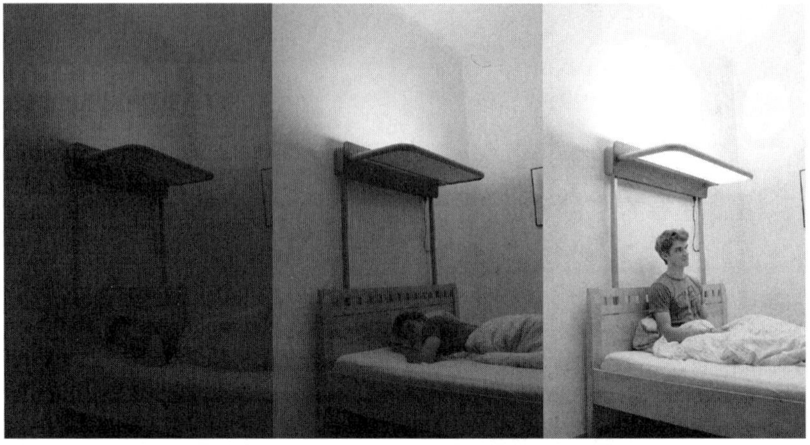

Figure 52–3. Stages of continuous incremental naturalistic dawn simulation.

Left-to-right: Twilight dawn onset beginning in darkness at approximately 0.001 lux 90 minutes before sunrise (upward whole-room projection); smoothly rising illumination approaching sunrise during sleep; bidirectional full sunrise illumination peaking at approximately 300 lux, anchored to wake-up time.

Source. Photo courtesy of Zeitgeber Lighting GmbH.

of naturalistic dawn simulation as a bedroom intervention that mimics bright light therapy during the final period of sleep in an otherwise darkened bedroom. The "dawn" intensity is adjusted so that the user awakens around the time of a simulated sunrise no brighter than typical room light, even though it may still be dark outside.

Clinical trials of naturalistic dawn simulation have produced remissions from winter depression equivalent to those using bright light therapy after waking, along with corrective circadian rhythm adjustment. This positive result caught public attention and prompted lighting manufacturers to market low-end dawn simulators (sometimes unfortunately termed "dawn alarm clocks") that do not replicate the naturalistic properties of outdoor dawns. The signals in these products lack the duration and full dynamic range of light intensity, which extends from the "crack of dawn" to sunrise. Created as a low-cost commodity, these commercial devices also undermine a central property of naturalistic dawn illumination by substituting narrow directionality of the light for a simulation of diffuse sky cover. A naturalistic dawn simulation system providing diffuse and full room illumination (Figure 52–3; see www.cet.org/dawn-simulators) is being prepared for release to the consumer public.

Conclusion

Bright light therapy is an effective treatment for SAD as well as non-seasonal depression and a variety of sleep disorders. Controlled research has proven that it can work as well or better than antidepressants for some patients when using light boxes at the optimal dosage, with potential side effects being very mild. Dawn simulation also shows promise of similar benefits, specifically for gradually easing patients' awakening and saving time at the start of day. Overall, light-based chronotherapeutic approaches provide a medication-free option that is gaining increasing use for mood and sleep issues tied to circadian rhythm misalignment.

Recommended Reading

Center for Environmental Therapeutics website: https://cet.org

Wirz-Justice A, Benedetti F, Terman M: Chronotherapeutics for Affective Disorders: A Clinician's Manual for Light and Wake Therapy, 2nd Edition. Berlin, Karger Publishers, 2013

53

Neuromodulation Treatments in Development

Joshua C. Brown, M.D., Ph.D.
Linda L. Carpenter, M.D.

Introduction

All psychiatric treatments must solve the same problem: accessing the brain. Just as medications are designed to access the brain from the bloodstream, neuromodulation treatments use various forms of energy to alter brain activity in a way that is beneficial and long-lasting. Neuromodulation methods discussed in this book so far have included transcranial magnetic stimulation (TMS), electroconvulsive therapy (ECT), deep brain stimulation (DBS), vagus nerve stimulation (VNS), phototherapy (light energy), and chronotherapy (based on manipulating the timing of biological systems). In addition to these, many other neurostimulation methods are being developed and tested by researchers to see whether they can benefit patients. Most are variations of the methods already established. We can place them into several categories based on the type of energy they use to treat the brain: electricity, magnetism, sound (ultrasound), mechanical (vibration), and light (phototherapy). Other chapters have described treatments that used most of these methods. In this chapter, we introduce several up-and-coming approaches that show promise for future use. These neuromodulation treatments are all still currently in development, which means they have no U.S. Food and Drug Administration (FDA)-approved indications for treating psychiatric disorders. The FDA approves or clears new medical devices only when research trials have proven clinical benefit and safety.

Transcranial Direct Current Stimulation

Electricity is the currency of the brain. The brain sends and receives signals with electricity. It should not be a surprise, then, that electrical stimulation can be used to change undesirable brain activity. How and where to change it is the challenge. Even knowing the rationale behind neuromodulation therapies, the idea of receiving electricity into your brain can be scary. We can be comforted by several things: First, as mentioned, the brain produces its own electricity (it runs on about 20 watts). Amazingly, it produces 80,000 times more electricity than what is delivered by ECT and 1 million times more than that given in TMS over a course of treatment. Second, only about 10% of the electricity actually reaches the brain because most of it is filtered out by the scalp and skull—or *cranium* (i.e., trans*cranial*)—before it gets to the brain.

What Is Transcranial Direct Current Stimulation?

Transcranial direct current stimulation (tDCS) delivers electrical energy to the brain in the form of *direct current* (think Thomas Edison). It is similar to ECT, except it uses only 1% of the energy of ECT (typically, a stimulation dose is a very weak electrical current of 1–4 milliamperes [mA] applied for up to 20 minutes), and as a result, tDCS does not produce seizures or require anesthesia. In fact, it is not even strong enough to cause brain cells to fire (called an *action potential*). Instead, tDCS can increase or decrease the charge of a brain cell to make it easier (or harder) to fire, sort of like how a fully charged car battery still requires the turn of the key to start the car, whereas a nearly dead battery can still start the car, but only after a struggle. tDCS gives the brain's neurons a bit of a "push" and tips the balance so they are more likely to fire. Like the car analogy, tDCS is thought to have the most impact when the stimulation is combined with some other brain activity to "turn the key," such as psychotherapy or memory training.

How Is It Done?

During tDCS, a small amount of electricity flows between two electrodes placed anywhere on the outside surface of the head. An *electrode* is a conductor of electricity—for tDCS, it is usually a small square or round object that makes contact with the scalp and has something to hold it in place, such as a rubber headband or elastic cap. Often the electrode is soaked with salt water or placed over a bit of gel to ensure the electricity spreads out evenly in the electrode and makes good contact with the scalp. The electrodes are positioned on the head so that electricity will flow through targeted brain regions (i.e., regions thought to contribute to symptoms or disorders). They are then connected to a small battery, and a control panel is used to select the intensity, frequency, and patterns of stimulation. tDCS treatment protocols typically involve application of stimulation at least once per day (around 20–30 minutes) for multiple days.

Side Effects

tDCS is considered very safe, with no permanent side effects. During stimulation, it can cause discomfort at the site of stimulation, skin redness, and tingling or itchy sensations. Other side effects reported in clinical trials include dizziness, headache, nausea, and insomnia, but these were reported just as often by those receiving sham tDCS as by those receiving real tDCS. *Sham* is the term used in neuromodulation clinical trials to describe a treatment that looks and feels like the real thing but does not actually deliver energy to the brain—just as a placebo pill in drug studies looks identical to the real agent but contains only sugar. More side effects can occur with higher-intensity stimulation, but these are not used with traditional tDCS because it becomes painful to the scalp.

Advantages

In addition to being very safe, tDCS is portable and cheap. This means that instead of traveling to a treatment center multiple times per week for many weeks, as patients must do when they receive TMS or ECT, patients can receive treatment at home. Accessibility is a major barrier for many people who live far away from specialty clinics or who have transportation limitations, but tDCS sessions can be delivered under the supervision of a clinician through remote control and telehealth services. A number of tDCS devices are safe enough for unsupervised self-administration once a patient has been trained to properly use the equipment. tDCS is also inexpensive, costing as little as $30 for commercially made devices. At this low cost, paying out-of-pocket becomes possible for most people. These advantages mean that once researchers can prove that tDCS is an effective treatment, it could have a tremendous impact.

Clinical Benefits

tDCS is being studied in many disorders including depression, anxiety, attention-deficit/hyperactivity disorder (ADHD), stroke, chronic pain, migraines, fibromyalgia, tinnitus, addiction, schizophrenia, and rehabilitation of speech and motor function, but as yet no devices have received FDA approval to treat any of these disorders because clinical studies have not yet proven they are sufficiently effective. tDCS systems are available on the market right now, and consumers can find them advertised as useful for promoting "relaxation," "positive mood," "learning," and "focus," but using such devices without information about their safe and effective application is not without risks. As we mentioned earlier, the benefits from tDCS are most likely to come when its use is combined with some other form of therapy to boost effects on desired brain activity.

Use in Depression

Clinical studies of tDCS for depression have reported mixed results. Some patients have experienced strong benefits, others have experienced weak effects, and still others have shown no antidepressant effects. We speculate about the reasons for these varied responses later (see "Challenges"). Despite these challenges, one scientific report reviewed all the studies that had met the standard of a *randomized, double-blind, sham-controlled clinical trial* (a trial in which participants are randomly assigned to receive either sham or real treatment, and neither the patients nor the researchers know which treatment the patients are receiving; this is the highest level of evidence in medicine). The combined effect from six of these studies found tDCS to be as effective as TMS. Among participants receiving tDCS, 34% reported meaningful improvement (defined as a 50% reduction of symptoms or better), and 23% had no more depression at all following treatment. This is compared with 19% and 13% of participants who received the sham treatment, respectively. Even more recently, a comparison of 30 trials in depression reported similar results. Thus, tDCS is clearly beneficial in the treatment of depression. These results from numerous small clinical trials collectively set the stage for a large double-blind, sham-controlled trial, which is what must be done—with affirming results—in order for tDCS to receive FDA approval.

Use in Anxiety

tDCS for anxiety is not as well studied as for depression. In a very recent analysis of 15 different trials for anxiety, tDCS had no overall effect, although some of the studies did see improvements. One group recently tested tDCS in the way many have envisioned: the patients took a tDCS device home with them and combined tDCS treatment with cognitive-behavioral therapy (CBT) through a phone application. In a small study of six patients, five showed consistent benefits for both depression and anxiety through 6–10 weeks of treatment. Side effects were minimal, as expected. This study was not a sham-controlled trial, so we cannot know for sure if the benefits were due to tDCS. However, it does show the potential of using tDCS at home, combined with therapy, over long periods of time.

Challenges

Variable clinical responses are not unique to tDCS, but there are several reasons why tDCS might have more than most. First, unlike TMS or ECT, there is no way to "dose" tDCS for an individual's brain. Everyone gets the same amount of energy (i.e., 2 mA). ECT and TMS do not have this problem because doctors can determine the lowest energy to cause a seizure or cause finger movement. tDCS does not cause neurons to fire, only to fire more easily, so there is no way to confirm that it is reaching the brain. Second, the doses may be too low. A study in cadavers suggested that 2 mA may not be strong enough to reach the brain—it stops at the skull. Other studies indicate that doses two to three times higher (i.e., 4–6 mA) are needed to reach the brain in most people, but such doses can be painful. Third, a lot of choices must be made about how and where in the brain to stimulate. In fact, the choices are infinite! Scientists must make educated guesses about what parameters to use, such as how intense, how frequent, or how long pulses should be. Many scientists are working to solve these challenges, and despite them, tDCS has growing evidence that it can benefit depressed and anxious patients.

A Note About Cranial Electrotherapy

You may find several devices advertised that seem *similar* to tDCS (Fisher Wallace, Alpha-Stim, CES Ultra, Neurocare, Caputron MindGear, and others) but instead fall into a category called "cranial electrotherapy." Despite a lack of research data to prove they were effective and safe for treating medical disorders, early versions of these devices were being sold before the FDA began regulating medical devices in 1976. Thus, these devices were "grandfathered" into the system when current standards for FDA approval were established. This means that these cranial electrotherapy stimulation devices can be legally marketed to consumers (for mood elevation, anxiety reduction, sleep improvement, and enhanced mental or physical performance) even though they were never required to undergo rigorous studies comparing the treatment outcomes between active and sham stimulation groups to demonstrate substantial therapeutic effects. The body of research that has been published to demonstrate their therapeutic and biological effects does not reflect a high level of scientific quality, so they have not been adopted into the standard of care. Cranial electrotherapy stimulation devices on the market today use a variety of waveforms and pulse rates to deliver low-intensity electricity through a pair of electrodes that attach to a person's ears, eyelids, or temples or with clips, sponges, gels, or stickers.

Ultrasound Therapy

Low-Intensity Focused Ultrasound

One of the major limitations of many established neurostimulation therapies is that they are either invasive, requiring surgery in the brain (i.e., DBS), or they cannot access deeper brain structures that need to be reached. Low-intensity focused ultrasound (LIFU) is unique in that it can target deep brain areas without surgery or anesthesia. It is also different from many other neuromodulation interventions because it does not use electrical or magnetic energy but instead uses sound waves called *sonications*.

What is Focused Ultrasound?

Ultrasound refers to sound waves with a frequency *above* that of human hearing. LIFU uses ultrasound waves like the kind used to see a fetus during pregnancy, except that the ultrasound devices used to create images of objects inside of a uterus deliver continuous sound waves, whereas LIFU devices emit sound waves in packets or pulses. LIFU is not the first type of sound wave treatment to be applied to the brain. High-intensity focused ultrasound (HIFU) has been utilized to destroy pathological brain tissue or interrupt pathological brain circuits in more than 160 different diseases, including various cancers and disorders such as obsessive-compulsive disorder (OCD), essential tremor, and Parkinson's disease. When the functions of small brain areas become permanently out of balance, destroying these areas with HIFU can provide lasting relief. Unlike HIFU, application of LIFU seems to merely alter the activity of brain cells without permanently damaging them.

How Is It Done?

LIFU uses a helmet or strap to secure one or more transducers to the head. A *transducer* acts like a speaker to send sound waves deep into the brain. A head magnetic resonance imaging (MRI) scan is performed first to give the exact dimensions of the patient's skull shape. The skull is used to focus the sound waves so they will target a spot in the brain that is in the desired location and is the desired size—as small as half of a millimeter or as large as several centimeters. Like other forms of neuromodulation using electrical or magnetic waves, LIFU sound waves are delivered with specific parameters that together define the stimulation "dose" for each application, including the number of sonications per second (e.g., 100 Hz), the duration of sonication "trains" (e.g., 30 seconds), the duration of rest periods between trains, and the total number of sonication trains per session (e.g., 10 trains). The use of LIFU technology for treating psychiatric disorders is so new that little is known about the best parameters, but insights from other neuromodulation therapies should be helpful to guide research. For example, the time it takes to send a single pulse (called *pulse width*, which is about half of a millisecond for LIFU) is similar across all forms of brain stimulation.

Clinical Effects

LIFU has not yet been tested for any clinical indications. We mention it here because it has remarkable potential and unique capabilities that suggest its likelihood as a future therapeutic modality. Currently, only a handful of very small LIFU studies are available, and these have been conducted in healthy humans. We learn a few important things from these studies. LIFU appears to be safe and is able to affect the brain. For example, LIFU was delivered to a deep region of the brain that receives pain signals, called the *thalamus*, in 19 healthy people to try to alter pain tolerance. Researchers were able to see a change of brain activity in the MRI machine during the stimulation. What is more impressive is that when subjects got real, but not sham, LIFU, their pain tolerance was higher. In another study, LIFU was also able to improve the mood ratings from 31 healthy people. In the first test of LIFU in a clinical patient, a man in a coma due to a severe brain injury became fully awake and alert 3 days after LIFU was administered, and he was understanding speech and attempting to walk after 5 days. Although it is possible he may have had a spontaneous recovery anyway (double-blind, sham controlled trials must be performed), this nonetheless is a very exciting outcome. At the time of this writing, at least one clinical trial is under way testing LIFU for treatment of depression.

Peripheral Nerve Stimulation Therapy

What Are Peripheral Nerves?

Twelve pairs of nerves (called *cranial nerves*) connect your brain to different parts of your head, neck, and trunk. These cranial nerves are considered "peripheral" nerves because they do not come out of the spinal cord. Some cranial nerves have smaller branches coming off of them that are easily accessible because they are relatively superficial—that is, they are not too far beneath the surface of the skin. For example, the *trigeminal nerve* has branches in the forehead, and the *vagus nerve* has branches in the ear. Because they carry information back and forth between the body and the brain, some peripheral nerves offer a "highway" for stimulation to travel to the brain. Researchers have developed various types of devices that are placed on the body in a location over one or more of these peripheral nerve branches. These devices are designed to send signals to the brain by delivering low-intensity electrical stimulation that penetrates the skin and travels through the nerve back to the brain to create therapeutic effects.

Trigeminal Nerve Stimulation

The trigeminal nerve has multiple branches on the forehead, so it is easy to access for noninvasive stimulation with external devices that deliver low-intensity electricity through the skin (*transcutaneously*). Devices that provide transcutaneous trigeminal nerve stimulation (TNS) have proven effective and have received FDA approval for relieving migraine headaches and treating childhood attention-deficit/hyperactivity disorder (ADHD). Clinical trials of TNS have demonstrated potential for reducing seizure frequency in people with medication-resistant epilepsy but also indicate positive mood effects. Several small pilot studies have also suggested TNS might be effective for depression as well as posttraumatic stress disorder (PTSD).

The side effects associated with TNS are consistently mild and include skin irritation, headache, fatigue, and (only in pediatric epilepsy) increased appetite. Studies are under way to evaluate a novel take-home device that stimulates both the trigeminal nerve branches on the forehead and the occipital nerve branches on the back of the head; this device was recently FDA-approved for migraine treatment and is currently being investigated to treat depression. Side effects are generally mild and include temporary discomfort or unpleasant sensations during stimulation, a sensation of scalp numbness, sleepiness or fatigue or disrupted sleep, dizziness, headache, and skin irritation beneath the electrodes.

External Vagus Nerve Stimulation

The vagus nerve has fibers that carry signals in two directions: up to the brain from many areas of the body and down from the brain to organs such as the heart and stomach. Stimulating the vagus nerve with electrodes surgically implanted right on the nerve in the neck area has already been shown effective for treating depression and epilepsy (see Chapter 50, "Vagus Nerve Stimulation"). Neuromodulation treatments in development include noninvasive, nonsurgical ways to stimulate this same nerve. Like TNS, external vagus nerve stimulation devices (eVNS) may rely on relatively weak electrical signals that pass through the skin and travel to the brain to produce their effects. Some versions of eVNS use "vibrotactile" stimulation, which is actually a mechanical form of stimulation from a small vibrating device placed on the skin overlying the nerve. Branches of the vagus nerve in the outer portion of our ears have been targeted with eVNS; stimulation has produced effects on heart rate and blood pressure that are considered a type of "relaxation" response (i.e., the opposite of an acute stress reaction). Growing evidence indicates that stimulating the vagus nerve may reduce inflammation chemicals circulating in the blood, and many brain disorders and pain syndromes are thought to involve such inflammation. Although some commercial eVNS devices are available, none has undergone clinical investigations to establish safety and efficacy in the treatment of any medical disorder. A wide range of stimulation parameters have been used in eVNS clinical trials.

Magnetic Seizure Therapy

Most people think of TMS when it comes to neuromodulation therapy using magnetic energy (see Chapter 49, "Transcranial Magnetic Stimulation"). Magnetic seizure therapy (MST) is very similar to TMS except that it uses much higher energy (more pulses per second for more seconds at a time) to generate seizures. MST is like TMS in the same way that ECT is like tDCS. In fact, because ECT is still considered by many to be the "gold standard" treatment for severe depression, results from studies with MST are often compared with those from ECT. Like ECT, MST is done under anesthesia. It takes a similar amount of time and similar number of treatments (see Chapter 48, "Electroconvulsive Therapy"). The results of 10 studies published up to this point suggest that MST is as effective as ECT. This is exciting because MST appears to have fewer side effects; compared with ECT, MST had fewer memory and cognitive side effects and better recovery times after treatment. Large trials are now under way seeking to demonstrate sufficient safety and effectiveness of MST in order to gain FDA approval. MST may soon hold a place in the United States as an alternative to ECT with reduced cognitive side effects.

Personalized Stimulation Therapy

This last section is not dedicated to discussing any particular form of energy or stimulation but to emphasizing the incredible potential of personalizing neuromodulation treatments. Personalized approaches can be thought of as having two components: specific types of data from the brain or body of an individual patient, and treatment interventions that specifically respond to those data. Personalized neuromodulation is already being utilized in epilepsy. A technology called *responsive neurostimulation* (RNS) continuously reads brain waves from an implanted electroencephalography electrode, and those data are sent wirelessly to a computer. RNS learns to recognize patterns in a patient's electroencephalogram (EEG), namely, what the brain wave data look like when a seizure is about to start. Once a pattern is recognized, RNS automatically delivers a burst of electrical stimulation to "reset" the brain rhythm and disrupt the seizure from developing—sort of like defibrillating the heart with an automated external defibrillator device. Researchers are working to recognize biological signatures of depression, anxiety, and other psychiatric disorders with the hope that, once the signature is recognized, stimulation therapies can be delivered in a way designed to change the abnormal brain activity patterns back into healthy states.

One group from the University of California, San Francisco, has shown that this is not just a theoretical possibility. They used DBS (see Chapter 51, "Deep Brain Stimulation") electrodes and EEG brainwave signals in order to create a brain "map" of networks controlling mood symptoms in a 36-year-old female with severe depression. They were then able to use RNS to respond to the patient's internal state and immediately eliminate her depression symptoms with 90 seconds of stimulation. As she described it, "I suddenly felt a genuine sense of glee and happiness, and the world went from shades of dark gray to just—grinning." These effects lasted for hours after only 10 minutes of stimulation. These improvements lasted up to 6 weeks following 10 days of stimulations. When describing the RNS experience, she stated, "It struck me so clearly in that moment that my depression wasn't something I was doing wrong or just needed to try harder to snap out of; it really was a problem in my brain that this stimulation was able to fix. Every time they'd stimulate, I felt like, 'I'm my old self, I could go back to work, I could do the things I want to do with my life.'" These researchers are now developing a small clinical trial to try to repeat these benefits in 12 participants long term.

Conclusion

Clinicians and researchers agree that depression is not the same for every patient. Like cancer, there are likely many different types of depression. The future of depression treatment will likely include using sophisticated technology, such as brain imaging with MRI, electroencephalography, and other modalities, to determine which networks are involved in depression and how to bring them back to a healthy state.

Recommended Reading

Higgins ES, George MS: Brain Stimulation Therapies for Clinicians, Second Edition. Washington, DC, American Psychiatric Association Publishing, 2020

Rhodes M: 3,000 Pulses Later: A Memoir of Surviving Depression Without Medication. Danbury, CT, The Pushpin Press, 2013

Part V

The Treatments

Psychological

54

Cognitive-Behavioral Therapy for Major Depressive Disorder

Steven D. Hollon, Ph.D.

Introduction

Cognitive-behavioral therapy (CBT) is one of several psychosocial interventions shown to be as efficacious as antidepressant medications in the acute treatment of major depressive disorder (MDD) and appears to have an enduring effect that reduces risk for subsequent symptom return following treatment termination. This may be true for other types of psychotherapy, but it has not been as well established as for CBT, and it is clearly not true for antidepressant medications, which only work for so long as they continue being taken.

Description of the Treatment

CBT is based on the premise that how someone interprets the events that happen to them determines (in part) how they feel about those events and what they try to do about them. That is not to say that some things are not worse than others, only that being able to think accurately about the difficulties one faces can reduce distress and facilitate coping. There is reason to think that depression is "species typical" in that anyone can become depressed if something bad enough happens to them (e.g., most of us would have a grief reaction if we lost someone close to us), but about 20% of all females and 12% of all males enter adolescence at elevated risk for becoming depressed in response to minor stressors.

CBT teaches skills for dealing with those depressions. Treatment typically starts with an emphasis on behavioral strategies and then becomes more cognitive as sessions proceed. Depression is more a "disease of expectations" than of the capacity to do what one would typically do or to enjoy it once it is done. People who get depressed often find that they stop doing the things that they used to enjoy or that added meaning to their lives, usually because they do not expect to enjoy these things or because they doubt their ability to carry them out successfully. In CBT, patients are encouraged to test the accuracy of their negative beliefs by doing whatever they would have done if they were not depressed and letting the outcome determine the accuracy of those beliefs. For example, someone who is depressed might be inclined not to go to a party because it seems like too much trouble or they doubt they will enjoy it; with CBT, they would be encouraged to suspend their disbelief and go anyway. What these individuals typically find is that they enjoy themselves more than anticipated—perhaps not as much as if they were not depressed, but more than staying home. Neuroscience studies indicate that different neurotransmitters underlie "wanting" versus "liking," and it appears that "wanting" is what is most disrupted in depression.

CBT becomes more explicitly cognitive over sessions, although it never loses its emphasis on encouraging patients to use their own behaviors to test their own beliefs. People who are particularly susceptible to multiple episodes (the "recurrence prone") tend to blame themselves when things go wrong in a manner that further worsens their mood and undercuts their efforts to cope. Clinical experience suggests that this propensity predates adolescence and serves as a predisposing diathesis (whether inherited or acquired) that increases risk for onset. Naturalistic studies suggest that people who are prone to recurrence tend to generate their own stress; they are no more likely to experience major stressors that are independent of their own actions (e.g., death of a loved one), but they are more likely to encounter negative life events to which their own behaviors could have contributed (e.g., being unemployed or single). People who have the core belief that they are incompetent are unlikely to apply for the job they want, and people who believe they are unlovable are unlikely to pursue a relationship with someone who sparks their interest. When these individuals do succeed in getting a job or forming a relationship, they are more likely to misinterpret minor events as major catastrophes for which they hold themselves responsible and that they subsequently mishandle because these events seem overwhelming.

CBT teaches people to be more systematic in how they evaluate the causes and implications of the stressors they face. Rather than string one negative inference after another, they are taught to ask themselves three questions about each negative inference: 1) what is the *evidence* for (and against) that belief; 2) is there any *alternative explanation* for that event; and 3) what are the real *implications* of that event, even if it turns out to be true? In effect, CBT teaches patients how to evaluate the accuracy of their beliefs in a more systematic fashion and to use their own behaviors whenever possible to test the competing interpretations. As previously noted, most people who are prone to recurrence enter adolescence with a latent predisposition to blame themselves when things go wrong, and treatment is often cast as a test between two competing theories: 1) something is deeply wrong with me (incompetent or unlovable depending on whether someone is oriented toward achievement or affiliation) versus 2) I simply chose the wrong strategies (perhaps as a consequence of overestimating the degree of difficulty or underestimating my own capacities). For less complicated patients, CBT keeps the focus on current life events but briefly explores the genesis of the core beliefs, usually some event in childhood or early adolescence that was misinterpreted or taken out of context. Even when the original event was not misinterpreted (e.g., an overly critical parent or cruel classmates), the perspective provided by greater maturity and systematic evaluation can help when questioning the original interpretation.

People with depressions superimposed on underlying personality disorders are even more likely to generate problems in their lives because they consistently act in ways that others find objectionable. For example, someone prone to paranoia tends to drive others away with their suspicions, and a narcissist wears their partners out with their insistent demands to be flattered. These behaviors are essentially compensatory strategies intended to protect the individual from the consequences of what they perceive to be their own weakness and foibles (incompetence or unlovability). What the person misses is that these compensatory strategies (intended to be self-protective) are what turns other people off. Someone who is just depressed may not go to a party because they do not expect to have a good time; they suffer in silence but do not poison their interpersonal relationships. Someone who has a depression superimposed on a narcissistic personality disorder may go to the party but may behave in a way that others find obnoxious, and interpret the others' reactions to them as slights. CBT can be extended to the treatment of underlying personality disorders via attending not just to current life events but also to childhood antecedents and the vicissitudes of their therapeutic relationship. Persons with underlying personality disorders are encouraged to test their core beliefs and underlying assumptions by dropping their compensatory behaviors to test whether they are truly protective, much as a patient prone to panic attacks is encouraged to drop their safety behaviors to test whether they are truly at risk of having a heart attack or psychotic decompensation.

Who Should Receive Cognitive-Behavioral Therapy?

The less self-protective a person's behaviors are and the less entrenched their beliefs, the more rapid the therapy process will be. Most people who are only depressed will respond within about 20–24 sessions over 12–16 weeks. For people with depressions co-occurring with underlying personality disorders, successful treatment typically requires a matter of months, if not years. An evolutionary perspective suggests that depression is not so much a disease or even a disorder but, rather, an evolved adaptation such as pain or anxiety that served a function in our evolutionary past. (There are "true diseases" in which mechanisms that evolved to serve a purpose have broken down; bipolar disorder, with its high heritability, low prevalence, comparable distribution across the sexes, and preferential response to medications is a high probability candidate.) Just what function depression evolved to serve is open to conjecture, but it is interesting to note that when someone gets depressed, their energy is directed to the cortex in a manner that facilitates slow and deliberate thinking. Most episodes of depression resolve on their own even in the absence of treatment (a process known as *spontaneous remission*), and neither psychotherapies nor antidepressant medications existed in our ancestral past. Given that unipolar depression is twice as common in females than in males and that initial incidence virtually explodes in early adolescence, an argument can be made that depression evolved to help people solve complex social problems that might otherwise get them excluded from the troop. Such individuals would be particularly likely to starve or be picked off by predators, and evolutionary selection pressures sit heaviest on females caring for offspring. If depression is an adaptation that evolved to help vulnerable adolescents resolve complex social problems and prevent ostracism from the troop, then any intervention that helps to resolve complex social issues in an accurate and effective way is likely to be preferred over one that merely anesthetizes the distress.

Conclusion

CBT has been shown to be as efficacious as and more enduring than antidepressant medications for the treatment of unipolar depression. Less complicated patients are likely to remit within a matter of weeks, whereas more complicated patients with depression superimposed on long-standing personality disorders will likely require months or even years. There is good reason to think that unipolar depression may be an adaptation that evolved to help people think carefully about their problems, and any intervention that helps patients think things through in a accurate fashion (e.g., CBT) is likely to be preferred over one that simply anesthetizes the distress (e.g., antidepressant medications).

Recommended Reading

Greenberger D: Mind Over Mood: Change How You Feel by Changing the Way You Think, 2nd Edition. New York, Guilford Press, 2015

Hollon SD: Is cognitive therapy enduring or antidepressant medications iatrogenic? Depression as an evolved adaptation. Am Psychol 75(9):1207–1218, 2020 33382283

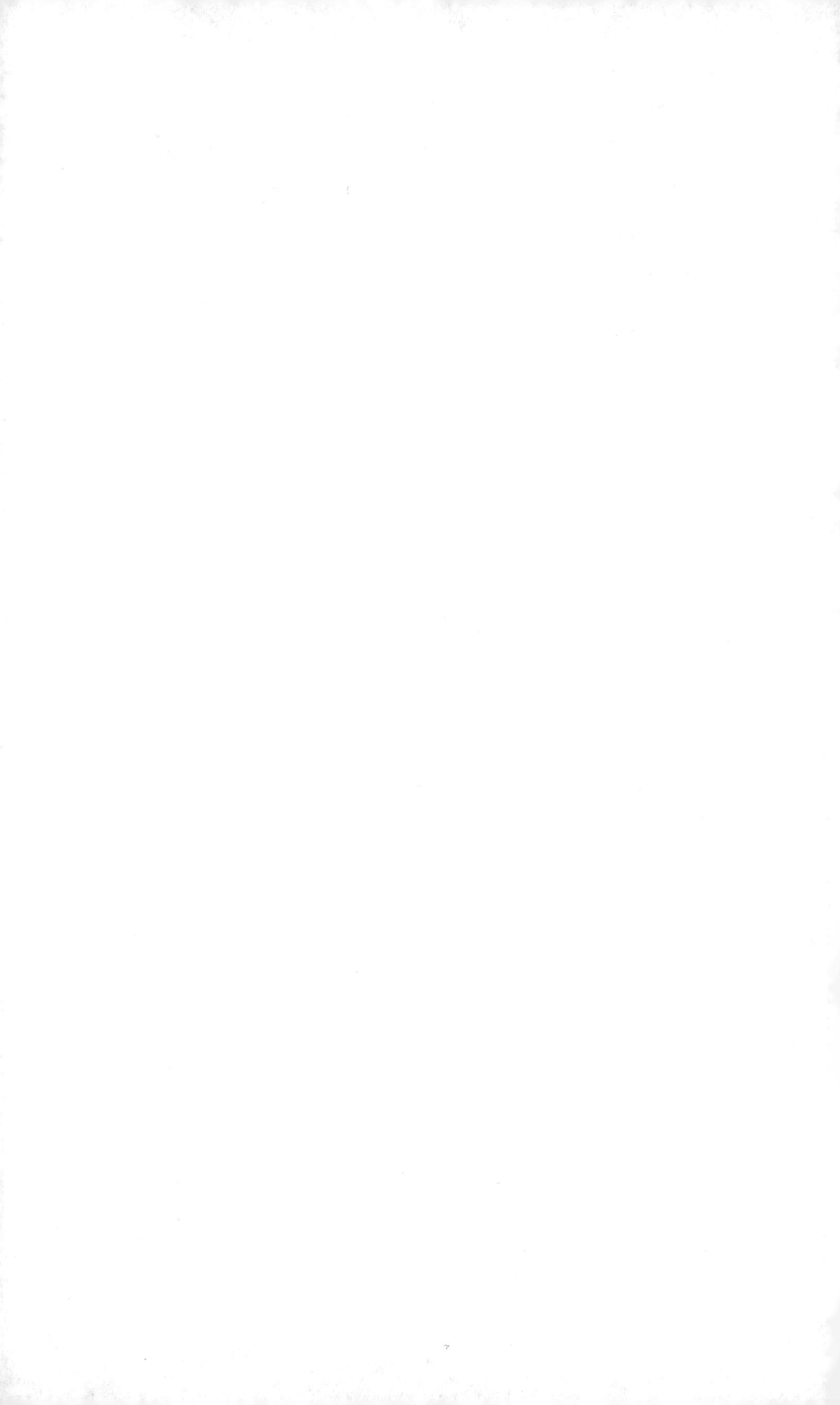

55

Interpersonal Psychotherapy for Major Depressive Disorder

Myrna M. Weissman, Ph.D.
Jennifer J. Mootz, Ph.D.

Introduction

Interpersonal psychotherapy (IPT) was developed in the late 1970s by Klerman and Weissman. Although many new medications for psychiatric disorders had demonstrated efficacy in order to obtain U.S. Food and Drug Administration (FDA) approval before they could be used, at the time, no clinical trials of any psychotherapy had been conducted. Psychotherapy nonetheless was the most common treatment used for depression—and some would say it was the preferred treatment. Thus, it was necessary to specify a psychotherapy—IPT—in order to train therapists and to conduct the first clinical trial establishing the efficacy of psychotherapy for managing symptoms of distress due to depression.

The first clinical trial compared IPT, then called "high contact," with use of the medication amitriptyline for the maintenance treatment of depression to prevent relapse and improve functioning. The surprisingly positive results of this trial led to the approach being named *interpersonal psychotherapy* and to many subsequent trials. More than 150 clinical trials have now been conducted that have established the efficacy of IPT for treatment of major depression, bulimia, posttraumatic stress disorder (PTSD), bipolar disorder, distress, and anxiety disorders in adolescents, adults, and elderly patients. Adaptations have been made and trials carried out to accommodate various disorders in diverse populations. Group and guided self-help versions of IPT are available, as are numerous translations, recommendations, and guidelines throughout the world. Modifications have been made to reduce cost, and brief versions have been developed for delivery by non-mental-health-trained community health workers. These developments are described in the 2018 paper by Weissman and colleagues cited in the "Recommended Reading" section at the end of this chapter. The 2024 book by Weissman and Mootz, also cited, describes the global reach and adaptations of IPT worldwide and in special populations in the United States.

Description of the Treatment

Despite the widespread use of IPT globally and its many translations, the core principles remain unchanged. The underlying concept of IPT is that regardless of the "cause" of the current depression—for example, genetic, biological vulnerability, past childhood experiences—the symptoms occur in a current interpersonal context. Understanding that context may help people change, improve, or leave the difficult situation and therefore reduce their symptoms and improve functioning. These ideas are simplified by the concept of the four core problem areas:

1. *Grief*—a loss through the death of someone important
2. *Disputes*—a disagreement with someone important; may be at an interpersonal impasse, a renegotiation, or dissolution of the relationship
3. *Transitions*—changes in life or relationships (positive or negative) that cause distress and reflection and require assessment
4. *Loneliness*—an absence of close relationships, which may be recent, the result of other problem areas, or lifelong

IPT is divided into three phases of treatment: initiation, middle, and termination. In the *initiation phase,* dealing with the problem area(s) begins with a series of strategies to understand patients' symptoms, problem context, and relationships. These strategies include

1. *The timeline*—explanation of symptoms and connection to interpersonal problems

2. *The sick role*—patient will feel better but for now should take care
3. *The interpersonal inventory*—survey of important people in the patient's life to understand who is helpful and who may cause more distress

The therapist works with the patient to identify the main problem area(s), which can change during therapy. This is followed by an explanation of the therapy and description of a set time limit. A time limit is important for evaluating progress, which is determined by tracking symptoms and functioning. Evaluation can help the therapist understand whether to terminate treatment if goals are met, continue treatment if there is progress but symptoms have not fully improved, or transition to an alternate approach if needed. IPT has been studied in a wide variety of durations.

The problem areas become the focus of the *middle phase*. These sessions begin with monitoring of the patient's mood and symptoms to track their progress and connect their mental health symptoms to their interpersonal problem and context. When the focus is on grief, IPT therapists work with patients to process their loss by encouraging conversation about the context of the loss (how it happened and the patients' relationship to that context). For example, a loved one might have been sick, and the patient became a caretaker, or the loved one's death may have been sudden, and the patient may not have had an opportunity to say goodbye. Patients' relationships with their lost loved ones can involve many emotions and be complex. Therapists strive to provide a safe setting for patients to discuss the positive and negative aspects of these relationships. Therapists work with patients to identify ways to honor their loved one, build or leverage interpersonal support while grieving, and consider ways to support their well-being going forward.

When dispute is the main interpersonal problem, IPT therapists guide patients to consider the stage of dispute, which could be in *renegotiation* (discussing or arguing), *impasse* (no further discussion), or *dissolution* (wanting to end the relationship). Therapists employ different strategies depending on the type of dispute. If patients are at an impasse, for example, therapists might work with them to decide whether they want to resume renegotiating the dispute or dissolve the relationship. If they are in a process of renegotiating, therapists can help them understand their style of communication and their role in the dispute through analyses of their communication during an argument. The next step is to identify strategies for more effective ways of communicating and to practice those strategies. Finally, if the dispute is at the *dissolution* stage, therapists can work with patients to emotionally process the end of the relationship and plan for the future.

Life changes, or transitions, could be another focus of the middle phase. Transitions in patients' lives can be the result of more obvious negative events (e.g., loss of employment, forced relocation, housing instability) or seemingly positive events (e.g., promotion, marriage, birth of a child). Therapists work with patients to understand the impact of the life change, especially how it relates to their distress and other relationships. For example, if someone just had a child, they may experience transitions in employment due to childcare responsibilities or develop a new sense of isolation. The focus is on understanding patients' conceptions of their old and new roles, what they like and do not like about each, and helping them learn to access or strengthen relationships to support them in their new role.

A fourth focus of the middle phase occurs when patients experience loneliness. Some patients experience lifelong loneliness that begins in childhood and have few attachments. Other patients might be experiencing loneliness because of another interpersonal problem (e.g., moving to a new city). In this case, focusing on a life transition might be more appropriate. Still others could have impaired relationships resulting from recurring disputes and difficulties relating with others. Strategies for addressing loneliness are to understand the patients' previous relationships, if any, and how they ended; identify patterns in their relationships; and help them practice forming or maintaining current relationships through in-depth roleplaying. Therapists and patients can emphasize resolving loneliness if it is difficult to identify another problem area.

The final phase of treatment is *termination*, or the ending phase of therapy. Termination includes processing feelings about ending therapy and no longer having the support of a therapist, reviewing progress, and deciding on options for future treatment, as needed and feasible.

The various adaptations of IPT for different disorders, ages, countries, and modalities can be found in a number of books. The core features described here are the same regardless of the adaptation. The therapist's role is active, encouraging the patient's advocations, directing them toward the strategies outlined above, and encouraging change in their lives. The patient is encouraged to consider the current problems that created the distress. The therapist views the therapy as an interpersonal relationship and as a way to help patients to find new strategies.

Who Should Receive Interpersonal Psychotherapy?

No treatment works for everyone, even when indicated by the results of clinical trials. IPT has been tested and shown to be efficacious for depression in people of all ages, beginning with adolescents. There are no data or indications of efficacy with any biological markers. No trials of IPT adaptations have been conducted for prepubertal children or for people with schizophrenia or psychotic disorders. Although best studied as a treatment for depression, IPT has been tested and shown to be efficacious with adaptations for individuals with distress, major depression, bipolar disorder, eating disorders, anxiety, PTSD, and comorbid medical illnesses. IPT has not been shown to be effective in primary substance abuse.

There are some cultures in which group therapy is more acceptable than individual therapy. We also have found the opposite to be true in other populations. In some cultures, group treatment must be separated by sex. In others, we found that parents had to be included in the treatment of unmarried women in their twenties. We cannot make any general statements, and we urge users to take into account their own comforts and what is standard practice and acceptable in their own social group and culture. The Weissman and Mootz book describes uses in 31 countries and some suggested adaptations.

Is This Treatment Effective?

Excellent evidence from clinical trials has shown that IPT is effective in reducing the symptoms of depression (i.e., the *response*). The treatment is also effective in helping patients stay in *remission*—that is, remain symptom-free or have reduced symptoms once response has been achieved. These studies have compared IPT with placebo, medication, and other psychotherapies. The magnitude of the response and effective remission depend on various circumstances, which are often unknown. Patients with depression may *relapse* (i.e., experience a return of symptoms after a period of remission), and, as with any treatment, a complete clinical evaluation is warranted to determine the factors involved in the relapse before a decision can be made regarding whether medication, IPT alone, a combination of both, or a new medication or psychotherapy should be tried. In general, if vegetative symptoms, sleep problems, or appetite problems are present, medication is indicated. If a new rupture occurs in a personal attachment, a course of IPT could be indicated, especially if it was successful in the past.

Are Other Treatments Used in Conjunction With This Treatment?

Since the first clinical trials, IPT has been considered a treatment that can be used alone or with medication. These treatments can alternate depending on patients' needs, wishes, and previous experience. Although there is no definite indication for using IPT in combination with medication, the general thinking and some data suggest that medication reduces the symptoms of depression, such as sleep disturbance, appetite changes, anxiety, and helplessness. IPT helps with the problem of interpersonal and social functioning, two domains that are highly intertwined. The patient's wishes and past experiences should be considered in this decision. In general, as mentioned earlier, if a patient is experiencing serious vegetative symptoms, loss of sleep, and weight loss, then a medication should be considered. In some conditions such as bipolar disorder, maintenance medication is almost always indicated. During pregnancy, medications may need to be stopped and IPT used alone.

Several studies have shown that patients receiving the combination of medication and IPT do better than those receiving either treatment alone, but many others have shown the efficacy of using either treatment alone. Clinical judgment, patient preference, and past experiences need to inform these decisions. No trials have tested the efficacy of IPT combined with other psychotherapies, but it is highly likely that therapists borrow techniques from other evidence-based treatments. It is good for therapists to be flexible and knowledgeable about the different evidence-based psychotherapies because, for example, following a course of IPT, a patient may be helped by concentrating on emotional regulation with a course of dialectical behavior therapy or other targeted therapy. As with medication, there are no strict guidelines for psychotherapy.

Conclusion

Psychotherapy has become a growth industry. Several excellent manualized psychotherapies have now been tested in controlled clinical trials. Psychotherapy is becoming increasingly more accessible, which has contributed to its many adaptations. The premise of IPT is that human attachments are essential to our well-being. Disruption of these attachments, through deaths, disputes, or life changes or the absence of attachments is associated with distress. IPT is one of several available evidence-based treatments to promote human connection.

Recommended Reading

Weissman MM, Markowitz JC, Klerman GL: The Guide to Interpersonal Psychotherapy: Updated and Expanded Edition. New York, Oxford University Press, 2018

Weissman MM, Mootz JJ: Interpersonal Psychotherapy: A Global Reach. New York, Oxford University Press, 2024 (open access available)

56

Psychodynamic Psychotherapy

Glen O. Gabbard, M.D.

Introduction

Psychodynamic psychotherapy is widely used for patients whose illness does not appear to respond to other psychotherapies. In this regard, it is a critically important part of the approach to the treatment of a person with depression. Research has shown that the average patient receiving brief dynamic therapy is better off than 86% of those on a waiting list who are wanting to start psychotherapy. Moreover, when follow-up measures are included in the research, patients who receive psychodynamic psychotherapy maintain therapeutic gains and often continue to improve after treatment has ended. The psychodynamic approach appears to have an "extended release" effect in that it sets in motion an ongoing internal process of self-reflection. Whereas the medical diagnosis approach may often be characterized as an experience of passivity, the dynamic approach involves actively engaging patients as collaborators whose knowledge and experience of themselves contributes to the ultimate diagnostic understanding. A skilled psychodynamic therapist engages in an exploratory process along with the patient in which both participants bring up possibilities about why the individual has fallen into depression.

Another distinction is that the *Diagnostic and Statistical Manual of Mental Disorders* (DSM) diagnosis of depression is considered simply one piece of a puzzle that both therapist and patient are pursuing. A key feature of psychodynamic psychotherapy is that the physician stays attuned to their own reactions to the patient. An aging doctor may feel sorry for their much younger patient and become overly empathetic in a way that discourages the patient from thinking for themself. During the treatment of this young patient, the physician may recognize that they are treating their patient like a version of their own daughter, who is about the same age. This overly sympathetic reaction is an example of what we call *countertransference*, in which the physician's strong feelings toward a patient may interfere with a carefully thought-out understanding.

Conversely, when a patient has powerfully negative feelings toward the doctor, such as viewing the doctor as a "know-it-all," this also may interfere with the treatment process. These feelings can be intensely positive or intensely negative toward the physician or psychotherapist, and an astute psychotherapist tries to tune into exaggerated emotional reactions and recognize them as *transference*. Both experiences are common, and the psychodynamic therapist will gradually become aware of these feelings and bring them up for discussion if they are interfering with the process.

Another central theme within psychodynamic psychotherapy is that much of one's daily experience is suppressed or avoided because it may lead to troubling thoughts and feelings. A basic notion in this approach is that we are consciously confused and unconsciously controlled. We go through our lives thinking that we are masters of our own fate. However, most of us end up spending a good deal of our time repressing or burying aspects of our past that still haunt us. Much of what we have lived is "forgotten," altered, or avoided; yet we are deeply affected by the past and cannot avoid flashbacks of old memories that distress us and feeling a degree of longing for those we have lost.

A wise psychodynamic psychotherapist is often able to identify those areas of the psyche that patients have suppressed or discarded. A compassionate observation from the therapist may help patients recognize something that has been repressed for a long time. Fragments of the patient's life that have been haunting them may become more available so that the sources of pain, loss, humiliation, and regret may be understood more completely by the therapist and the patient. Practitioners of psychodynamic psychotherapy spend time with their patients in a psychodynamic interview that covers their childhood development and its difficulties as well as what factors have made the patients' *adult* life challenging. In addition, the psychodynamic therapist looks for aspects typically avoided in the routine investigation of a patient's past. Cultural and religious background may be of considerable importance for some patients, to the point that they avoid these topics. The therapist also listens for slips of the tongue, such as when a patient means to say "mother" but says "murder" instead.

Description of the Treatment

The result of a thorough psychodynamic assessment is that one obtains valuable information about the patient's interpersonal relationships in three contexts: 1) childhood relationship patterns, 2) the real and transferential aspects of the relationship between the patient and the clinician, and 3) the patient's current relationships outside of the doctor-patient relationship. This constellation of factors leads to a psychodynamic formulation with three components: 1) a sentence or two that describes the clinical picture and the associated stressor or stressors precipitating the reason for seeking help; 2) a process of formulation that develops hypotheses about how the biological, intrapsychic, and sociocultural factors contribute to the clinical picture; and 3) a brief statement about how the first two features of the formulation may inform the treatment and the prognosis.

Psychodynamic psychotherapists identify biological factors that can be genetic or based on environmental influences, such as an early trauma or a head injury. In addition, sociocultural factors may include a history of immigration, religious and/or cultural practices, and longstanding family patterns. Psychodynamic psychotherapy is not meant to explain everything about patients. Rather, it should succinctly highlight major issues, especially their relevance to treatment planning.

Who Should Receive Psychodynamic Psychotherapy?

Few rigorous studies have examined which patients are likely to benefit from psychodynamic psychotherapy. However, clinicians must take individual preference into consideration when deciding how to proceed with a particular patient. A substantial number of individuals regard their depressive themes as growing out of a psychological matrix that requires understanding and mastery. Patients in this category may refuse medication—many already have tried medications designed to improve depression that failed in their case. Some patients with depressive symptoms may hold negative attitudes about taking antidepressants, and they may even regard such medications as ineffective. Still others may have prejudicial thinking about medication and imbue these agents with specific unconscious meanings.

Are Other Treatments Used in Conjunction With This Treatment?

Despite the lack of systematic studies, most experts would agree that psychodynamic psychotherapy is generally *not* indicated as the exclusive treatment for patients in the acute phase of major depression. However, these approaches may be useful with some patients whose depression has failed to respond fully to pharmacotherapy or to re-educative psychotherapies. For example, some data indicate that highly perfectionistic and self-critical patients with depression are not likely to respond to either brief pharmacological or psychological treatments; this subgroup may be particularly suited to more extended psychodynamic approaches. Patients with significant characterological pathology in addition to major depressive episodes may have significant obsessive-compulsive or narcissistic traits that will require longer treatments.

Conclusion

We must keep in mind the fact that each patient's compliance with any medication regimen will be affected by their characterological substrate. Moreover, one must never forget that psychodynamic assessment of patients will assist in all aspects of treatment planning, including that of those with multiple problems.

Recommended Reading

Gabbard GO: Textbook of Psychotherapeutic Treatments. Washington, DC, American Psychiatric Publishing, Inc, 2009

Gabbard GO: Psychodynamic Psychiatry in Clinical Practice. Washington, DC, American Psychiatric Publishing, Inc, 2014

57

Behavioral Activation

Anahi Collado, Ph.D.
Laurel Hicks, Ph.D.
Sona Dimidjian, Ph.D.

Introduction

In the 1970s, a new way of thinking about depression was suggested that viewed depressive behavior as being shaped and maintained by rewards and punishments. It also suggested that depression originates when individuals have limited access to rewarding or pleasant events in their lives *and* habitually engage in escape behaviors to avoid negative events. Despite initial scientific support, this behavioral theory of depression was eclipsed in the 1980s by cognitive theories proposing that negative thoughts were pivotal agents maintaining depression. As a result, behavioral techniques used to treat depression, such as scheduling enjoyable activities, were employed primarily in the support of techniques designed to counter negative thoughts in cognitive-behavioral therapy (CBT). Two decades would pass before interest was renewed in behavioral techniques as a stand-alone approach to depression treatment. Then, a team of researchers compared CBT with behavioral therapy (referred to as *behavioral activation*, or BA), and they found that BA performed just as well as CBT (and even better for some people), which lent support to the more straightforward and potentially more scalable BA approach.

Description of Behavioral Activation

The modern applications of BA are guided by the belief that recovering from depression and living a meaningful life require engaging in activities that are enjoyable, foster connection, and promote the experience of mastery or accomplishment. Also central to BA treatment is the importance of approaching rather than avoiding problems and challenges in one's life. With guidance from a BA therapist, patients complete a depression or anxiety "map" in which they identify three elements: 1) challenges or problems in the context of their lives that limit their experience of reward, 2) feelings related to this context, including the affective and somatic aspects of depression (or anxiety), and 3) actions (or inactions) connected to the feelings. Next, the therapist and patient identify the links between these elements and, in particular, the ways in which action (or inaction) maintains or exacerbates both feeling states and contextual challenges, eliciting what many experience as a downward spiral of depression. The depression map (Figure 57–1) allows for a clear depiction of *why* one started to feel a certain way, *what* one feels, and *how* those feelings may have persisted for a prolonged period. It also provides a clear direction for how to begin to make changes to alleviate depression. Although the exact reason why individuals begin to feel depression may be elusive, the connection between how their feelings lead to activities or behaviors and vice versa is a primary target of BA.

Once the association between the person's feelings and their activities becomes clearer, they and their therapist collaboratively work to identify behaviors and activities that can reverse the existing negative feedback loops. These activities can be enjoyable, important, or increase connection with others. Patients are asked to track activities throughout the day and how they felt during these activities, using monitoring forms. The objective of tracking is to gain awareness about the activities that relate to mood in both the short and long term, with the end goal of identifying a personalized "behavioral antidepressant" consisting of activities that are enjoyable, provide a sense of accomplishment or connection, and are aligned with personal values. In this way, the main ingredient of BA has been hypothesized to be the extent to which individuals increase their engagement in such "antidepressant" activities, the reward they experience as a result, and the changes they make in their life context.

Throughout their work together, the therapist encourages the patient to act from the "outside in" and not from the "inside out," which means that instead of waiting to feel "better" to engage in an activity, the patient is supported in following a schedule and engaging in the planned activity to feel better. Also important to BA is a focus on establishing or reengaging routines that may have supported positive mood in the past. This is especially important in cases in which things may be outside of a person's control or in which contextual chal-

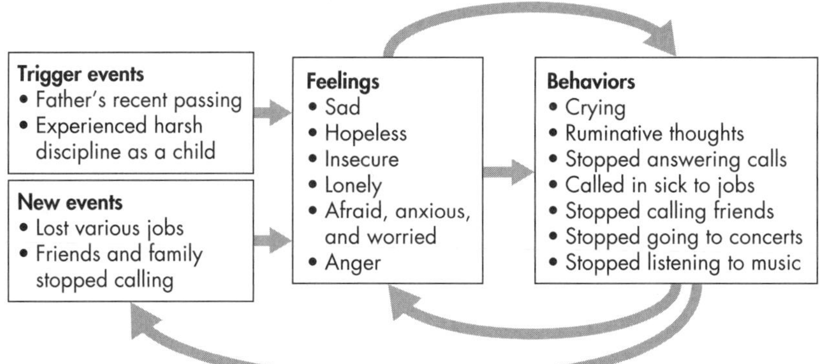

Figure 57–1. Example of a depression map created in collaboration with a therapist.

lenges are unlikely to change quickly. Therapist and patient also work together to set realistic goals and activities by selecting, scheduling, and structuring them in a gradual, stepped manner in order to increase their attainability and the person's motivation. For example, if an individual wants a new job, the steps may be to update their résumé, gain knowledge of the job market, apply for the job, and go on an interview. Frequently, the person works with their therapist on additional skills, such as problem solving and communication skills, to help remove any barriers that deter them from completing the scheduled activities and are necessary to address contextual challenges or problems. The length of BA typically ranges between 6 and 24 sessions, depending on the setting and the patient's needs.

Who Should Receive This Treatment?

BA continues to be heavily researched, and results from several research studies have found it to be effective in treating depression, treating anxiety, and increasing general well-being. Emerging research also supports its use as a stand-alone treatment for symptoms of posttraumatic stress disorder (PTSD). This approach is also incorporated into other effective interventions to treat substance use disorder and depression. For example, BA was integrated into a standard behavioral treatment intervention for smoking cessation and nicotine replacement therapies and found to be more effective than traditional treatment.

BA also has shown benefits across developmental age groups, including adolescents, new and expectant parents, and older adults. Because BA is present-focused and flexible, various contexts can be highlighted during the sessions. For example, new parents may focus on their new role, including the lack of time and increased expectations, whereas older adults may be moving through a transition in which they have more time and are more focused on their health and mortality. For adolescents, BA is further adapted to involve their parents in the treatment, and materials and worksheets are adapted to be more visually appealing and developmentally appropriate. Because BA is a person-centered approach, it has garnered strong enthusiasm and support as an intervention that is naturally responsive to many different cultures and beliefs. Specifically, through BA, patients identify important personal values and work together with a therapist to schedule activities that correspond to those values.

Given BA's defined targets of intervention and brevity, many studies suggest that it can overcome traditional barriers to accessing mental health care. Promising research has explored its efficacy when delivered by non-clinicians, such as community health workers and peer specialists, who share lived experience with the people they serve. Other studies have examined the delivery of BA using technology, including applications and Web-based platforms. These studies highlight the potential of addressing mental health treatment disparities for individuals who do not have access to a therapist or who do not want to engage in therapy.

Conclusion

BA is an effective, brief intervention that has a long history of clinical use. It is acceptable, effective, and accessible across a variety of treatment settings. Furthermore, its strength as an intervention is that it is adaptable to various clinical, cultural, and individual needs given its person-centered focus, theoretical framework, and clear targets for change.

Recommended Reading

Dimidjian S, Barrera M Jr, Martell C, et al: The origins and current status of behavioral activation treatments for depression. Annu Rev Clin Psychol 7:1–38, 2011 21275642

Martell CR, Dimidjian S, Herman-Dunn R: Behavioral Activation for Depression: A Clinician's Guide, 2nd Edition. New York, Guilford Press, 2022

58

Trauma-Focused Cognitive-Behavioral Therapy for Posttraumatic Stress Disorder in Youth

Cody G. Dodd, Ph.D.
Claire L. Kirk, Ph.D.

Introduction

What Is Trauma, and How Is It Treated?

Potentially traumatic events are experiences that a person considers to be life-threatening. Although most children and adolescents exposed to trauma show resilience over the long term, some go on to experience a range of physical and mental health reactions for months or years following the event. Trauma-focused cognitive-behavioral therapy (TF-CBT) is a group of treatments for posttraumatic stress disorder (PTSD) and other forms of prolonged trauma reactions. Commonly used and evidence-based TF-CBT protocols include prolonged exposure for adolescents, TF-CBT, and trauma and grief component therapy. The treatments are based on the cognitive-behavioral therapy (CBT) model, which emphasizes the impact of learning processes, the environment, and patterns of thinking on an individual's recovery following a traumatic event. Compared with other therapies, CBT is more structured, time-limited, and focused on the development of skills for managing symptoms. TF-CBT introduces youth and family education specific to PTSD and pairs it with CBT interventions for mood and anxiety disorders that have been adapted for trauma-related problems. For children and adolescents, CBT is supported by more than five decades of research and hundreds of clinical trials. TF-CBT builds on this base of research support.

Since the 1990s, there has been an expansion in research supporting TF-CBT as the primary treatment for youth affected by traumatic events. Although several approaches to TF-CBT have been developed, most contain a similar series of phases, including psychoeducation, emotion regulation, exposure, cognitive coping, and relapse prevention. Treatment is usually completed over 3–6 months of weekly sessions lasting 60–90 minutes each. Homework is assigned to ensure that the skills learned in therapy are practiced and applied in daily life. Practice between sessions is critical to making progress in therapy, and it helps prevent symptom relapse once therapy ends. In earlier sessions, children are often asked to practice relaxation techniques and other coping skills at home. Later, therapy homework focuses on facing feared or avoided situations associated with the trauma, taking time to recount memories of their traumatic experiences, and "taking back" other aspects of their lives that might have been given up after the trauma.

Throughout treatment, the TF-CBT therapist works to integrate the family into therapy. This means that caregivers and other family members are viewed as natural helpers and are encouraged to join portions of therapy to help support the child or to learn therapy skills to use themselves. Trauma affects the entire family, and research has shown there are significant benefits to involving caregivers throughout the course of TF-CBT. Family involvement depends on the youth's age, developmental stage, and relationship with their family. Parents of young children in TF-CBT may be heavily involved in treatment, whereas many adolescent patients take a more active and independent role.

The management of safety issues is another common focus of TF-CBT. Youth who have experienced trauma may be at higher risk for suicidal ideation and additional traumatic experiences, such as maltreatment. Taking steps to reduce their risk for suicide and further traumatization is critical to overall treatment success. Suicide safety planning includes both youth and families and results in a step-by-step guide of what to do during a suicidal crisis. Addressing the risk for further traumatization can differ based on the young person's current circumstances. Typically, therapists work with the parents separately in order to reduce the likelihood of future traumatic events, improve the safety of the home environment, and increase child monitoring and supervision.

What Is the History of Trauma-Focused Cognitive-Behavioral Therapy?

Early research on TF-CBT utilized protocols adapted from CBT for adults affected by trauma. Deblinger and colleagues conducted one of the first of these studies, demonstrating preliminary support for CBT in a small group of sexually abused children and adolescents with PTSD. At that time, TF-CBT primarily consisted of gradual exposure strategies designed to help the child to habituate to distressing memories and situations related to their trauma. Their approach also included other core components of CBT, including educating the child and family about trauma and PTSD, teaching basic coping skills, taking steps to reduce the risk for future trauma exposures, and coaching parents to model and reinforce skills learned in treatment.

Over the next two decades, studies were conducted examining variations of this basic framework in different formats, with youth affected by different types of traumas and in different settings and with therapists who had differing training backgrounds. Several studies have examined ways in which TF-CBT components can be adapted or expanded to make them more effective in reducing youth PTSD symptoms or to be more easily delivered by therapists. To date, more than two dozen controlled clinical trials have examined the effects of TF-CBT on PTSD in children and adolescents. Based on this research, several manuals for treatment have been developed and are used in real-world mental health settings today. These manualized approaches are rooted in cognitive-behavioral principles but differ in how they emphasize certain components of treatment. For example, whereas some therapies begin with a number of sessions dedicated to education, parent training, and emotion regulation skills, others move more quickly through this phase and emphasize exposure.

Description of the Treatment

Navigating life after trauma can be difficult and confusing for everyone involved. As a result, TF-CBT usually starts with a *psychoeducation* phase, which involves teaching youth and families about traumatic stress reactions and helping them identify how their trauma has impacted them. One goal of this portion of therapy is to help caregivers understand what their child is experiencing so that they can better support the child. Another goal is to help youth understand and express what they are experiencing and feeling. Children and adolescents are often relieved to learn that there are names for the symptoms they are experiencing and that others have felt the way they do after frightening and confusing events. The psychoeducation phase of treatment also prepares youth and families for therapy by explaining how CBT works, establishing goals for therapy, and describing the other components of treatment that will be used to achieve treatment goals.

Following the education phase, therapists teach youth and families *emotion-regulation skills* needed to manage reactions to stressful situations that occur in daily life. Some of the most common skills taught in this phase of treatment are relaxation techniques such as diaphragmatic breathing or progressive muscle relaxation. Depending on the youth's preferences and needs, therapists may teach other strategies, such as using mindfulness meditation, increasing their engagement with enjoyable activities, or seeking support from trusted loved ones or friends. Usually, emotion-regulation strategies are taught to manage stressful thoughts and feelings occurring in response to everyday situations, such as arguments with friends or family or receiving "bad" news. However, with practice, these strategies can often be used to manage symptoms of PTSD and other mental health problems, such as anxiety or depression.

Once the youth becomes competent in basic emotion-regulation skills and their safety issues have been well managed, the therapist begins guiding them through the process of *exposure*. This phase of therapy takes many forms but typically involves supporting the patient in facing stressful situations and memories associated with the trauma. Exposure works by reversing the cycle of avoidant coping that drives other trauma reactions, such as intrusive thoughts and hypervigilance. This cycle often involves avoiding talking or thinking about the trauma or avoiding situations that are reminders of the trauma. In the short term, avoidant coping may provide relief from painful feelings and memories. However, in the long term, it can interfere with important aspects of life, such as relationships, school, work, or health. By interrupting the cycle of avoidance, youth and their therapists can begin to "take back" activities, relationships, and responsibilities that brought meaning to their life before the trauma.

The two most common types of exposure used in TF-CBT are in vivo and imaginal exposure. *In vivo exposure*, also known as "real life" exposure, involves confronting situations that trigger stressful thoughts and feelings. These situations are known as *trauma reminders*, and they can relate to the trauma through any of the five senses. Trauma reminders can be people, places, smells, tastes, thoughts, feelings, or sounds, among other things. For example, a child who is a domestic violence survivor may become very scared when people speak with loud voices because this reminds them of their parents yelling at each other during violent episodes at home. An in vivo exposure for this child may involve going to a busy restaurant to practice being around loud voices in a safe setting. Youth are often encouraged to start with exposures that feel more manageable and less overwhelming. Later, as their confidence and tolerance build, they can take on situations that are more challenging. For many children and adolescents affected by trauma, in vivo exposure exercises are a critical step toward a return to healthy developmental activities, such as going to school, engaging in academics, making friends, and participating in sports or other extracurricular activities.

Imaginal exposure involves facing painful thoughts, feelings, and memories associated with the trauma. Through repeated imaginal exposures, youth begin to relieve the stress and negative impact that the memories of the event have on their daily life. Usually, therapists guide the child or adolescent through this process by having them tell the story of their traumatic experience in detail, several times, over the course of multiple sessions. The therapist typically asks for details, such as what the individuals saw and experienced as well as what they were feeling and thinking during the traumatic event. Imaginal exposure works for two main reasons. First, it helps the youth organize their memories of the traumatic event in a less-stressful way. Second, by repeatedly and purposefully remembering the trauma, youth habituate to trauma reminders. Put simply, with practice, youth can learn to retell their story or be reminded about the trauma without becoming overwhelmed.

Another benefit of exposure is that it often reveals unhelpful beliefs, attitudes, or "rules" developed in reaction to the trauma. For example, a survivor of sexual abuse might come to believe that they are "broken," "unworthy of love," or that "nobody can be trusted completely." Beliefs such as these may promote the use of avoidant or unhelpful coping strategies and cause problems in relationships and other aspects of life. In these cases, therapists may introduce a cognitive coping phase of treatment designed to promote more helpful patterns of thinking. This may involve perspective-taking exercises, challenging trauma-related beliefs, or learning to accept thoughts and feelings without acting on them. In the case of the sexual abuse survivor, a TF-CBT therapist might encourage them to reflect on how their beliefs conflict with the advice they would give to a loved one in a similar situation. In doing this, the therapist could help them explore and develop other ways to think about the trauma, themselves, or their relationships.

The final phase of TF-CBT is referred to as *relapse prevention*. Typically, therapists begin this transition out of treatment once the youth can tell the story of their trauma from start to finish with minimal distress and once most of their PTSD symptoms have reduced. This phase involves reviewing skills learned in therapy and making plans to continue using them in the future as challenges and stressful events occur. Often, therapists begin by helping youth identify stressful events that may lead to a temporary return of symptoms, such as changes in family circumstances, school-related issues, anniversaries related to the trauma, or upcoming legal events related to the trauma. Once these events have been identified, a plan for coping can be developed based on strategies learned in prior treatment phases.

Therapists also usually help youth and families develop a safety plan that specifies what to do if they cannot manage symptoms on their own or if they experience a crisis. Such a plan might specify which problems require professional help and which problems are "normal" for children and adolescents to face using their own coping skills and the support of loved ones. It can be helpful to involve caregivers in the relapse prevention planning so that they too can be on the lookout for warning signs and encourage their child to seek mental health care again when needed. Similarly, many therapists plan for long-term check-ins or booster sessions to review skills, assess symptoms, and help youth and families feel confident they can get help if needed.

Who Should Receive Trauma-Focused Cognitive-Behavioral Therapy?

TF-CBT is most appropriate for children and adolescents experiencing some or all of the four primary features of PTSD. These include 1) *reexperiencing* or reliving the event, often through upsetting thoughts about what happened or in nightmares and flashbacks; 2) *avoiding* reminders of the event or attempting to suppress or distract themselves from thoughts, feelings, and memories related to the event; 3) experiencing unhealthy *changes in their thinking and mood*, often represented by overly blaming themselves for what happened and feeling guilty or shameful all the time; and 4) *hyperarousal* symptoms, which include constantly being on the lookout for danger and being startled easily. Research has shown that it is typical for youth to experience some level of distress and some PTSD symptoms in the days and weeks following a traumatic experience. However, not all youth who experience traumatic events develop PTSD. In fact, for many, the symptoms of PTSD tend to resolve naturally, without intervention, within up to half a year or more after a trauma. For this reason, it is important to wait at least 1 month before beginning treatment for PTSD.

For youth who continue to have symptoms of PTSD or any other significant changes in mood or behavior after a traumatic event, an assessment from a qualified mental health professional is the first step in determining whether trauma-focused therapy is appropriate. A trauma-focused assessment will help identify the traumatic events the child has experienced, evaluate their reactions to those events, and determine which event is currently causing the most distress (also known as the *index trauma*). For youth to engage in TF-CBT, they must have some memory of the traumatic event, which the therapist will also determine during the assessment. Through interviews and surveys, the therapist will assess whether the child is experiencing impairing symptoms of PTSD beyond what is typical based on their age and the time since the trauma. As part of the initial evaluation, the therapist will also determine whether the child is experiencing other problems or difficulties that may require treatment, beyond their posttraumatic stress symptoms. In cases in which children are experiencing multiple problems, the therapist determines which problems should be prioritized in treatment. Sometimes, treatment of PTSD is the primary focus; in other cases, treatment may target other concerns first, such as severe behavior problems, before TF-CBT commences.

Is It Effective?

Research support for TF-CBT as a treatment for child and adolescent PTSD includes more than a dozen clinical trials, many of which were conducted with large groups of youth in real-world clinics, both in developing and developed nations. Studies of TF-CBT have included youth who have experienced different types of traumatic events, including physical and sexual abuse, disaster exposure, accidents and medical trauma, and exposure to war-related events. Most of the research has been conducted with older children and adolescents, and more studies are needed to further examine the usefulness of TF-CBT with children younger than 8 years of age.

Studies show that most children and adolescents who receive TF-CBT experience reductions in symptoms of PTSD, anxiety, and depression before the end of treatment. Youth treated with TF-CBT have also been found to maintain their progress for longer than 1 year. Some youth may experience symptom relapse, and, in these cases, booster sessions may be scheduled in the months after they graduate from therapy to promote maintenance and reduce the need for additional treatment.

Although TF-CBT is mostly used as an individual therapy, research has shown that it is effective when delivered in group and Web-based formats. However, these approaches are usually recommended only when face-to-face therapy is impractical because research indicates that individual TF-CBT leads to a better treatment response. Group TF-CBT has most often been implemented and studied in the aftermath of large, shared traumatic events (e.g., natural disasters, terror events, or wars), when individual therapy is often impractical due to the sheer number of potentially affected youth. Similarly, Web-based TF-CBT, conducted over telehealth applications, has been used to address barriers to treatment such as geographical limitations or the quarantine protocols of the coronavirus disease 2019 (COVID-19) pandemic. The feasibility of this option depends on various factors, including the child's or adolescent's developmental level and motivation.

Are Other Treatments Used in Conjunction With This Treatment?

TF-CBT is widely recognized as the first-line treatment for young people with PTSD. Clinical trials have not consistently shown that the effects of TF-CBT on PTSD symptoms can be improved by combining it with medication or other therapies. Consequently, alternative therapies or combinations of TF-CBT with other treatments for PTSD should not be considered before first trying a full course of individual TF-CBT. However, youth affected by traumatic events may experience a variety of problems not directly tied to PTSD, such as depression, anxiety, angry or defiant behavior, school problems, running away from home, using drugs and alcohol, self-harm, or suicidal thinking. In such cases, families should discuss options for treatment with a qualified mental health provider.

Caregivers of youth with PTSD and other problems should be cautious about enrolling their child in multiple therapies at once. Research has not rigorously evaluated the potential positive or negative effects of combining TF-CBT with many other common medications or types of therapy. Integrating TF-CBT with other treatments has the potential to be overwhelming for a young person and to result in slowed progress or worsening of symptoms. Thus, it is generally not recommended that youth begin medication or other therapies during a course of TF-CBT, although it may be beneficial for youth to *continue* treatment for pre-existing problems while in TF-CBT. One common example of this is medication treatment for attention-deficit/hyperactivity disorder (ADHD) that the child or adolescent was taking prior to the trauma.

Conclusion

Trauma is unfortunately something that many young people encounter across childhood and adolescence. Although most youth recover spontaneously after a traumatic event, some develop lasting symptoms of posttraumatic stress and could greatly benefit from professional intervention. In those cases, TF-CBT is an effective and approachable treatment for helping youth and their families recover after a traumatic event. TF-CBT is backed by many years of research and involves several steps, along with homework and caregiver involvement, to bolster effectiveness. TF-CBT involves education about trauma, coping skill building, exposure, and cognitive restructuring to help decrease posttraumatic stress symptoms and increase the individual's ability to return to functioning well in all areas of their life.

Recommended Reading

Cohen JA, Mannarino AP, Deblinger E: Treating Trauma and Traumatic Grief in Children and Adolescents, 2nd Edition. New York, Guilford Press, 2017

National Child Traumatic Stress Network: Families and caregivers. Available at: https://www.nctsn.org/audiences/families-and-caregivers

59

Prolonged Exposure Therapy for Posttraumatic Stress Disorder

Anna E. Wise, Ph.D.
Sheila A. M. Rauch, Ph.D.

Introduction

Posttraumatic stress disorder (PTSD) may develop after one experiences or witnesses a traumatic event that includes death, threatened death, loss of bodily integrity, or sexual violence. Although most survivors of trauma recover naturally over time, some may develop PTSD or other mental health issues. Trauma survivors with PTSD often describe feeling stuck in the traumatic memory experience as though it is haunting them. With PTSD, the traumatic event comes back to the survivor in thoughts, nightmares, and strong emotional or physical reactions to reminders, often called *intrusive symptoms*. In addition, survivors with PTSD try to avoid thinking about the trauma and people, places, and situations that may remind them of it, and they may have problems with sleeping and concentration, increased irritability, and feeling "on guard." Although having some or many of these symptoms is normal shortly after a trauma, some trauma survivors may notice that their symptoms remain or even worsen over months following the traumatic event. *Prolonged exposure* (PE) is an effective treatment option for people with PTSD who want to take their lives back from trauma.

More than 35 years of clinical practice and research support PE therapy as effective in reducing PTSD and the related mental health impacts of trauma. PE reduces PTSD, which has been identified across various cultures and trauma types. Furthermore, it can be used in many settings, including specialty mental health and primary care, and new research has even expanded PE for use in nonmedical settings.

Description of the Treatment

Typical Length

PE treatment is an individualized, flexible, and manualized therapy. Treatment duration is typically 8–15 weeks of 60- or 90-minute sessions. Additional models have now been developed and shown effective as well, including massed models (daily sessions for 2 weeks) and a brief model (weekly 30-minute sessions for 4–8 weeks) for embedded mental health providers in primary care. In addition to sessions with the therapist, patients complete practice between sessions to move what they are learning in sessions into real-life practice.

Outline of Course of Therapy by Modules

PE has three components: psychoeducation, in vivo exposure, and imaginal exposure with processing. *Psychoeducation* focuses on providing a shared patient and therapist foundation about trauma, PTSD, and how PE works. *In vivo* and *imaginal exposure* focus on approaching the trauma memory or memories and reminders in a relatively safe and therapeutic way to confront avoidance and reduce the symptoms of PTSD. The first two or three sessions include an overview of the treatment program, discussion of common reactions to trauma, and information about in vivo and imaginal exposure. Intermediate sessions consist of completing imaginal exposures with the therapist and identifying in vivo exposures to be completed for home practice. The final session includes an imaginal exposure, review of treatment progress, and discussion of relapse prevention strategies.

The imaginal exposure phase includes revisiting the trauma memory by going back in the mind's eye and talking through the trauma memory aloud as though it is happening now with the therapist present. During imaginal exposures, patients repeatedly go over the story of the traumatic memory. They begin to notice their distress associated with the trauma memory decreasing over time as they learn to tolerate their trauma memory and the difficult emotions related to it. As a result, they develop a new understanding about the meaning of the trauma and what it says about them as a person, both at the time of the trauma and now.

Many trauma survivors have experienced more than one traumatic event, and the therapist works with these individuals to identify which trauma memory should be targeted first in treatment. In some cases, more than one trauma memory may be processed using imaginal exposure during a course of PE therapy.

The second type of exposure exercise in PE is in vivo exposure. Individuals work with their therapist to create a list of situations, places, and people that they have been avoiding or enduring with distress because these things remind them of the traumatic event. In vivo exposures involve gradually approaching situations that are relatively safe in order to learn that their distress and fear will decrease if they remain in the situation and experience it repeatedly. Together, imaginal and in vivo exposures provide an opportunity for trauma survivors to gain new perspective about their traumatic experience and challenge unhelpful beliefs about themselves, others, and the world.

PE includes daily and weekly home practice. Patients are asked to listen to a recording of their imaginal exposure every day in between sessions. They and their therapists also work together to identify weekly in vivo home practices. Completing home practice is a critical part of engaging in PE therapy because these home exposures integrate the learning that occurs in therapy with the patient's daily life.

Roles of Therapist and Patient in Therapy

In PE therapy, the therapist and patient collaborate to identify exposure targets and ultimately reduce the patient's PTSD symptoms. During in-session exposures, the therapist's role is to provide supportive guidance and encourage patients as they approach trauma memories and situations. The therapist provides support during imaginal exposure and processing, and guidance for planning exposures for home practice. PE is individualized to each person and how they experience trauma and PTSD, and the therapist and patient work together to overcome any obstacles that arise in treatment.

Hypothesized and/or Empirical Mechanisms of Change

PE was developed from applying emotional processing theory to PTSD. Emotional processing theory suggests that avoiding trauma-related reminders and developing negative beliefs regarding yourself, others, or the world maintain the symptoms of PTSD and create a problematic fear structure or *trauma memory structure*. This trauma memory structure includes everything that was present at the time of trauma: the stimuli (e.g., people, things), the responses (e.g., what the survivor did at the time, what others did), and the meaning associated with those stimuli and responses (e.g., "I am a bad person," "I am at fault," "No one loves me"). A trauma survivor with PTSD reacts to the world as though threat is present whenever anything in the environment "cues" this trauma memory structure. They react to the world as though the trauma situation is ongoing at all times. Consider the following example: A person is crossing the street and sees a red car speeding in their direction (*feared stimuli*), so they quickly jump back onto the sidewalk. They notice that their heart is racing and that they are perspiring (*fear responses*). They then consider that speeding cars are dangerous (*meaning associated with stimulus*) and that their quick action, racing heart, and perspiration indicate fear (*meaning associated with response*). The fear structure is helpful for the person to provide information regarding how best to respond to the threat. However, it can become problematic when the trauma stimuli and responses become generalized to innocuous cues (e.g., the person develops a fear response anytime they see a red vehicle) and lead to subsequent avoidance of or strong emotional responses to those cues. Avoidance of trauma memories or trauma cues maintains PTSD symptoms because it prevents new learning.

PE therapy works to reduce PTSD symptoms via *emotional engagement*—connecting with the trauma memory and feeling the strong emotions connected with it. In PE, patients intentionally bring up emotional responses to the trauma memory in a safe, therapeutic environment and learn that the emotions become less intense or that negative emotions can be handled. In addition, PE works to reduce PTSD symptoms by shifting unhelpful trauma-related beliefs. Specifically, through both in vivo and imaginal exposure with processing, patients learn that 1) fear, anxiety, or other difficult emotions will not continue forever, and they can tolerate difficult trauma-related emotions; 2) revisiting the memory is not the same as reliving the trauma; and 3) the trauma is different from similar but safe situations.

Who Should Receive Prolonged Exposure Therapy?

Age and Developmental Level

Research shows that PE is an effective treatment option for PTSD in adults and adolescents (age 12 years and older), with growing research supporting adaptations for use with younger children. Because PE therapy is individualized, the protocol can be adapted for developmental or functional issues, such as comorbidity, cognitive impairment, or other concerns.

Psychological Indications or Biomarkers

Many people seeking treatment for PTSD have additional psychological concerns as well, such as depression, anger, general anxiety, or panic attacks. PE often works to reduce the symptoms of other co-occurring psychological disorders in addition to reducing PTSD symptoms. Sometimes people with PTSD are also abusing alcohol or other substances; in fact, they may be using these substances to avoid or reduce their distress related to the trauma. Depending on the severity and level of alcohol or substance use, the therapist may recommend that the individual engage in substance use treatment prior to or concurrently with their PE treatment.

PE is safe and effective for most people with PTSD; however, it may not be recommended in a few specific situations, for instance, someone who is having a strong urge to harm themself or someone else or who is currently at high risk for being physically abused or harmed (e.g., in an abusive relationship with ongoing physical or sexual abuse). In these instances, the therapist may recommend other treatment to meet the person's immediate safety needs before engaging in trauma-focused therapy.

Researchers have begun investigating possible biomarkers that may help predict who is likely to have the largest reduction in symptoms from PE treatment. This research is in the early stages and aims to provide more individualized care by suggesting possible additions or augmentations to PE treatment in the future.

Is It Effective?

Remission Versus Response

Excellent evidence has supported that PE is effective at reducing symptoms of PTSD in people with various trauma histories (e.g., military/combat trauma, sexual assault, accident, childhood trauma). Most patients see a significant reduction in their symptoms after attending 6–15 sessions of PE, and many no longer meet the criteria for PTSD after completing an entire course of treatment. The last session of PE focuses on learning strategies that help the person maintain the benefits of treatment going forward. Research examining people who completed PE therapy shows that benefits remain even up to 10 years after treatment completion.

Relapse and How to Deal With It

Relapse is rare for individuals who complete PE. When it does occur, it is most often associated with either a change in how the person views the trauma or entry into a period of generally higher life stress (e.g., new job, becoming a parent). Although relapse is rare, patients will experience the normal increases and decreases in stress and anxiety that we all have in life, and if these stresses remind the person of their trauma, they may experience an increase in symptoms. PE therapists encourage patients to take their life back from PTSD using the tools they learned in PE to approach reminders and any associated difficult emotions that may arise in daily life. Patients who completed PE but are having difficulty confronting trauma reminders on their own are encouraged to contact their therapist for support. The PE-trained therapist can schedule maintenance treatment sessions with the person if needed.

Are Other Treatments Used in Conjunction With This Treatment?

Pharmacology (Helpful or Interfering?)

Prior research comparing participants receiving PE therapy alone with those receiving PE therapy plus psychiatric medication suggests PE therapy alone is as effective at reducing PTSD symptoms as combination treatment. Benzodiazepines may interfere with PE, and anyone taking these medications should talk with their PE provider about how to best use them while doing PE. Aside from benzodiazepines, medications do not appear to interfere with PE therapy, although research is ongoing to examine the optimal sequencing and specific medications that may facilitate PE-related learning.

Other Therapies

Previous research combining PE with stress inoculation and cognitive therapy has not shown additional benefits to adding other psychotherapies to PE, such as cognitive-behavioral therapy (CBT) and attachment theory, CBT and problem solving, individual and group therapy, or individual and family therapy. Some research has even shown less good end-state function when additional interventions are added to PE. In general, research suggests that focusing a period of care on PE alone may provide the best benefits for PTSD reduction.

Adaptations of PE to address co-occurring disorders simultaneously have shown benefit for treatment of alcohol and substance use disorders. PE therapy has been used in combination with relapse prevention for individuals with PTSD and substance use disorder in a therapy called Concurrent Treatment of PTSD and Substance Use Disorders Using Prolonged Exposure, or COPE. This approach integrates these two therapies into a single treatment provided by one therapist. COPE provides all components of PE, educates patients about the relationship between PTSD symptoms and substance use, and teaches them techniques to help manage their cravings for drugs or alcohol and skills to prevent relapse of substance use.

Conclusion

PE is a robust and effective treatment for PTSD with more than 35 years of research supporting its effectiveness and efficacy in patients with varying degrees of PTSD severity and those with PTSD comorbid with other diagnoses. It is individualized, flexible, and adaptable to address the many ways in which people experience PTSD. Research continues to further adapt PE to increase retention (get more patients to an effective "dose"), response (get more people to remission), and efficiency (get people to remission more quickly).

Recommended Reading

Rothbaum BO, Foa E, Hembree E, Rauch SAM: Reclaiming Your Life From a Traumatic Experience: A Prolonged Exposure Treatment Program—Workbook, 2nd Edition (Treatments That Work Series). New York, Oxford University Press, 2019

Rothbaum BO, Rauch SAM: PTSD: What Everyone Needs to Know. New York, Oxford University Press, 2020

60

Cognitive Processing Therapy for Posttraumatic Stress Disorder

David C. Rozek, Ph.D., ABPP
Patricia A. Resick, Ph.D., ABPP

Introduction

Cognitive processing therapy (CPT) was developed in 1988 to treat posttraumatic stress disorder (PTSD). Following years of pilot work, an open trial, and the publication of a therapist manual, controlled research began and continues to this day. CPT was first implemented as a group treatment with rape victims, most of whom had extensive histories of trauma, including child sexual abuse. Individual and/or group CPT then was used for other survivors of forms of interpersonal violence and for veterans and active duty military personnel. In the early 2000s, the U.S. Department of Veterans Affairs (VA) chose CPT as the first treatment to be disseminated for combat veterans with PTSD and began training thousands of VA therapists in this approach. Since then, it has been translated into 12 languages and is used throughout the world.

Description of the Treatment

Typical Length

Originally CPT was developed as a 12-session therapy, but more recent research and practice indicate that, rather than a set number of sessions, the therapist and patient are looking for a good *end state*, meaning the patient's PTSD symptoms are reduced and their quality of life has improved. Some people complete therapy very quickly (i.e., 5–6 sessions), but others (e.g., those with complex trauma histories) may need more than 12 sessions.

One of the many strengths of CPT is that it can be provided in multiple formats. Although often conducted in sessions that occur once or twice per week, it has been adapted to more intensive programs in which sessions occur daily or multiple times per week (i.e., three or more times per week), and all of these sessions can be done in person or via telehealth. Treatment can be in individual or group format or a combination of both. CPT also may or may not include a written account of the trauma. Smartphone applications, such as CPTCoach, are available to support treatment. Different CPT formats all have been shown to be effective for treating PTSD.

Outline of Course of Therapy by Modules or Ideas

CPT has a predictable structure for each session. Sessions begin with a general check-in, followed by setting an agenda. Each session includes a specific goal, a review of the previous practice assignment, learning/practicing a skill, and a new practice assignment. Treatment begins with identifying the patient's PTSD symptoms, providing an overview of PTSD symptoms (e.g., intrusive memories, avoidance, negative thinking and mood, hypervigilance), and explaining how individuals may get stuck in their recovery. As part of their reflection on PTSD and its impact on their life, patients are asked to write an impact statement regarding their thoughts about the causes and consequences of the traumatic event. This assignment is different than other therapies for PTSD because it focuses on the person's *beliefs*, not on the details of the event, which allows patients to concentrate on the impact of the trauma and begin identifying potential *stuck points* (ideas that keep them stuck in their PTSD).

The second component of CPT is to provide a stepwise process for learning to redefine and reappraise these stuck points. Patients are taught how to identify negative thoughts and how these thoughts are connected to and feed negative emotions. Often, these stuck points are related to guilt and shame (e.g., I should have…, If I had…), negative self-views (e.g., I'm worthless), or negative views of the world (e.g., the world isn't safe; I can't trust anyone). Patients learn to challenge their negative thoughts through open-ended questions and worksheets that identify patterns of problematic thinking (e.g., mind reading, jumping to conclusions) and learn to develop more balanced and realistic thoughts. These skills are practiced through daily worksheet assignments.

The third phase of CPT focuses on recovery through practice and mastering the skills learned. Patients apply their skills to common themes that trauma impacts, including

- *Safety:* inability to protect oneself; thinking other people are dangerous
- *Trust:* inability to trust oneself to make decisions; cannot trust others
- *Power and control:* feeling helpless in situations; thinking others are trying to control them
- *Esteem:* negative beliefs about self-worth and respect; thinking others are uncaring
- *Intimacy:* difficulty with self-comforting; cannot connect with others

Roles of Therapist and Patient in Therapy

CPT is a very collaborative therapy. In the beginning, the therapist asks many questions to try to understand how the patient became stuck in their recovery from the trauma—whether avoidance of negative emotions or unhelpful thinking has kept them from adapting to the traumatic memory. As therapy proceeds, the therapist teaches the patient to examine their thoughts and look for more balanced ways of thinking. Over time, as skills become easier, the patient gradually takes the lead throughout sessions, and the therapist acts more as consultant and guide. At the end of CPT, the patient has developed a skill set that shifted their thinking back to a more realistic view and now has tools that can be applied to other stressful situations in the future.

Hypothesized or Empirical Mechanisms of Change

When someone experiences a trauma, they may develop a new way of thinking because coping with that trauma may disrupt or modify their preexisting beliefs. Typically, beliefs changed by the trauma are unrealistic, inaccurate, and improbable and are directly tied to negative emotions (e.g., anger, guilt, shame). Previous negative beliefs held by an individual may also be reinforced by the trauma. CPT focuses on challenging unrealistic thinking that stems from the traumatic experience and helps create a more realistic and balanced way of thinking. It focuses on how a person's thoughts, feelings, behaviors, and physiological responses are interconnected. Changing these thoughts plays a critical role in the recovery from PTSD and allows natural emotions about the event (e.g., sadness, anger, fear) to decrease gradually.

Who Should Receive Cognitive Processing Therapy?

Age and Developmental Level

CPT has been studied mostly in adults, with a few studies supporting its use for adolescents. CPT works for various trauma types (e.g., combat, sexual assault, vehicle accidents, physical assault) and for different people (e.g., military, civilians). Individuals struggling with a combination of trauma and other conditions, such as substance use, depression, or suicidal thoughts and behaviors, may also benefit from CPT.

Psychological Indications or Biomarkers

Psychological assessment includes scales to measure the severity of a person's PTSD symptoms as well as their depression, substance abuse, and other co-occurring conditions. Although not employed in general clinical work, CPT has been shown to decrease heart rate and startle response and to inspire changes in the brain, particularly in executive functioning (thinking and reasoning).

Is It Effective?

Remission Versus Response

Remission from a PTSD diagnosis among civilians is particularly high, up to 80% if they complete treatment. Among individuals included in study analyses, more than half remitted from a PTSD diagnosis even if they dropped out or never started treatment. CPT has undergone more than 40 randomized clinical trials, consistently demonstrating one of the largest effect sizes for symptom and clinical improvement. It has been extensively tested across various populations, traumas, and settings, revealing high remission rates—up to 80% in civilians if treatment is completed—from a PTSD diagnosis. Similar positive outcomes are observed in military personnel with slightly lower remission rates from a PTSD diagnosis. Furthermore, the majority of individuals participating in CPT report meaningful reductions in PTSD symptoms, including trauma-related depression, and an improvement in overall quality of life.

Relapse and How to Deal With It

Several CPT studies have followed participants for 9–12 months and found they experienced little to no relapse of symptoms. In a study in which rape was the primary trauma experienced, patients were followed for an average of 6 years and showed no relapse. Once PTSD has been treated, relapse is highly unlikely. Booster sessions are recommended for anyone who does experience an increase in symptoms.

Are Other Treatments Used in Conjunction With This Treatment?

Pharmacology (Helpful or Interfering?)

Many people try medication first, so it is common for patients to already be taking antidepressants. If this is the case, we ask the patient to remain stable in their dosage until they have completed CPT. However, medication is not a first-line treatment for PTSD, so we encourage patients to start CPT without starting new medication.

Other Therapies

CPT is a stand-alone treatment and does not usually include other therapies. Family members may participate in a session prior to treatment to explain CPT. If someone has symptoms of another disorder that remain after CPT is completed, then they should be treated for the other disorder.

Conclusion

CPT is an effective treatment for PTSD that is personalized for each individual. Clinicians work collaboratively with patients to reflect and identify how traumas have negatively impacted their ways of thinking and feeling. Patients learn to reappraise their negative thoughts to make them more realistic and balanced using a structured and tailored process. Through practice and mastery of these skills, patients target their beliefs about the trauma and the common areas affected by trauma and work toward recovery. Ultimately, CPT provides patients with a skill set that can be used to help with their trauma-related thoughts and to manage other stressful events in the future.

Recommended Reading

Resick PA, Stirman SW, LoSavio ST: Getting Unstuck From PTSD: Using Cognitive Processing Therapy to Guide Your Recovery. New York, Guilford Press, 2023

WBEZ Chicago: Episode 682: Ten sessions. This American Life (podcast), August 23, 2019

61

Exposure and Response Prevention for Obsessive-Compulsive Disorder

Rebecca L. Schneider, Ph.D.
Alyssa L. Faro, Ph.D.

Introduction

Exposure and response prevention (ERP) is a cognitive-behavioral therapy (CBT) grounded in decades of scientific research on fear learning. The first clinical study conducted in the 1970s established ERP as an effective treatment for obsessive-compulsive disorder (OCD). ERP is distinct from exposure therapy for other anxiety disorders because it includes both exposure *and* response prevention. *Exposure* involves facing whatever is feared, including *obsessions* (i.e., thoughts, feelings, urges) and *triggers* (i.e., objects, people, places). *Response prevention* involves resisting *compulsions* (i.e., repetitive behaviors that reduce distress). For example, someone who worries about contaminating others might practice exposure by touching a doorknob and practice response prevention by refraining from wiping it down afterward.

Until recently, ERP traditionally was conducted using a habituation approach. This involved gradually working up a *fear hierarchy* (i.e., ranked list of fears) and conducting each exposure in that hierarchy until anxiety reduced enough that the person *habituated* to each fear. Newer research has led to the development of the *inhibitory learning model.* According to this model, fear-based associations cannot be unlearned, but new associations can be learned that, if strong enough, can successfully *inhibit* the original learning. Imagine a sandcastle with a moat that overflowed and created a stream back to the surf. This stream is like the initial fear-learning; ERPs create new paths from the moat that you pour water into again and again until there are deeper paths than just that first one. Eventually, more water travels the new paths—"doorknobs can be safe" and "I can handle this anxiety"—than the original path—"doorknobs are contaminated." Inhibitory learning shifts the focus of ERP to tolerating anxiety and strengthening this new learning, such as by increasing surprise (e.g., noting unexpected outcomes) from the exposure, doing exposures in multiple settings and with varying fear levels, and emphasizing tolerance of anxiety rather than anxiety reduction.

Description of the Treatment

Having learned the theory behind ERP, you may be asking yourself, "So what does this really look like in the therapist's office?"

Here is some great news: human brains are wired to learn information! This means that many people have significant success with ERP after a few months of treatment, with ongoing booster sessions to keep the new knowledge fresh. Although many factors contribute to how long an individual will be in therapy, many get significant relief from their symptoms with 12–16 sessions.

When you begin treatment with an ERP therapist, the therapist will likely start with an assessment to help identify all the different areas of your life that OCD has crept into and how it is interfering. Often, OCD is so sneaky that a person may not even recognize a subtype as OCD until they discover that other people have the same worries or behaviors. By labeling the triggers, obsessions, and compulsions, the patient and therapist can work together to develop a plan for how they will target OCD.

Next, the patient and therapist begin crafting ERPs together, practicing first in their sessions. Then the therapist assigns homework for the patient to continue practicing their ERPs at home, school, or wherever the new information needs to be learned. During an ERP, the individual will practice facing their fear while resisting the urge to perform a compulsion. For example, a new parent who is worried about accidentally harming their baby might practice carrying the baby without anyone else present, or someone who is afraid of harming a family member might practice looking at pictures of knives, holding a butter knife, and eventually cooking dinner using sharp knives. In the hours and days following an ERP, the brain sorts through the new information it has gathered and figures out how to make sense of it all: "Wait a minute! I can both feel anxious and have fun?"; "I can do this hard thing and handle it?" Over time, the once-feared stimulus becomes increasingly ambiguous in its meaning.

Who Should Receive Exposure and Response Prevention Therapy?

One of the best things about ERP is that it really works. Most people with OCD will benefit from ERP. This is true across the life span, with children as young as 2 years of age successfully completing treatment, although in younger patients, there is greater emphasis on behaviors with less focus on thoughts. The younger the child, the more their parents should be involved, but parents and loved ones can (and should!) be involved in treatment of youth at any age.

Levels of motivation and willingness affect who will have the greatest success with ERP. The more motivated someone is, and the more willing they are to perform exposures as homework outside the therapy room, the more successful their treatment will be. Just as with any new skill, practice makes a difference. Imagine playing a piano recital without ever practicing outside of the lessons!

Other factors that impact treatment success include severity level, insight, and presence of comorbidities (other diagnoses). Individuals whose OCD causes more distress and interference, and those with less awareness of the illogicality of their obsessions and compulsions (*insight*), often benefit less or need a longer treatment course than those with less severity and better insight. Comorbidity is the norm in OCD, with most individuals having multiple diagnoses. The presence of these additional diagnoses predicts increased OCD severity, decreased response rates to ERP, and increased relapse rates. However, several studies have found that increasing the treatment "dose" (e.g., having more frequent sessions) can be enough to erase this difference in treatment response. Family accommodation also predicts treatment response; the less family members accommodate the patient's OCD, the more responsive to treatment that patient will be.

Is It Effective?

ERP is considered the "gold standard" treatment for OCD, which means it has the most evidence supporting its effectiveness in treating OCD. Studies have revealed that most people experience a reduction in symptoms following treatment, with many no longer meeting the diagnostic criteria for OCD.

OCD is considered to have a "waxing and waning" course, which means it is sometimes easier and sometimes harder to manage throughout one's life. Although ERP does not "cure" OCD, it can lessen symptoms to the degree that they are no longer interfering or distressing. Often, patients will notice that their symptoms return or worsen during times of stress, transition, or other big life events. In some cases the content of the symptoms will stay the same, but in other cases symptoms will present in a different way than previously expressed. Relapse prevention helps individuals identify the clues that OCD is present and learn how to respond to intrusive thoughts, no matter what form they take, without getting caught up in the content of those thoughts.

Are Other Treatments Used In Conjunction With This Treatment?

ERP outperforms medication in the treatment of OCD, but a combination approach (ERP plus medication) can be helpful for people with moderate to severe OCD. Selective serotonin reuptake inhibitors (SSRIs) are considered the *first-line* medication treatment for OCD, meaning they are the first-choice medication with which to start.

ERP also can be combined with other treatment approaches. Acceptance and commitment therapy (ACT) has good evidence supporting its use in OCD and often is used in conjunction with ERP. Exposure done from an ACT framework emphasizes increasing flexibility, reducing avoidance, and doing things that matter to the person regardless of whatever thoughts, feelings, or urges might arise.

Family involvement is an important part of ERP at all ages. A key aspect of treatment involves teaching family members about OCD and how they can support their loved one without providing reassurance or accommodating the OCD, both of which perpetuate the OCD cycle and ultimately exacerbate the condition. If someone has contamination-themed OCD, they may ask a relative to take out the trash for them or may seek the relative's assurance that they will not get sick if they touch the trash. Through treatment, the relative might learn to respond, "I can tell this is hard for you, and I know you can handle it" rather than saying, "Don't worry, you won't get sick." Parents of children with OCD can work with their child's therapist independently or alongside their child as part of the treatment team. The goal of parent work is to reduce accommodation while increasing support to help their child face their fears even when the child's motivation is low.

In some cases, a person might benefit from more frequent ERP sessions. ERP can be delivered in person or virtually, in a group setting, or in higher levels of care, including intensive outpatient, partial hospitalization, and residential programs. Speaking with your therapist about your needs and rate of progress will help you figure out what intensity of treatment is right for you.

Conclusion

ERP is the best-studied treatment for OCD with the strongest evidence supporting its effectiveness across all ages. It involves facing fears and obsessions while resisting compulsions. ERP is usually delivered as weekly individual therapy but can also be delivered more frequently or in a group setting. Family members are often involved in treatment. ERP is highly effective alone or in combination with medication or other therapeutic approaches.

Recommended Reading

Abramowitz JA: The Family Guide to Getting Over OCD: Reclaim Your Life and Help Your Loved One. New York, Guilford Press, 2021

Hershfield J, Bell J: When a Family Member Has OCD: Mindfulness and Cognitive Behavioral Skills Affected by Obsessive-Compulsive Disorder. Oakland, CA, New Harbinger, 2015

62

Cognitive-Behavioral Therapy for Social Anxiety

Cynthia L. Turk, Ph.D.
Jordan M. De Herrera, M.A.
Kimberly B. Day, M.A.

Case Vignette

Jasmine was a 25-year-old Black female who sought treatment for lifelong social anxiety. When she presented for treatment, Jasmine was married to Theo, expecting her first child, and working as a paraprofessional in a school. She aspired to go back to college to get the credentials to become a full-time teacher but had not taken steps toward doing so because of the profession's social and public speaking demands. Jasmine described her social anxiety as a barrier to closeness with family because she actively avoided family gatherings. Jasmine feared that people would notice her anxiety, that she would not be skillful in social situations, and that others would judge her negatively as a result.

Jasmine sought treatment because she was distressed by her social fear and avoidance, which were preventing her from living a life consistent with her values and goals. Jasmine met the *Diagnostic and Statistical Manual of Mental Disorders* (DSM) diagnostic criteria for social anxiety disorder.

Introduction

Jasmine was not alone in her suffering. Approximately 12% of people meet the diagnostic criteria for social anxiety disorder at some point in their lives. Cognitive-behavioral therapy (CBT), developed by psychiatrist Aaron T. Beck in the 1960s–1970s, is a research-based short-term psychological treatment approach shown to be effective in treating various psychological disorders. The idea for CBT originated when Beck noticed specific patterns in his patients' thoughts during therapy. These thought patterns were typically negative, lacked validity, and influenced the patients' behaviors and emotions. In CBT, individuals learn how to identify and change the distorted thoughts that negatively impact their behaviors and emotions. Studies have shown that CBT is the most effective psychological treatment for social anxiety disorder.

Description of the Treatment

The most effective versions of CBT for social anxiety disorder include a combination of cognitive restructuring and exposure. *Cognitive restructuring* helps people recognize negative thoughts that increase their anxiety and often promote avoidance. *Exposure* typically involves helping them gradually face their fears in a therapeutic way that allows for new learning. The cognitive-behavioral therapist's role is to help their patients identify and change the thoughts and avoidance behaviors that are maintaining their symptoms. The therapist offers support, listens, coaches, and ultimately teaches patients to be their own therapist. According to cognitive models, social situations trigger negative beliefs and distorted thought patterns that contribute to the maintenance of anxiety.

> Jasmine consented to participate in CBT. Early in treatment, she learned to use anxiety as a signal to attend to what she was saying to herself. Jasmine identified automatic thoughts such as "I will not know what to say," "I am not interesting," and "If there is a pause in the conversation, they will think I am boring." Jasmine learned not to accept her automatic thoughts as facts. She practiced actively considering realistic alternatives such as "I can always ask about their weekend," "Most conversations are about routine things like the weather," and "Pauses are a normal part of conversations."
>
> Later in treatment, Jasmine came to appreciate that she held certain core beliefs about herself, others, and the world that stemmed from some of her early life experiences. For example, Jasmine's family taught her that people who were depressed, anxious, or had other mental health problems were "unacceptable." Therefore, she believed that anyone noticing her anxiety would judge her as unacceptable. She identified core beliefs including "Anxiety equals incompetence" and "I am unworthy." She began to question these fundamental beliefs and consider alternatives. For example, she considered whether it was possible to simul-

taneously be a competent teacher and become anxious at times with colleagues or in the classroom. She questioned her very limited definition of *worth* (unworthy = experiencing anxiety) and considered evidence that she was both worthy and deserving (e.g., she was a good, kind person). She opened herself to the possibility that other people might not automatically judge her negatively if they noticed her anxiety or if she made a social mistake. Instead of elaborating on her anxiety-provoking beliefs and hiding her anxiety, she actively considered alternatives such as "It's okay to get anxious" and "Anxiety does not equal incompetence."

Seeing social situations as less dangerous and adopting a more compassionate view of herself made it easier for Jasmine to engage in exposures. In turn, the exposures provided her with evidence contrary to her automatic thoughts, making it easier for her to change her beliefs. Jasmine completed exposures that included disagreeing in conversations, making "small-talk" about things such as the weather, breaking pauses during conversations, asking questions during conversations, and conversing with an authority figure such as the school principal. She did eight exposures in session, during which her therapist played the role of someone in Jasmine's life, such as a coworker, and they would have a 10-minute conversation. Jasmine also did many exposures outside of session. She started with one challenging weekly exposure but progressed toward challenging herself almost daily with exposures outside of session during the course of her therapy.

At the beginning of treatment, Jasmine believed that disagreeing with someone was dangerous (e.g., "I will be disliked if I disagree with someone"). She did exposures in her daily life wherein she practiced disagreeing with people, such as coworkers or her mother-in-law, about various things such as the best place to eat Mexican food or how good a particular movie was. These exposures and the associated cognitive restructuring allowed Jasmine to learn new things (e.g., my feared outcome rarely occurs) and develop less anxiety-provoking alternative beliefs (e.g., "If I disagree with someone, it's unlikely they will dislike me"; "Disagreements can help people to get to know each other better"). As a result, she became less anxious about disagreeing with others and stopped avoiding expressing her opinion, which allowed her to be truer to herself. Like most patients, Jasmine started with exposures that did not represent her greatest fear and gradually approached more difficult situations over the course of therapy.

The focus toward the end of therapy is relapse prevention and termination. The therapist and patient review progress, what has been learned, how to maintain and build on gains, and what to do if a setback arises.

Over the course of treatment, Jasmine learned that anxiety is a cue to challenge her negative automatic thoughts and to approach what she fears. By the end of treatment, she reported less avoidance at work. She reported engaging with relatives she had not spoken to in years and feeling closer with her own family and less anxious when interacting with her husband's family and friends. Jasmine looked forward to involving more people in her child's life now that she was no longer avoiding so many social situations. Treatment terminated at the time her daughter was born, but she believed she had the skills to address future social challenges, such as returning to school.

In most research studies, good results have been shown with 12–16 weekly CBT sessions, but individuals outside of research studies may be seen for more or fewer sessions. For example, Jasmine was seen for 20 sessions. Treatment is delivered in either 1-hour individual sessions or 2.5-hour group sessions. Group sessions typically comprise two therapists and four to six participants.

Who Should Receive Cognitive-Behavioral Therapy?

CBT for social anxiety is helpful for individuals of all ages, but it is modified for children and adolescents to be suitable for their developmental level. Individuals who are willing to gradually approach feared their social situations in order to build the life they desire will benefit the most. An openness to examining one's thoughts and feelings is also quite helpful.

Is It Effective?

Like Jasmine, many individuals with social anxiety disorder who are treated with CBT respond well to treatment. *Response rates* reflect a meaningful decrease in symptoms, whereas *remission rates* indicate an absence of the disorder. Studies have reported response rates of 58%–75% after 12–16 sessions. These improvements appear to be durable; one study examining efficacy immediately after the end of treatment and 6, 12, and 24 months later found response rates of 63%, 72%, 70%, and 69%, respectively. Remission rates were 38%, 44%, 44%, and 39%, respectively.

After treatment, some individuals may experience social anxiety disorder symptoms when facing new situations that were previously impossible due to fear and avoidance (e.g., getting a new job). Facing a goal-consistent novel social situation is a sign of treatment success. In this situation, the individual needs to use skills such as cognitive restructuring that were acquired during treatment. If their anxiety persists or intensifies, the individual should schedule a booster session with their therapist. Typically, one or two sessions will help them get back on track. During a booster session, the therapist and patient discuss the symptoms and stressors, review skills, and engage in problem-solving.

Are Other Treatments Used in Conjunction With This Treatment?

Individual in-person CBT that includes cognitive restructuring and exposure is the first-line recommendation for social anxiety disorder treatment, given its efficacy and lack of side effects. Studies examining pharmacotherapy (most commonly selective serotonin reuptake inhibitors [SSRIs]) and CBT generally have found similar benefits in the short term (e.g., 3 months). Pharmacotherapy may lead to faster improvements (e.g., several weeks) relative to CBT (e.g., a couple of months). However, the effects of CBT are longer-lasting, with less relapse after treatment cessation. Pharmacotherapy may also produce unwanted side effects for some patients. Although one might think combined treatment would be superior to either CBT or medication alone, the very limited available research on combined treatment does not support this idea. If a person chooses to do both CBT and medication, it may be helpful to stagger the treatments to clarify which intervention is producing which results. For most patients, we recommend starting with CBT and adding a medication later if needed.

An alternative to traditional in-person CBT is internet-based CBT, which shows promise in initial research. Although most socially anxious people do not need social skills training, some people benefit from combining this intervention with CBT. Although the research base is not as extensive, other CBT techniques that may be helpful may include relaxation training, mindfulness practice, and acceptance-based interventions.

Conclusion

Jasmine's journey through CBT for social anxiety disorder not only highlights the effectiveness of this evidence-based intervention but also underscores the profound impact it can have on a person's life. Through cognitive restructuring and exposure, Jasmine reshaped her responses to social situations and her beliefs about herself and other people. CBT for social anxiety disorder offers hope for those grappling with social anxiety disorder. Like Jasmine, many individuals experience lifelong suffering and subsequent improvement with treatment such that they can lead fulfilling and authentic lives.

Recommended Reading

Fleming JE, Kocovski NL, Segal ZV: The Mindfulness and Acceptance Workbook for Social Anxiety and Shyness: Using Acceptance and Commitment Therapy to Free Yourself From Fear and Reclaim Your Life. Oakland, CA, New Harbinger, 2013

Hope DA, Heimburg RH, Turk CL: Managing Social Anxiety: A Cognitive-Behavioral Therapy Approach, 3rd Edition (Treatments That Work Series). New York, Oxford University Press, 2019

63

Dialectical Behavior Therapy

Shireen L. Rizvi, Ph.D., ABPP
Jesse Finkelstein, Psy.D.

Introduction

Dialectical behavior therapy (DBT) was originally developed by Marsha Linehan, Ph.D., at the University of Washington to treat individuals diagnosed with borderline personality disorder (BPD) who were experiencing chronic suicidality and nonsuicidal self-harm. Through her clinical practice with women with BPD, She had determined that "standard" cognitive-behavioral therapy (CBT) was not effective with this group of individuals. She believed that it was not as effective because people with BPD struggle with pronounced emotion dysregulation that was not being addressed in the standard therapy of that time.

When Linehan first began her research into treating individuals with BPD, she applied cognitive-behavioral change strategies, including ways in which individuals could think differently about their experience or engage in more effective behaviors than with suicidal or self-harm thoughts or behaviors. She found that all this emphasis on change was not working; her patients were not improving and found the focus on change to be deeply invalidating. They reported that change strategies oversimplified the ease of solving problems and did not work for the depth of problems they experienced. In addition to her background in psychology, Linehan was also a budding practitioner of Zen Buddhism. It occurred to her that maybe she should forgo behavioral change strategies and instead apply Zen-Buddhist principles of acceptance to see if that would help her patients find success. Although her patients did find these strategies validating, they now felt frustrated because they were not receiving the help they needed to reduce the causes of their suffering and move closer to their life goals.

Over time, Linehan arrived at the notion of dialectics to inform the development of her treatment. *Dialectical philosophy* (i.e., holding two contradictory views as true simultaneously, such as accepting life exactly as it is while also working to make it different) functioned as the glue that these seemingly oppositional approaches of behaviorism and Zen-Buddhist principles needed to facilitate change in this difficult-to-treat population.

The core dialectic of DBT is the balance of acceptance and change: "You have to change—and you're perfect as you are." We are all perfect as we are. We are exactly as we should be, as the result of the billions and billions of things that brought us to this moment. Yet we can always do better. We can always grow. We can always increase our capacity to love and to care for ourselves and for others. Dialectical thinking allows us to hold these contradictory views at the same time, validating where we are now while still pushing us to do things differently and expand our awareness. Beyond balancing the primary dialectic of acceptance and change, the concept of dialectics informs treatment in multiple ways. Dialectical philosophy teaches us that tension and conflict are inevitable and cannot be avoided. This tension can occur between ourselves and others or within ourselves. For example, people frequently think in black-and-white terms such as "This is awful" versus "This is wonderful" or "That person is terrible" versus "That person is the best." *Dialectical thinking* involves the willingness to hold multiple perspectives at once, with the goal of moving toward a synthesis of these apparently opposing perspectives that will allow us to form a new understanding.

After Linehan formed the foundations of DBT and then published her treatment manual in 1993, DBT began to be taught, researched, and offered throughout the world.

Description of the Treatment

The ultimate goal of DBT therapy is to help people build a life worth living. Rather than being a "suicide prevention" program, DBT is designed to help individuals build a life such that they no longer want to die. In its standard form, it is an outpatient treatment with four "modes" or components: 1) weekly one-on-one therapy between the patient and therapist; 2) weekly skills training; 3) phone coaching, which includes opportunities for patients to contact their therapists as needed; and 4) team meetings for therapists. DBT may also involve as-needed family sessions or consultation with medication prescribers in order to provide comprehensive mental health care.

In practice, these modes mean that people in DBT have at least two appointments per week—individual therapy and skills training. The length of treatment can vary but usually lasts at least 6–12 months. DBT is often referred to as a year-long treatment because that was how long it was conducted in the initial studies of its effectiveness. However, Linehan often said that the length of treatment was largely dictated by the confines of research funding and that DBT was never intended to be capped at 1 year; some individuals with longstanding patterns of difficulties may need more time in DBT.

Individual therapy follows a prescribed target hierarchy. Therapists address life-threatening behavior (e.g., suicide attempts, suicidal ideation, self-harm), followed by therapy-interfering behavior (e.g., not showing up for sessions or not doing homework), and then quality-of-life-interfering behavior (e.g., employment problems, substance use, depression). A motto of DBT to explain this hierarchy is "first save life, then save treatment." DBT therapists use a combination of acceptance, change, and dialectical strategies to address these treatment targets. The DBT therapist holds multiple roles, including cheerleader, coach, collaborator, teacher, and problem solver, which circulate around the broader mission of helping patients achieve their goals of creating a life worth living. A crucial assumption in DBT is that the therapeutic relationship is a relationship between equals. Often, individuals with emotional vulnerability arrive to treatment experiencing an enormous amount of shame; countless loved ones, coworkers, and providers have told them that who they are and how they behave are somehow wrong and abnormal. By establishing that DBT is a relationship of equals, the treatment recognizes the reality that we are *all* suffering and struggling at times and that there is nothing intrinsically wrong with any of us. Everyone is on their own path toward emotional freedom, and some people just need help along that path. A DBT therapist can be radically genuine with their patient rather than adopt a role.

In skills training, DBT focuses on providing skills in four main areas: *mindfulness*, which aims to help us remain in the present moment and attend to our thoughts and emotions without judgment; *interpersonal effectiveness*, which consists of strategies to communicate effectively without losing our cool or our self-respect; *emotion regulation*, which addresses our ability to manage, change, and reduce our vulnerability to difficult emotions; and, *distress tolerance*, which teaches us how to manage intense emotions and crises without making the situation worse or harming ourselves. These skills are taught in weekly group sessions, typically lasting 2 hours, in which the first half is devoted to reviewing the homework of skills taught the previous week and the second half is focused on teaching new skills. It takes about 6 months to complete one round of all four skill modules. Many comprehensive DBT clinics offer two rounds of skills training to help ensure that individuals fully digest the material and have ample opportunity to practice the skills.

The third mode of treatment is on-call phone coaching. In DBT, therapists work with patients to use skills to increase effective emotional regulation, distress tolerance, and interpersonal communication. It is one thing to teach and practice these skills in a therapy session, but it is another to use them in the "real world." By offering phone coaching, therapists help their patients generalize skills use to all aspects of their lives, especially when they most need it. Sometimes these calls may focus on urges to engage in suicidal or self-harm behaviors, but the principle is the same: using skills to engage in effective behaviors without resorting to ineffective ones.

The fourth mode of treatment is DBT team sessions. These sessions are colloquially known as "therapy for the therapists." Linehan found that, because of the severity of patient behaviors, DBT therapists needed support from a team of therapists to help maintain their motivation and reduce burnout. The team sessions have the additional benefit of combining the collective wisdom and experience of a team of therapists to help individual therapists develop treatment plans for their respective patients.

Who Should Receive Dialectical Behavior Therapy?

DBT is often the first choice of treatment for individuals who engage in chronic self-harm behavior for emotion regulation purposes. As mentioned, it was originally developed for adults with BPD. However, almost immediately after the treatment manual was published, clinicians and researchers began to use DBT with other populations due to its focus on concrete, tangible skills and its underlying premise that emotion dysregulation was the driver of many problems. Although most of the research on DBT has focused on BPD, adaptations have been developed that include using DBT to treat other, or co-occurring, psychological disorders such as substance use, posttraumatic stress disorder (PTSD), and eating disorders. Adaptations have also been made to include other developmental groups, including adolescents and children.

Is It Effective?

Hundreds of peer-reviewed publications on DBT are now available in the research literature, including dozens of randomized controlled trials, multiple review papers, and meta-analyses. The vast majority of the research indicates that it is effective for reducing suicidal behavior and nonsuicidal self-injury. Newer research on DBT has focused on issues related to making the treatment more efficient as well as on how to implement it effectively in large systems. A growing body of literature suggests that skills training "alone"—that is, without accompanying weekly individual therapy—can be effective for certain problems and disorders.

Conclusion

Since the first study of DBT was published more than 30 years ago, DBT has grown in use across a wide variety of settings and populations and for a number of psychological conditions. DBT may be especially appropriate for individuals who experience chronic suicidal thoughts and behaviors or who meet criteria for BPD. However, a growing body of research suggests that it can also be helpful for those with other psychological conditions. DBT is a flexible treatment that appeals to many people due to its nonjudgmental, validating stance and its focus on teaching concrete skills to cope with life's difficulties. Making DBT more broadly accessible is a goal of many clinicians and researchers.

Recommended Reading

Chapman AL, Gratz KL: The Borderline Personality Disorder Survival Guide: Everything You Need to Know About Living With BPD. Oakland, CA, New Harbinger, 2007

Manning SY: Loving Someone With Borderline Personality Disorder: How to Keep Out-of-Control Emotions From Destroying Your Relationship. New York, Guilford Press, 2011

64

Cognitive-Behavioral Therapy for Eating Disorders

Sean Kerrigan, M.D.

Introduction

Treaters have long grappled with the unique thoughts and behaviors that maintain eating disorders. For some time, with less clinical insight, patient behaviors were reduced to a "hysterical" temperament or even a failure of parenting. Treatments in this mold often lasted months to years and rarely achieved resolution.

An application of cognitive-behavioral therapy (CBT) for eating disorders, helmed by Christopher Fairburn, Ph.D., did not emerge until the late 1970s and was initially focused only on bulimia nervosa (BN), a disorder defined by persistent bingeing and purging. At that time, BN was seen as extremely difficult to treat, and more than half of all patients treated with traditional "talk" therapies experienced relapse. With CBT, patients began to report relatively quick improvements with their eating and feeling empowered by its practical, action-oriented approach.

Efforts over time have shifted to develop a "transdiagnostic" approach that expands the scope of CBT beyond BN. Fairburn described frequent symptom overlap among BN, binge-eating disorder (BED), and even restricting disorders such as anorexia nervosa (AN), and some patients have been seen to "migrate" among diagnoses over the course of a single treatment. The result that emerged from years of research was an enhanced CBT for eating disorders that is effective for core behavioral symptoms across a diagnostic spectrum.

Description of the Treatment

At its core, CBT for eating disorders is intended to highlight (and later restructure) the connection between a patient's unstable eating patterns and their distorted thoughts about their body or shape. Once this link is established, it may be easier to see why eating is heavily influenced by pre-set beliefs and how attempts to restrict, binge, or purge to gain bodily control can ultimately reinforce a cycle of hopelessness.

CBT therapists work in tandem with patients to better understand their unique pattern of disordered eating and how it perpetuates itself. Therapy may start by crafting a "formulation" to help visualize the path from specific body distortions to food habits (Figure 64–1). A patient's system of beliefs can have its own logic that defies real-world feedback; however, the formulation offers an opportunity to challenge such beliefs by assessing the impact of these beliefs on day-to-day decisions. Because the roots of a patient's thoughts about their body can be elusive and be influenced by a lifetime of unique experiences, it is often fruitful in CBT to focus on the most visible and impairing eating behaviors themselves and work backward.

What Can I Expect From a Typical Treatment?

Although CBT can work well in various settings and contexts, it is commonly used first as an outpatient, "self-directed" therapy that relies on a workbook or manual with a standard set of treatment exercises. Although some patients appreciate the flexibility of working on their own timetable or do not feel ready to discuss their body with a stranger, most ultimately benefit from supplemental sessions with a therapist (as an individual or within a group) to help guide the use of a manualized treatment, troubleshoot difficulties, and provide more accountability along the way.

A course of therapist-led CBT for eating disorders can be broken down into two main phases:

Phase 1: Changing meal behaviors

- *Education:* The therapist offers insights into the medical and psychological effects of remaining malnourished, in part to motivate and to set realistic expectations for what therapy can achieve if the patient has other acute medical problems, excessive fatigue, fluctuations in blood sugar, and so on.

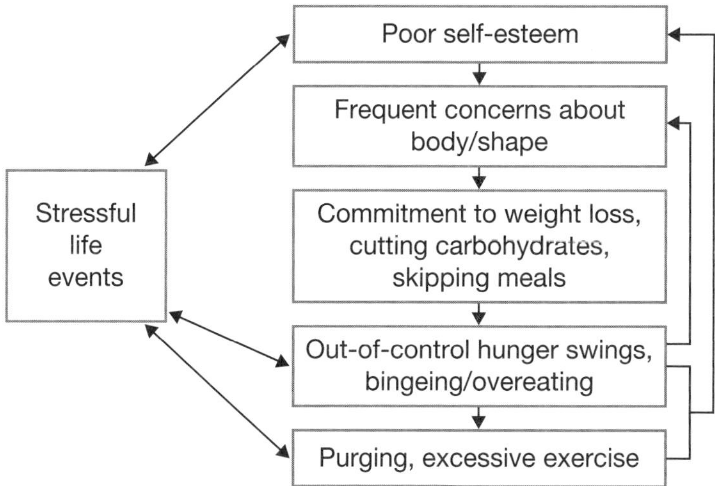

Figure 64–1. Typical formulation of binge/purge cycle in bulimia nervosa.

- *Food diary* (Table 64–1): Patients are asked to document their food intake consistently and with great detail. This attempts to draw a clearer connection between food choices, specific feelings, and triggering situations. The activity encourages the patient and therapist to work together with shared data to target eating behaviors and track progress.
- *New eating pattern:* Use of a "prescribed" eating plan that typically involves three meals and two snacks each day, with a focus on consistency. This aims to reduce daytime restriction, reduce ebbs and flows of intense hunger that motivate binges, and help the patient regain normal fullness cues.

Phase 2: Reducing triggers and addressing thought distortions

- Therapist and patient work to broaden the patient's food choices by creating a list of their avoided or "feared" foods. This stage typically involves gradually exposing the patient to new eating experiences, sometimes even during sessions for one-to-one support.
- A bulk of the therapy involves challenging specific body/shape distortions by studying real-world evidence, particularly experiences that do not support the patient's body narrative. The therapist introduces the patient to a more flexible vision of "healthy eating" and the appropriateness of different body shapes and sizes.
- The therapist pursues strategies to reduce the patient's compulsive body, mirror, or calorie checking throughout the day and carefully analyzes interpersonal triggers that repeatedly lead the patient to episodes of restriction, bingeing, or purging.

Table 64–1. Sample food diary used to monitor intake and associated feelings/behaviors

Time/Date	Intake	Setting	Binge	Vomit	Emotion/Behavior
7:20 A.M.	Milk (1 cup); omelet w/ham	Home before work			No issues. Anxious about a lunch meeting.
10:15 A.M.	Snickers bar, trail mix	Bathroom		X	Struggled waiting for lunch, not ready for a presentation.
1:00 P.M.	Salad with grilled chicken, cucumbers, tomato, carrots, feta, balsamic (medium)	Desk at work			Completed 50% of meal, still felt guilty after snacking on chocolate earlier.
7:00 P.M.	Half a turkey sandwich; hummus and celery	Pacing, on the phone			Worked out for 65 minutes on the elliptical before dinner to help unwind.
11:00 P.M.	Chips Ahoy, 1 sleeve; Ben & Jerry's ice cream, 1.5 pints; box of frozen mozzarella sticks with marinara	Watching television in bedroom	XX	X	Too hungry, couldn't stop until it was all gone. Really hopeless, passive suicidal thoughts again.

A formal CBT treatment can span from 6–8 weeks in accelerated form (usually longer in more intensive treatments that include groups) to 20–24 weeks in its most typical form with an individual therapist. Treatments can extend much longer depending on one's severity of illness, the presence of other psychiatric problems such as depression or obsessive-compulsive disorder (OCD), and the need to address acute medical needs that arise when people reach a low weight or vomit repeatedly.

There are no specific age requirements for using CBT when it comes to eating disorders, although younger patients may benefit from some modifications to the typical approach (which was initially developed with adults in mind). It is often necessary to involve the patient's family members to combat their child's particularly regressed behaviors at the dinner table or to find ways to reduce the patient's blame and guilt by "externalizing" their illness. This works by helping the child recognize the eating disorder as something with an opposing, harmful agenda that is separate from their baseline thoughts and feelings. It can even be helpful to give the disorder its own name or identity and to introduce game or play elements to better "fight the foe" alongside the parents as a team.

Is It Effective?

The short- and long-term benefits of CBT for eating disorders have accrued an abundance of support for use in patients of different ages and life situations, although the level of clinical impact can vary depending on the diagnosis. Currently, the strongest body of evidence supporting the use of CBT is for BN and BED. For BN, studies have demonstrated that completing a full therapy course can effectively eliminate binge/purge cycling in roughly 30%–50% of patients and lead to sustained remission at 5- to 10-year followups. CBT also leads to a profound 50%–60% reduction in binge frequency and intensity for patients with BED, and, in many cases, the positive results in patients with BED have eclipsed those of behavioral weight loss programs or medications alone.

In AN, data are more limited but suggest that patients who use CBT after first reaching some initial weight stabilization see the most impact. This would be expected because malnourished patients have a higher rate of dropping out of therapies prematurely when they need a higher level of medical care or after deferring treatment during the height of their body distortions.

In a few landmark studies, the rate of remission at 1 year for weight-restored individuals with AN was promisingly high (estimated at 65%) compared with that for less-structured therapies, and time to relapse (body mass index [BMI] <17.5, resuming bingeing/purging) was significantly longer in the CBT group. Although the number of consistent research participants with AN has historically been lower compared with that of participants with BN or BED, these data suggest some optimism about the use of behavioral therapies for these patients, especially those with greater treatment motivation and fewer medical crises.

What About Relapse?

In CBT, the last phase of treatment for eating disorders not only acknowledges a strong potential for relapse (given the tenacity of these disorders) but also takes steps to develop a preemptive response with the patient's unique challenges in mind. This process starts with an honest dialogue between patient and therapist about the interventions and coping strategies found to be most helpful during the course of therapy. Special attention is placed on recognizing "cues" or first signs that a relapse may be imminent and creating a stepwise plan of action to find support that the patient feels is realistic. This could involve maintaining their food diary to stay mindful of eating patterns, having a designated "comfort space" in the home that allows temporary distance from a trigger, or having a list of supportive people to text or call who are prepared and waiting to help.

It should be emphasized that the goal of CBT is not to "solve" or remove all problematic eating behaviors or thoughts but to solidify new skills that help patients manage expected obstacles to healthy eating more flexibly in the future. Impulsive thoughts to purge or a drive to thinness may be persistent and never within a patient's complete control, but how the patient chooses to respond to these experiences (or slip-ups) will ultimately determine their ability to sustain recovery.

Are Other Treatments Used in Conjunction With This Treatment?

CBT has been shown to be quite effective and leads to impressive remission rates as a sole intervention for eating disorders. However, CBT is not always preferable over other evidence-based treatments or for use in isolation. It is extremely common to augment CBT with medication or to complement it with another type of therapy to achieve optimal results, especially if the patient has other psychiatric diagnoses needing attention.

Medications

Antidepressants

Antidepressants (e.g., selective serotonin reuptake inhibitors [SSRIs]) can be extremely effective in reducing the frequency and severity of binge/purge episodes in BN and BED patients, likely in part because eating disorders are strongly linked to depressive disorders. Although many assume that these medications would also be useful in AN (because people with AN often struggle with the same anxiety, mood swings, and OCD features that SSRIs target), a significant amount of data suggest a lack of any real benefit for that patient population.

Atypical Antipsychotics

When patients with AN, in particular, struggle with sleepless nights, restless activity, and agitation around meals, atypical antipsychotic medications such as olanzapine or risperidone have been used to help calm behaviors and ease the refeeding process. The side effects of weight gain and sedation with these medications can be a plus in this situation, although this can also lead to treatment dropout. Of note, these medications demonstrate no clear reduction in "delusional" thoughts around food or body as we might expect in patients with a primary psychotic disorder such as schizophrenia.

Appetite Stimulants

Medications such as mirtazapine and cyproheptadine can improve appetite and potentially aid weight restoration for motivated CBT patients. Cyproheptadine in particular is easy to tolerate and can work well for younger patients who struggle with nausea or have an aversion to specific food textures.

Therapies

Family-Based Therapy

Family-based therapy (FBT) is the leading evidence-based approach for children and adolescents with AN. This strategy is focused primarily on weight stabilization and empowering parents to take more control of the refeeding process under the supervision of a therapist. FBT is often vital after a young patient's rapid weight loss and can help reduce their risk of hospitalization. In the late phases of FBT, after the patient has achieved some medical stability, CBT strategies are often employed to help address the patient's body/shape distortions and aid in the transition to more independent treatment goals.

Dialectical Behavior Therapy

Many patients report poor self-image (that often transcends body/shape), unstable relationships, and persistent thoughts of self-harm when feeling isolated. These symptoms may precede the eating disorder and reflect longstanding attachment problems, or behaviors such as restriction or purging may morph into a form of self-injury when other coping skills repeatedly fail. For these patients, dialectical behavior therapy can be a useful addition to nutritional stabilization and may even supersede the use of CBT.

Group Therapies

Eating disorder patients usually encounter group therapy when they enter higher levels of care (e.g., inpatient units, residential treatment, day programs) that typically include a supervised dining room, post-meal processing, and peer discussions regarding body image that incorporate CBT principles. Local outpatient groups are also available that are modeled after Alcoholics Anonymous in that they are patient-driven and offer additional mentorship opportunities.

Recommended Readings

Fairburn CG, Cooper Z, Shafran R: Enhanced cognitive behavior therapy for eating disorders ("CBT-E"): an overview, in Cognitive Behavior Therapy and Eating Disorders. Edited by Fairburn CG. New York, Guilford Press, 2008

Lock J: An update on evidence based psychological treatments for eating disorders in children and adolescents. J Clin Child Adolesc Psychol 44:707–721, 2015

65

Acceptance and Commitment Therapy

Fredrick Chin, Ph.D.
Steven C. Hayes, Ph.D.

Introduction

Acceptance and commitment therapy (ACT, which is said as a single word, not as initials) is an evidence-based and process-oriented form of modern cognitive-behavioral therapy (CBT). ACT uses acceptance and mindfulness methods and commitment and behavior change methods to increase psychological flexibility.

Origins and History

Unlike most evidence-based methods, ACT did not begin as a treatment focused on particular disorders or psychiatric syndromes, such as panic disorder or major depression. Rather, it began more than 40 years ago as an effort to identify the smallest set of *psychological processes* (ways of adjusting to the world and one's role in it) that could be scientifically shown to do the most good in the most areas of life, from mental health to behavioral health to social wellness.

Based on insights that emerged from the senior author's (S.C.H.) own panic disorder and on a research program on human cognition called *relational frame theory*, ACT targets six radically transdiagnostic processes of change. The first two, *emotional acceptance* (experiencing feelings fully, with neither needless defense nor clinging) and *cognitive defusion* (noticing thoughts as they arise without entanglement), are designed to foster greater psychosocial openness. The next two, *flexible attention to the now* and *perspective-taking* or noticing sense of self, are designed to foster greater psychological awareness. The last two, *chosen life values* and *commitment to values-based actions*, are meant to foster greater life engagement. The first four processes taken together are considered - *mindfulness processes*. The last two processes taken together are considered *behavior change methods*. Together, the three pillars of openness, awareness, and active engagement and the six specific processes they contain make up the concept of *psychological flexibility*.

These six flexibility processes are argued to function like the sides of a box—that is, each relates to the others, and it takes six strong sides for the box itself to be strong. Research evidence supports this idea in that each element has been shown to be useful and to combine with the others in a synergistic way. These flexibility processes are transdiagnostic because they are known empirically to apply to almost every area of human functioning, not just to mental health disorders. An advantage of this approach for patients who improve with ACT is that when other issues arise, the skills they acquired to deal with, say, anxiety or depression, will—with some modification—apply to, say, maintaining an exercise program, stopping smoking, or dealing with the stress of running a business.

In terms of its basic theory, ACT is among the most "behavioral" of modern psychological interventions. However, its emotional and values focus and emphasis on the therapeutic relationship sometimes lead to it being categorized as a humanistic therapy. ACT was developed from a pragmatic philosophical perspective that views concepts as tools; thus, all ideas in ACT are held lightly and are viewed as "true" only insofar as they are shown to be helpful. This quality makes it easy to combine ACT with a range of ideas, cultural views, or perspectives, and, perhaps as a result, this approach has readily spread around the world. It is not hard to find ACT therapists in virtually any country or language community, and the World Health Organization distributes free ACT self-help materials in 21 different languages, describing it is as helpful "for anyone who experiences stress, wherever they live and whatever their circumstances."

Description of the Treatment

Arguably, more consistent evidence is available on how ACT works than for any other specific type of psychotherapy. ACT works primarily by increasing psychological flexibility—that is, the degree to which people are able to contact the present moment as conscious human beings, fully and openly, and to change or persist in behaviors in pursuit of chosen values. Because of its process focus, ACT is a very flexible intervention, and specific variations exist for virtually any problem or population. Nevertheless, given that this particular book comes from the Anxiety and Depression Association of America, in this chapter we describe how ACT is generally conducted when addressing anxiety or depression.

Typically, ACT protocols for anxiety and depression range from 10–12 sessions, although more may be necessary for patients with complex problems or who present with multiple problems. Briefer protocols (2–4 sessions) have also been developed and have been scientifically shown to significantly reduce distress. Substantial research evidence exists for ACT in virtually every modality, such as individual therapy, group therapy, computer applications, books, websites, or peer programs. If people are "stuck," ACT often begins with examining what else has been tried and noting if any of the attempts are actually linked to *inflexibility* processes, such as experiential avoidance, rigid attention, or maintaining a story of oneself even if it is harmful to chosen values and goals.

Once the therapist and patient agree on a new agenda, each of the six flexibility processes are targeted and then combined. The use of exercises, guided meditations, metaphors, and homework is common. The exact sequence varies with patients' problem areas and clinician preference; although all elements are known to be helpful, current evidence has not identified a specific sequence as being relevant to outcomes. It is common for the behavioral commitments of treatment to involve exposure methods, especially in patients with anxiety disorders, but, in such cases, the exposure is intended to expand the patient's values-based action and help them practice openness and awareness skills, not to get rid of their anxiety, per se. Ironically, ACT still does well in reducing anxiety despite this not being the primary goal of treatment.

ACT therapists are asked to work on their own psychological flexibility and to target these ACT processes toward themselves. This means that therapy using the ACT model tends to feel accepting and nonjudgmental, with a conscious connection in the present between two people facilitating the patient's values and values-based habits of action. The ACT therapeutic relationship is not hierarchical, and the therapist may feel more like a coach than an authority.

Who Should Receive Acceptance and Commitment Therapy?

Currently, more than 1,050 randomized controlled trials (see bit.ly/ACTRCTs) and thousands of studies of other kinds have been conducted on ACT. It has been found to be superior to non-treatment or to treatment as usual and is at least as good as any other form of evidence-based therapy. ACT is not appropriate for nonverbal populations, but its methods do apply, with minor adjustments, across age and developmental levels. Compared with other evidence-based therapies, such as more traditional CBT, ACT appears to be better for people who have multiple mental health concerns and who show problems with psychological flexibility. Some evidence suggests, however, that individuals who are *extremely* experientially avoidant may do better with traditional CBT. Although ACT is generally combined with exposure in the treatment of anxiety, it is known to be helpful even without exposure and is sometimes used with patients who refuse exposure methods or who drop out of other evidence-based treatments.

Is It Effective?

ACT is considered to be evidence-based across the various anxiety and depressive disorders, with outcomes at least as good as those of other evidence-based methods. One way of measuring the effectiveness of a treatment is by measuring the *response rate,* or the degree to which patients show some marked improvement in their symptoms over the course of treatment. Although no standard method for categorizing response rate in psychotherapy treatment has yet been developed, studies indicate that response rates for individuals with depression range from 50% to 58%, and response rates for individuals with anxiety range from 56% to 75% following treatment. These rates compare favorably with those of other forms of treatment, including other therapies and medication-based interventions.

Another way of characterizing treatment effects is by evaluating *remission rates,* the percentage of patients who no longer exhibit clinical levels of symptoms or no longer meet the criteria for diagnosis. These data may vary widely depending on the characteristics of the study (e.g., some focus exclusively on people with severe symptoms, whereas others focus on mild to moderate presentations). Recovery rates for patients with depression range from 24% to 82% across studies, and rates for those with anxiety disorders range from 44% to 62%. Again, these are comparable with those of other evidence-based treatments.

If relapse occurs and the individual's previously acquired levels of psychological flexibility were good, a refresher course is commonly attempted. If the person did not become more psychologically flexible following an initial course of ACT, relapse will usually lead to referral to practitioners who use other treatment methods.

Are Other Treatments Used in Conjunction With This Treatment?

In general, long-term outcomes with ACT are better than those for medications alone, but research does not yet suggest that medications are helpful or hurtful long-term when used in combination with ACT, except with regard to their having a negative impact on ACT-based exposures. Preliminary evidence suggests that ACT can be helpful when used in combination with psychedelic medication, and vice versa.

Broadly speaking, ACT is compatible with a number of other treatments, especially those that target mindfulness and behavioral processes. For example, it can be used to target avoidance behaviors that may otherwise interfere with behavioral activation or prolonged exposure treatments. Indeed, the emphasis on psychological processes in ACT may make it especially appealing, simple, and sensible to use in combination, either in part or in whole, with other established, empirically supported treatments.

Conclusion

ACT is a modern form of CBT that implements acceptance and mindfulness strategies, in conjunction with traditional behavioral change methods, to encourage patients to experience their difficult thoughts, feelings, and events in order to pursue valued life directions. Compared with other treatments, ACT is unique because it is derived from a basic scientific account of human language and cognition, developed within a pragmatic philosophical perspective, and intended to be utilized across psychiatric diagnoses and across individuals with a diverse array of presenting concerns. ACT itself is composed of six distinct but related processes of change, all of which independently foster healthy and adaptive functioning. Research indicates that ACT outperforms both no-treatment and treatment-as-usual conditions and that it is at least comparable in efficacy with other forms of evidence-based therapy. Moreover, ACT is suitable for people from diverse cultural and ethnic backgrounds, across age and developmental levels, and among individuals who hold differing perspectives, viewpoints, and ideologies. It can be used on its own as a stand-alone intervention or used in conjunction with other treatments, including other empirically supported psychotherapies.

Recommended Reading

Hayes SC: Get Out of Your Mind and Into Your Life: The New Acceptance and Commitment Therapy. Oakland, CA, New Harbinger, 2005

Hayes SC: A Liberated Mind: How to Pivot Toward What Matters. New York, Avery, 2019

66

Positive Affect Treatment

Alicia E. Meuret, Ph.D.
Michelle G. Craske, Ph.D.

Introduction

"I just want to feel happy again." This treatment goal is understandably common among people who no longer look forward to or experience joy in things they previously found rewarding. Remarkably, most pharmacological and psychological treatments focus on decreasing unwanted negative thoughts and symptoms but not on increasing the degree of positive mood that individuals experience. Although it is normal to struggle to feel positive emotions such as pride, joy, interest, or a sense of mastery or accomplishment, persistent difficulty with looking forward to or enjoying aspects of one's life is harmful.

Anhedonia (*A* [Latin for without] *hēdonē* (Greek for pleasure) or "the reduced ability to experience pleasures" as defined initially by Théodule-Armand Ribot in 1896, describes a psychological condition characterized by an inability to experience pleasure in normally pleasurable acts. Deficits in hedonic functioning affect a person's ability to experience positive emotions in the moment and can also affect anticipation, drive, or motivation to obtain and learn from positive outcomes in the future. For example, the capacity to joyfully anticipate and imagine a get-together with a friend will drive our effort to arrange a meeting (*wanting*). The capacity to savor the occasion—appreciating the conversation, feeling the connection, enjoying the tastes of the foods (*liking*)—will also engage our capacity to learn what is most likely to bring about reward so we can feel positive emotions again in the future (*learning*).

Anhedonia, or deficits in wanting, liking, or learning of reward, is associated with a wide range of mental, physical, and social consequences. These deficits can make it challenging to look forward to positive events, uphold a job, savor a friendship, and understand how to make oneself feel more positive. Feeling that very little gives one joy or meaning can contribute to a loss of purpose, a sense of hopelessness, or even the desire to end one's life. With this in mind, we developed a new psychological treatment called *positive affect treatment*, or PAT, incorporating theory, research, and clinical experience to target anhedonic reward deficits.

Description of the Treatment

Typical Length

PAT follows the rationale, components, and structure of traditional evidence-based psychotherapies. The treatment protocol in our clinical studies specifies 15 weekly sessions over nearly 4 months. Our published PAT workbook encourages tailoring treatment to patients' needs; whereas some patients may struggle to get motivated for rewarding activities, others may lack a sense of joy or mastery while engaging. Determining patient needs may shorten or lengthen treatment times.

Outline of Course of Therapy by Modules

PAT is composed of three modules. The first module (sessions 2–7) targets behavioral activation augmented by savoring exercises. The second module (sessions 8–10) teaches cognitive tools for increasing attention to positive stimuli. The third module (sessions 11–14) focuses on the cultivation of positive emotions through mood-boosting exercises of appreciative joy, gratitude, generosity, and loving-kindness. Session 15 is a relapse program.

Psychoeducation (session 1) teaches patients about the nature of low positive affect, including its impact on behavior, thoughts, and feelings (*mood cycle*). The concept that experiencing positive emotions facilitates positive thoughts and actions (*upward spiral*) is central. Another key goal is expanding a patient's vocabulary to describe positive emotions.

Our first module, *Actions Towards Feeling Better*, encompasses three skills: monitoring daily activities and mood, designing and practicing new positive activities, and savoring the moment. Like behavioral activation, an empirically validated approach for treating depression (see Chapter 57, "Behavioral Activation"), the scheduling and completion of positive activities aims to strengthen patients' well-being or their sense of mastery and accomplishment. Such activities might include taking a warm bath, connecting with a friend, or organizing a closet. Changes in mood related to these activities are closely monitored, and patients are encouraged to identify and name the positive emotions involved. "Savoring the moment" is a novel skill whereby activities are retroactively recounted in the first-person present tense to allow patients to reexperience their positive activities, thereby increasing positive mental imagery (e.g., using all senses) and positive self-representation (e.g., pride, mastery).

Attending to the Positive, our second module, teaches participants to notice positive aspects of past ("Finding the Silver Lining"), current ("Taking Ownership"), and future ("Imagining the Positive") experiences. Individuals with emotional disorders frequently struggle to recognize positive aspects in everyday situations, find it challenging to give themselves credit, and have trouble envisioning positive events in the future. Challenging one-way attention to the negative by turning the focus toward the positive allows patients to anticipate and appreciate the outcome of their actions.

The final module, *Building Positivity*, teaches a set of thinking and behavioral skills—loving kindness, gratitude, generosity, and appreciative joy—that engage with the emotions that arise when one wishes for the happiness and well-being of others. These skills aim to increase positive mood by cultivating social connections, prosocial behavior, empathy, and genuine appreciation.

As is standard in evidence-based psychological interventions, between-session practice is fundamental to skills mastery and symptom improvement. Practice worksheets accompany each PAT skill to help monitor mood and activity. The final relapse-prevention session reflects on treatment gains and troubleshoots anticipated barriers to facilitate continued skills implementation.

Roles of Therapist and Patient in Therapy

Therapists who administer PAT should be familiar with the principles of cognitive-behavioral therapy (CBT). Therapists need to understand that the very nature of anhedonia is a lack of drive, effort, and ability to enjoy or appreciate positive change—at least at first. Motivation is thus not a prerequisite to treatment success but the treatment target itself.

Hypothesized Mechanisms of Change

Drawing from affective neuroscience and experimental psychopathology research, PAT is composed of therapeutic techniques that directly target one or more reward system components (i.e., liking, wanting, learning) to improve positive affect.

Who Should Receive Positive Affect Treatment?

PAT is designed to facilitate improvement in low positive mood. Sustained reductions in the frequency, variety, and intensity of positive emotions are experienced as difficulties feeling joy, pride, or excitement; noticing the positive in a situation or oneself; getting motivated or excited about things; or connecting with others. Low positive affect can be present in most psychiatric conditions but can also be experienced by individuals without diagnoses. As such, it is likely widely applicable and beneficial when tailored to the needs of the individual. To date, the therapeutic benefits of PAT have been studied in adults presenting with depression, anxiety, and low positive affect. Preliminary findings from our PAT trials suggest equal benefits for younger and older patients. Likewise, efficacy does not differ for patients taking stable dosages of psychotropic medication.

Is It Effective?

The efficacy of PAT as a treatment program has been evaluated in two randomized controlled intervention trials. A third trial is ongoing. Close to 200 patients with clinically significant and impairing anxiety or depression, functional impairments, and severely low positive affect were assigned randomly to PAT or to a matched intervention called *negative affect treatment* (NAT). NAT uses traditional cognitive-behavioral skills to reduce the negative affect associated with emotional disorders, including exposure to distressing and avoided situations; cognitive restructuring to reduce catastrophizing, overestimates of threat, and self-blame attributions; and arousal regulation through respiratory training. We theorized that PAT would be more effective in improving positive affect, while NAT would be more effective in reducing negative affect. Findings from our first clinical trial showed that low positive affect at pretreatment increased to near-normative levels in people receiving PAT but remained clinically low in those receiving NAT. Surprisingly, the PAT group also had greater improvement in and lower levels of negative affect and symptoms of depression, anxiety, and stress than the NAT group and had a seven-times-lower probability of suicidal ideation following treatment. Our second trial replicated the superior effects of PAT over NAT in improving positive and negative affect. We also examined what may drive these effects (i.e., treatment mechanisms) and found that PAT led to more significant changes in selective reward sensitivity measures, such as greater heart rate accelerations in response to receiving a monetary reward.

Together, our empirical studies strongly suggest that PAT improves positive affect and aspects of reward hyposensitivity. Efforts to examine who would benefit the most from PAT (i.e., moderators) and from which treatment skill (i.e., dismantling studies) are in progress. Such information will be crucial to combat relapse and nonresponse through optimized treatment selection.

Are Other Treatments Used in Conjunction With This Treatment?

Engaging in multiple treatments to address the same problems simultaneously can make it challenging to identify the effects of individual therapies. As such, we recommend only employing one psychological treatment at a time. Notwithstanding, no evidence has shown that interventions directed toward other problems (e.g., family or couples therapy) would interfere with PAT.

Many patients in our PAT trials were receiving a stable dosage of psychotropic medications. For the same reasons just noted, we do not recommend making changes (i.e., changing dosages or beginning new medications) during treatment. Future studies are needed to determine the benefits of combining PAT with psychotropic medication.

Conclusion

Taken together, PAT offers a conceptual and empirical alternative to traditional CBT for treating symptoms of depression, anxiety, and low positive affect/anhedonia. Patients' treatment goal is both the reduction of negative symptoms and the restoration of positive mood and so they can live a meaningful, valuable, and joyful life. PAT provides ample opportunities to meet these goals and has been well received by patients who experience a lack of rewarding experiences and emotions, along with symptoms of depression and anxiety.

Recommended Reading

Craske MG, Meuret AE, Echiverri-Cohen A, et al: Positive affect treatment targets reward sensitivity: a randomized controlled trial. J Consult Clin Psychol 91:350–366, 2023

Meuret AE, Guinyard AL, Craske MG: Positive Affect Treatment for Depression and Anxiety: Workbook (Treatments That Work Series). New York, Oxford University Press, 2022

67

Family-Focused Therapy for Bipolar Disorder

David J. Miklowitz, Ph.D.

Introduction

Family-focused therapy, or FFT, is an outpatient treatment for bipolar disorder in children, adolescents, and adults. It was derived from the behavioral family therapy for schizophrenia, with first publications appearing in the early 1990s. It was developed in conjunction with literature on familial expressed emotion, which showed that individuals with bipolar disorder whose parents or spouses are highly critical, hostile, or emotionally overprotective are at greater risk for illness recurrences (new episodes) over time than those with lower-key, more benign family members.

Description of the Treatment

FFT typically consists of weekly or biweekly 1-hour sessions with a bipolar disorder patient and their family members, which can include parents, a spouse, siblings, or other caregivers. It is offered during the aftermath of an acute manic or depressive episode, when the individual may still have active symptoms that may be confusing to them and their family members. FFT is not recommended for patients who are in the middle of a manic episode. Its purpose is to reduce stress in the family or marriage and to increase the protective effects of family relationships by acquainting family members with the nature and causes of bipolar disorder and emphasizing healthy family communication and problem-solving.

The length and frequency of treatment depends on the severity of the disorder. Adults or adolescents with full bipolar I or II disorder are seen for 21 sessions over 9 months (12 weekly, 6 biweekly, and 3 monthly sessions). Children and adolescents who are at high clinical and familial risk for bipolar disorder—typically those with depression and brief or subthreshold manic episodes who also have family members with bipolar disorder—are seen for 12 sessions over 4 months, with sessions offered weekly for 8 weeks and biweekly for 8 weeks.

FFT consists of three main stages or modules. In the first, *psychoeducation*, individuals and families are provided with information about bipolar disorder, such as early warning signs of new episodes; the differences between depressive, manic, hypomanic, or mixed episodes; the prognosis of the disorder over time; the role of genetic, biological, and stress factors; and illness management strategies. Individuals and families learn to recognize when new episodes of mania or depression are developing and to implement relapse prevention plans consisting of strategies for minimizing the impact of symptoms or changes in functioning. For preventing mania, relapse prevention plans may include calling the treating psychiatrist for a medication adjustment, helping the individual to regulate sleep/wake cycles, taking breaks from or adjusting work or school schedules, and keeping family conflicts to a minimum. Relapse prevention for depression may include exercise, behavioral activation (scheduling pleasurable events), or meditation. Importantly, the psychoeducation module appoints the person with the disorder as the "expert" in bipolar disorder and emphasizes that person's subjective experience of the illness as being potentially more informative than facts about the disorder. The individual is encouraged to track their mood states and sleep/wake patterns using online or paper-and-pencil diaries.

In the second FFT phase, *communication enhancement training*, individuals and their family members are encouraged to rehearse structured ways of talking and listening to each other. They are also provided handouts illustrating communication skills such as offering positive feedback for specific behaviors, using active listening, making positive requests for changes in others' behaviors, communicating clearly, and expressing negative feelings. This leads into the final module, *problem-solving skills training*, in which families are taken through the steps of defining existing or anticipated family or individual problems, generating and evaluating solutions, choosing one or more of those solutions, and implementing the chosen solutions to reduce familial stress. In adults, problems often center on regaining functioning after an illness episode by resuming their work, parenting, or social roles. In youth, problems often have to do with school performance, peer relationships, sleep/wake habits, use of social media, and respectful behaviors. Less commonly, families will discuss strategies for addressing problems related to the patient's adherence to medication, exercise, or dietary regimens. Sometimes, the issues are about how much to tell others in the patient's social network about the disorder.

Therapists, who have a minimum of a master's degree, are trained in several ways. First, they must be comfortable working with families and know how to engender interactions between family members instead of focusing on the bipolar patient's intrapsychic conflicts or cognitions. Second, they must know a substantial amount about bipolar disorder so they can explain its presumed etiological pathways, risk and protective processes, and treatment regimens to families with varied educational attainment. Third, they must be able to work from a treatment manual, given the structured skills-training agenda of most sessions. On the flip side, people with bipolar disorder and their family members must be willing to practice skills with each other between sessions.

Is It Effective?

FFT is usually combined with standard medication for bipolar disorder, such as mood stabilizers (e.g., lithium, lamotrigine, divalproex) and second-generation antipsychotic agents (e.g., quetiapine, risperidone, aripiprazole). Antidepressants and anxiolytic agents or psychostimulants are sometimes prescribed, especially when the patient has comorbid disorders such as generalized anxiety disorder or attention-deficit/hyperactivity disorder (ADHD).

In a network meta-analysis of 39 randomized psychotherapy trials with adult or adolescent participants with bipolar disorder, psychoeducational treatment in a family or group format was associated with lower recurrence rates over 1 year compared with psychoeducation in an individual therapy format. In randomized trials, FFT combined with medications has been associated with reductions in recurrence rates, faster resolution of depressive symptoms, and improved family functioning among adults and adolescents with bipolar disorder who received FFT with medications compared with adults and adolescents who received brief psychoeducation and medications. In two randomized trials of youth at high clinical and familial risk for bipolar disorder, faster recovery from mood episodes and lower rates of depressive recurrence over 1–4 years were observed in those receiving FFT compared with those receiving less intensive forms of psychoeducation.

FFT appears to improve the symptoms of bipolar disorder by improving family functioning, including the degree of positive emotions expressed during family interactions and the individual's perceptions of family conflict or available support. Early evidence in youth at high risk for bipolar disorder indicates that FFT has effects on brain circuits related to emotional processing and emotion regulation, including the ventral and dorsolateral prefrontal cortex and its connections with lower brain structures.

Conclusion

FFT is recommended as an adjunct to standard medication management for patients with bipolar disorder during the stabilization and maintenance phases of care. It is limited by the required involvement of family members, although it can be administered by telehealth to families who live apart. Much is still to be learned about the subpopulations who respond best to FFT as well as its active components.

Recommended Reading

Miklowitz DJ: Bipolar Disorder: A Family-Focused Treatment Approach, 2nd Edition. New York, Guilford Press, 2010

Miklowitz DJ: The Bipolar Disorder Survival Guide: What You and Your Family Need to Know, 3rd Edition. New York, Guilford Press, 2019

68

Cognitive-Behavior Therapy for Bipolar Disorders

W. Edward Craighead, Ph.D., ABPP

Introduction

Origins of Cognitive-Behavior Therapy

During the 1970s, behavior therapy and cognitive therapy were amalgamated to form cognitive-behavior therapy (CBT). Behavior therapy had developed after World War II primarily to treat anxiety disorders and posttraumatic stress disorder (PTSD). During the mid-1960s and early 1970s, behavior therapy's breadth expanded, and it was demonstrated also to be an efficacious treatment for mood disorders. Cognitive therapies, developed by Albert Ellis and Aaron T. Beck in the 1960s, focused on treating mood disorders from their inception. It became clear, especially in their treatment of mood disorders, that these two approaches to psychotherapy shared much of the same conceptual backgrounds and had the same goals and thus could be integrated into one set of therapeutic interventions. Beck became the foremost spokesperson for this integrated model of psychotherapy.

Bipolar Disorders

At the time CBT originated, it was widely thought that bipolar disorder types of mood disorders did not emerge until mid-life. Indeed, it was strongly argued that the first episode of bipolar disorder rarely emerged before the age of 20. More recent studies, however, indicate that two-thirds of individuals who are diagnosed with bipolar disorder experience their first episode between the ages of 15 and 25 years. Although some variations exist, bipolar disorders comprise the specific diagnoses of bipolar I and bipolar II, bipolar disorder not otherwise specified (NOS), cyclothymic disorder, and bipolar disorder induced by another health condition or by substances, including some medications.

As described in Chapter 2 ("Bipolar Disorder") in this book, bipolar I disorder is diagnosed when an individual either has an episode of mania that occurs for about 1 week (if depression presents first, then the depression must have lasted 2 weeks) or is hospitalized for the episode. Bipolar II disorder is diagnosed when a person either has had an episode of depression and experiences a hypomanic episode (a milder and usually shorter form of mania) or has been hypomanic for a period of time but was not diagnosed when that occurred and subsequently experiences a depressive episode for 2 weeks. Cyclothymia is diagnosed when an individual experiences mild hypomanic or mild depressive symptoms over a period of 2 years (1 year for those younger than 18), but the symptoms are not severe enough to warrant a diagnosis of bipolar disorder. Bipolar disorder NOS is diagnosed when a person is experiencing distress and life disruptions resulting from milder forms of mania and depression, neither of which otherwise meets full criteria for diagnosis as another psychiatric disorder.

Bipolar I disorder occurs in about 1% of the population, whereas bipolar II and bipolar NOS occur in about 3% of the population. Both latter forms of the disorder have the potential to develop into bipolar I disorder, although, somewhat counterintuitively, the NOS form has a higher likelihood of this occurring. Notably, the diagnosis of disruptive mood dysregulation disorder, which appears quite similar to bipolar disorder, occurs only among youth who do not yet meet the diagnostic criteria for bipolar disorder but very well may in the future.

Bipolar disorders are chronic psychiatric conditions with high rates of recurrence and an average number of nine manic and/or depressive episodes during the person's lifetime. Fortunately, nearly one-half of individuals with bipolar disorder are largely symptom free between episodes; yet the other half continue to experience symptoms, mostly depression, that do not fully meet the diagnostic criteria for the disorder but are nevertheless disruptive to a high quality of life. Because of their chronic and episodic nature, bipolar disorders have the fourth-highest burden of all psychiatric disorders, including days lost from work due to the disorder. The risk of death from suicide is extremely high among people with bipolar disorder, with most estimates being near 15%—almost 1,000 times the rate in the general population. This high rate is at least partially attributable to patients' attempts to regulate their mood with potentially lethal substances, including excessive and frequent alcohol abuse combined with medications or other substances, such as opioids.

Very effective treatments are currently available for bipolar disorders, especially when they are detected and treated earlier in life. Treatment can produce essentially full recovery between episodes. Although typically slow to accomplish, recovery is quite often achieved, providing relief from the disorders for patients and for those associated with them. Despite effective treatments, the rate of recurrence remains as high as approximately 90%, on average, thus showing the chronic and episodic nature of bipolar disorders and their negative impact on the lives of individuals who have them. A major cause of recurrence is the failure of patients to adhere to their effective treatment regimen, including medications, even when they have achieved relief from the distress of the disorder.

Early Treatments for Bipolar Disorder

For many years, it was widely accepted that the only treatment for bipolar disorder was some form of medication, typically resulting in the prescription of lithium (or other mood stabilizers) or an antipsychotic medication when patients first presented with symptoms of severe mania, and treatment with both antidepressants and antipsychotic medications when patients were initially diagnosed with bipolar disorder because of a severe depressive episode. Gradually, alternative medical treatments, especially the use of anticonvulsants, were employed and found to result in a fairly high rate of successful treatment. Nevertheless, the rate of recurrence remained high, so research investigators began to seek alternative and adjunctive treatments to enhance and sustain the effects achieved with medications. The most successful of these new endeavors was the combining of the effective medications with psychosocial interventions, including CBT.

Description of the Treatment

CBT is typically a short-term psychotherapy that can be used alone or in conjunction with psychiatric medications. Most evaluations of its efficacy comprise 16–20 sessions conducted over 12–16 weeks, with the sessions occurring twice per week during the first 4 weeks of treatment. Research studies employing CBT as an augmentation to medications for bipolar disorder have used 20 or more sessions of CBT. CBT for bipolar disorder has also incorporated daily activity and mood monitoring from social rhythm therapy.

CBT begins with a review of the patient's history and symptoms. When CBT is judged to be an appropriate treatment, its starts with a psychoeducational component that describes the course of treatment and how it is believed to work for the specific disorder being treated. The therapy continues with a review of problematic behaviors and focuses on increasing the patient's positive activity level. The ultimate goal of CBT is to correct fundamental faulty beliefs about oneself. This initially is done by teaching patients to identify things they spontaneously say to themselves that produce specific negative and positive feeling states. This "self-talk" is then related to cognitive errors the person might be making, such as *overgeneralization* (e.g., taking one piece of corrective feedback from work and concluding that "I'm no good at anything I do at work") or *misattribution* (e.g., "I might have done this task well, but most good things I do are just good luck").

During approximately the middle of the course of the therapy sessions, the focus becomes psychologically deeper as the therapist guides the patient toward understanding that these cognitive errors are tied to fundamental negative beliefs (e.g., "I am worthless," "I am unlovable") and that the ultimate goal of therapy is to counteract these beliefs. At all levels (i.e., self-statements, cognitive errors, and underlying beliefs), the goal of CBT is to move cognitive awareness and activity from a negative view of the self, the world, and the future to a more adaptive level. Although the content of the self-statements, cognitive errors, and underlying beliefs differs in many ways during a hypomanic or manic episode compared with a depressive episode, the principle of modifying the behavior and cognitive patterns to a more adaptive level still applies.

Although research studies have typically been conducted in a 12- to 16-week paradigm with specifically diagnosed disorders, it is fairly common when treating bipolar disorders and also in general clinical practice (especially with complicated and co-occurring disorders) for CBT to require many more sessions over a longer period of time. This is particularly true for patients with a chronic disorder such as bipolar I disorder or cyclothymia.

Who Should Receive Cognitive-Behavior Therapy?

CBT was developed to treat anxiety disorders and major depressive disorder, and excellent clinical trial data demonstrate that it is a first-line treatment for those clinical problems. CBT may also be a first-line treatment for the approximately 33% of bipolar disorder patients who initially present with depressive disorders, although such patients are likely eventually to need appropriate complementary medications, especially if they experience severe hypomania or manic symptoms.

For patients diagnosed with bipolar I disorder and, typically, bipolar II disorder, CBT serves as an adjunctive treatment to an appropriate medication regimen. In a series of excellent studies in the United Kingdom, Scott and colleagues showed that CBT was most effective if used as an adjunctive treatment for earlier bipolar episodes and appeared to be of little value to patients with bipolar disorder who have had 12 or more episodes of either mania or depression. CBT may also be used as a recurrence-prevention strategy once a particular episode has been successfully treated—that is, "booster sessions" can be initiated in an early intervention fashion when the patient, their family or associates, or their general physician notes the beginning of a potential recurrence of either a manic or depressive episode.

Is It Effective?

As noted in the preceding paragraphs, CBT is most often used in combination with medications prescribed by a physician to treat bipolar I and usually bipolar II disorders. The primary effects of CBT seem to be on improvement of the depressive symptoms associated with the disorders, although there appear to be substantial improvements in manic symptoms as well, primarily through increasing adherence to the prescribed medication regimen.

CBT may be used alone when treating bipolar II disorder (especially if person is in a depressive phase) and for the longer-term treatment of cyclothymia. However, the therapist must have a strong working knowledge of bipolar disorder and remain sensitive to the potential need to combine the therapy with referral to a psychiatrist for appropriate medications when CBT alone is providing inadequate treatment for the presenting symptoms.

Holmes and her colleagues have suggested that imagery be included in CBT for bipolar disorder, which seems especially likely to be helpful given the creative and imaginative capabilities frequently characteristic of individuals diagnosed with these disorders. Because of the frequent entanglement of families in the lives of bipolar individuals, I have found it very valuable to incorporate various aspects of attachment theory (insecure and disorganized attachment styles) as well as family-focused therapy (see Chapter 67) when conducting CBT, especially long-term CBT in patients with bipolar I disorder.

Conclusion

CBT is an evidence-based psychotherapy for mood disorders, and it has been found to be effective as an adjunctive therapy with appropriate medications in the treatment of bipolar I disorder. It may sometimes be used as a monotherapy for treatment of the other types of bipolar disorders or an initial depressive episode, but even then it may need to be implemented concurrently with an appropriate physician-prescribed antidepressant or mood stabilizing medication. CBT treatment of patients with one of the complex patterns of bipolar disorder may also include augmentation procedures such as social rhythm therapy, principles from attachment theory, and mental imagery.

Recommended Reading

Miklowitz DJ: The Bipolar Disorder Survival Guide: What You and Your Family Need to Know, 3rd Edition. New York, Guilford Press, 2019

Otto M, Reilly-Harrington N, Knauz RO, et al: Managing Bipolar Disorder: A Cognitive Behavior Treatment Program Workbook (Treatments That Work Series). New York, Oxford University Press, 2009

69

The Unified Protocol for the Transdiagnostic Treatment of Emotional Disorders

David H. Barlow, Ph.D.
Lauren S. Woodard, B.A.

Case Vignette

Zeke has always been a worrier. Despite having a stable career and no physical ailments, he is preoccupied with thoughts about his health, job performance, and financial standing. Zeke also worries about what others think of him and finds it difficult to interact with anyone outside of his small social circle. Within the past year, Zeke has experienced periods of intense fatigue, lack of interest in his hobbies, and feelings of hopelessness about his future.

Prompted by these recent episodes, he meets with a therapist for a diagnostic assessment, an interview used to determine his possible diagnoses and to formulate a treatment plan. The therapist informs Zeke that he meets criteria for three disorders: generalized anxiety disorder (GAD), social anxiety disorder, and major depressive disorder (MDD). Learning he is struggling with multiple diagnoses overwhelms Zeke. "How will I have the time, energy, and money to obtain treatment for three separate disorders?" he wonders. The therapist assures him that his diagnoses are related, all falling under the general category of *emotional disorders* (disorders associated with neuroticism and maladaptive responses to emotional experiences), and that it is possible to reduce his symptoms using a single, relatively brief, evidence-based treatment—specifically, the Unified Protocol for the Transdiagnostic Treatment of Emotional Disorders (UP).

Introduction

When it comes to the diagnosis and treatment of mental disorders, Zeke's presentation of more than one disorder represents the norm rather than the exception. Most people diagnosed with a specific anxiety or depressive disorder meet criteria for at least one other emotional disorder, a phenomenon known as *co-occurring* or *comorbid* disorders. In addition, the same symptoms are often found across disorders, although they present in different ways. Furthermore, when individuals with multiple diagnoses undergo successful treatment for one disorder, the severity of their other diagnoses tends to decrease as well.

In the 1980s, Dr. David Barlow and his colleagues became interested in the symptom overlap across emotional disorders, noting that the disorders had more in common than standard approaches to diagnosis and treatment would suggest. They began researching the underlying features that appeared across these disorders and determined that a subset of disorders were associated with a temperamental feature called *neuroticism*—a tendency to experience frequent and intense negative emotions, accompanied by a sense of uncontrollability over the emotions and the circumstances that generate them. Individuals who have high levels of neuroticism tend to avoid or suppress intense emotional experiences, which can reduce negative emotions in the moment but make them more frequent and intense in the future. Such avoidance can ultimately contribute to the development of one or more psychological disorders.

Given the association between neuroticism and emotional disorders, Barlow and colleagues developed the UP, a manualized treatment that could be utilized to treat a range of emotional disorders by targeting neuroticism directly instead of focusing on the symptoms of a given disorder. The first edition of the protocol, including both a therapist guide and patient workbook, was published as part of Oxford University Press's *Treatments That Work* series in 2011. A second, revised and updated edition of the protocol was released in 2017 and is available through Oxford University Press.

Description of the Treatment

The UP is an emotion-focused cognitive-behavioral therapy (CBT) that targets the thoughts, feelings, and behaviors associated with intense emotional experiences. It helps individuals develop adaptive responses to their emotions, which in turn reduces their anxiety and depressive symptoms and improves their overall functioning. The transdiagnostic nature of this treatment means it can be applied in a range of emotional disorder diagnoses (including anxiety, depressive, obsessive-compulsive and related disorders, trauma- or stress-related disorders, and others) in adults. The UP for children and adolescents is available as a separate protocol published within the *Treatments That Work* series. This protocol is an ideal treatment for individuals who are experiencing comorbid disorders.

The UP is composed of eight treatment modules that target neuroticism by emphasizing adaptive skills for responding to aversive or intense emotions. Aligned with best practices in CBT, therapists teach patients a series of discrete skills through semistructured therapy sessions that incorporate the presentation of new information, discussion of how the information applies to the patient's experience, in-session practice of new skills, and systematic exposures to feared sensations and experiences. Patients generally work through the protocol over 12–16 weeks, meeting weekly with their therapist for 50- to 60-minute sessions and completing assigned homework between sessions.

Module 1: Setting Goals and Enhancing Motivation

In the first module of the UP, patients generate specific and attainable goals for treatment and consider the pros and cons of making changes in their lives. These exercises help them contemplate the implications of treatment, facilitating an increased commitment to therapy and confidence in their ability to change.

Module 2: Understanding Emotions

The second module explores the nature and function of a range of positive and negative emotions (e.g., anxiety, guilt, excitement). Patients apply this information to their own emotional experiences, exploring their common triggers and subsequent emotional reactions to increase awareness of their emotional states.

Module 3: Mindful Emotion Awareness

In the third module, patients practice nonjudgmental awareness of their emotions. They are led through a series of exercises, including a mindfulness practice, that allow them to observe the thoughts, physical sensations, and actions that accompany their emotional states rather than avoid these experiences.

Module 4: Cognitive Flexibility

Module 4 explores how patients' thoughts and emotions interact and examines how *automatic thoughts* (thoughts that occur without reflection or intention) influence the patients' emotional experiences. Two unhelpful thinking patterns, referred to as *thinking traps*, are introduced. One such trap is the tendency to "jump to conclusions" or to overestimate the probability of a bad outcome, and the second is to "think the worst" or to catastrophize the outcome. In response to these thinking traps, patients are encouraged to apply strategies that promote more balanced, flexible attributions and appraisals.

Module 5: Countering Emotional Behaviors

In module 5, patients acknowledge and challenge behaviors that enable their avoidance of uncomfortable emotions. They explore their various overt and subtle avoidance behaviors before generating *alternative actions* (actions that directly oppose existing, unhelpful tendencies). One example would be initiating a conversation at a party rather than avoiding it.

Module 6: Understanding and Confronting Physical Sensations

In the sixth module, patients explore the physical component of emotional experiences and the relationship between their physical sensations, thoughts, and feelings by evoking the physical sensations associated with strong emotional experiences. They complete a series of interoceptive exposures (e.g., hyperventilating to elicit feelings of dizziness or unreality; doing jumping jacks to elevate heart rate). Over time, the exposures lead to increased tolerance of, and ability to cope with, physical sensations that accompany emotional experiences.

Module 7: Emotion Exposures

In module 7, patients confront triggers and situations that generate strong emotional reactions, facing increasingly difficult situations over time, and use the skills developed in previous modules to cope with these emotional exposures.

Module 8: Recognizing Accomplishments and Looking Forward

In the eighth and final module, patients review their progress and develop plans for continued practice. They are encouraged to remember that treatment is a long-term commitment and that lasting change requires continued practice of the skills learned through the UP.

Is It Effective?

A large and ever-growing body of research literature suggests that the UP is as effective as protocols that target only one disorder (*single-disorder protocols*) in the treatment of anxiety and depressive disorders. The largest randomized controlled UP trial to date found that 63% of individuals who completed treatment with the protocol no longer met criteria for their primary (i.e., most significant/impairing) diagnosis, compared with 57% of participants treated with a single-disorder protocol, but the UP was associated with significantly less attrition. Research has shown that improvements are maintained for up to 3 years following treatment with the UP at rates that are similar to those observed following treatment with single-disorder protocols.

Nonresponse or Relapse

As with any treatment, some patients will not experience a full reduction of their symptoms following treatment with the UP or may struggle to maintain their improvements. In such cases, additional treatment may be warranted. Some individuals may benefit from scheduling "booster sessions," infrequent therapy appointments focused on refreshing previously learned skills and strategies. Such sessions have demonstrated value in maintaining progress achieved with CBT.

Some evidence suggests that treatment with the UP is beneficial for people who do not respond well to initial rounds of alternative treatment, such as pharmacotherapy or other psychotherapeutic interventions. Whether the protocol is more or less effective when implemented in conjunction with other treatments requires additional research, but general clinical wisdom would advise forgoing concurrent treatment unless the treatments would have no potential overlap in their effects. In that instance, communication and coordination among therapists is strongly recommended.

Many patients experience unease or uncertainty as they approach the conclusion of their treatment. Such feelings are a natural and expected part of the treatment process and should not be confused with a lack of progress. Treatment is a process with natural ebbs and flows, and symptoms are likely to fluctuate in response to various life stressors and events. Furthermore, the goal of treatment with the UP is not to eliminate negative emotions but rather to provide skills for responding to emotions in adaptive ways. On concluding treatment with the UP, patients are encouraged to use these skills as they face the emotional challenges inherent to the human experience.

Are Other Treatments Used in Conjunction With This Treatment?

The relationship between CBT and pharmacotherapy is not fully understood, but most clinical practice guidelines recommend choosing one method to start and then incorporating an alternative approach if progress is not satisfactory. UP patients are encouraged to continue taking their stable dosage of current psychotropic medications and are discouraged from increasing their dosages or adding additional medications. Nevertheless, many patients reduce or stop their medication during or following treatment, which should be done only under the guidance of a medical professional.

Conclusion

The UP is an effective and efficient treatment for people struggling with symptoms of one or more emotional disorders, including anxiety, depressive, and related disorders that are characterized by emotion dysregulation. Throughout the 12–16 semistructured therapy sessions, participants learn skills for effectively responding to their dysregulated emotional states and are guided to confront situations and emotions they typically fear or avoid, enabling increased engagement in important daily activities. Those who continue to implement the core strategies taught in the UP following their time in therapy are most likely to experience lasting results from the treatment.

Recommended Reading

Barlow DH, Farchione T (eds): Applications of the Unified Protocol for Transdiagnostic Treatment of Emotional Disorders. New York, Oxford University Press, 2018

Sauer-Zavala S, Barlow DH: Neuroticism: A New Framework for Emotional Disorders and Their Treatment. New York, Guilford Press, 2021

70

Self-Compassion-Based Psychotherapy

Christopher Germer, Ph.D.
Kristin Neff, Ph.D.

Introduction

Compassion is a feeling that arises when we see others in distress and spurs us to try to alleviate their suffering. In Latin, *compassion* literally means "to suffer with." We have all experienced compassion. Just think back to a time when you were really struggling, perhaps with anxiety or depression, and someone looked at you with kind eyes, listened carefully to what you were saying, spoke in a comforting or supportive manner, and perhaps put an arm around your shoulder. What effect did that compassion have on you? Chances are that you felt a lot better, began to think more clearly, and had some energy to go forward.

What Is Self-Compassion?

Self-compassion is a lot like compassion for others. It's a U-turn—offering ourselves the same kindness and understanding we might give to a dear friend who is struggling. Most people are more compassionate toward others than toward themselves. However, we ignore self-compassion at our own peril. Burgeoning research shows that self-compassion is strongly associated with happiness and emotional well-being, lower levels of anxiety and depression, better physical health, and more satisfying personal relationships. Fortunately, self-compassion can also be learned, including during psychotherapy.

There are various misconceptions about self-compassion, including the notion that it will make us weak or selfish or decrease our motivation. Research shows, on the contrary, that it results in more emotional strength and resilience, that learning self-compassion actually *increases* our compassion for others, and that self-compassionate people are *more* motivated to reach their goals.

A formal definition of *self-compassion* was created by Kristin Neff in 2003, along with a scale to measure it—the Self-Compassion Scale. In Neff's model, self-compassion involves three components: 1) mindfulness versus rumination, 2) common humanity versus isolation, and 3) self-kindness versus self-criticism. If you are experiencing anxiety or depression, imagine what it would be like if you could recognize and validate your feelings (*mindfulness*) rather than getting lost in rumination; felt connected with others in the midst of anxiety or depression (*common humanity*) rather than feeling isolated and alone; and were reassuring and supportive of yourself (*self-kindness*) rather than blaming and self-critical. With these mental habits, it is quite possible you would not feel anxious or depressed anymore.

History of Self-Compassion in Therapy

During the past two decades, interest in compassion in therapy has grown exponentially. Prior to that, compassion was hidden under the umbrella of "empathy," a crucial aspect of any therapeutic relationship. (Whereas *empathy* refers to emotional resonance, *compassion* is the desire to alleviate suffering. Resonating with another's suffering does not always involve caring about it.) Self-compassion in therapy has primarily taken the form of self-acceptance and nonjudgmental understanding. Leaders from different schools of therapy from Sigmund Freud to B. F. Skinner to Carl Rogers all considered self-acceptance to be psychologically beneficial.

In 2000, Paul Gilbert explicitly brought compassion into therapy. He had a revolutionary insight while he was treating depressed patients using cognitive-behavioral therapy (CBT). Gilbert realized that his patients could readily identify their cognitive distortions and replace them with more balanced thoughts, but they remained depressed as long as they spoke to themselves in a harsh and demeaning manner. He concluded that the *tone* of patients' inner dialogue was more important than the *content* of their thoughts for alleviating depression. In other words, we needed to "warm up the conversation." This insight led to compassion-focused therapy, which is the most empirically supported compassion-based treatment today. The primary focus of compassion-focused (or compassion-based) therapy is helping people become more self-compassionate, and in this chapter we seek to explain how self-compassion operates in therapy.

Description of the Treatment

There are three levels in which self-compassion can be integrated into therapy: 1) *therapeutic presence*—how therapists relate to their experience of themselves and the patient, mostly nonverbally; 2) *therapeutic relationship*—how therapists engage with patients, verbally and nonverbally; and 3) *therapeutic interventions*—how patients relate to themselves, especially by practicing self-compassion exercises at home.

Therapists can have a positive effect on patients by their *presence* alone. This is because human beings are hardwired to feel the experience of others within themselves. For example, if a patient describes a traumatic event and their therapist listens in a kind and understanding manner, the sense of warmth and safety created will inevitably impact that patient's experience of themselves and their trauma. The therapeutic *relationship*, or how the therapist actively engages with patients, can also alter patients' relationship to themselves. When treated in a respectful, compassionate manner, people internalize those conversations and may start to treat themselves in a similar way. Finally, self-compassion *interventions*, or practices, can be taught in therapy to cultivate self-compassion. When people think about self-compassion in therapy, they tend to think about practices such as meditation. However, meditation practices are just one part of the whole package. Ideally, the resource of self-compassion offers some of the benefits of the therapeutic relationship, and when self-compassion is practiced between sessions, it makes therapy "portable."

What Is a Self-Compassion Practice?

A *self-compassion practice* is any intentional effort to bring kindness and understanding to ourselves when we suffer, fail, or feel inadequate. Such efforts cultivate qualities of warmth, care, and connection. We can practice self-compassion *mentally*, such as by imagining how we might speak to friend in a similar situation and then speak to ourselves in the same manner. We can also practice *behaviorally*, such as by asking ourselves, "What do I need right now?" and then giving that to ourselves. Self-compassion practices can be *tender*, such as soothing ourselves when we are upset, or *fierce*, such as learning to say "No!" when we are treated unfairly. Anyone can practice self-compassion—the main question is *how* we practice.

The most widespread self-compassion training program at present is Mindful Self-Compassion, which we developed. This program contains a wealth of home practices that can be customized for personal or professional use. These practices can also be integrated into existing therapeutic interventions. For example, a person can practice compassionate encouragement during exposure therapy (e.g., "You've got this! You can do this!") or evoke a compassionate attitude during cognitive restructuring (e.g., putting a hand over their heart).

Mechanisms of Change

Self-compassion is a *transdiagnostic* mechanism of change in therapy and improves mental health across diverse clinical populations. A meta-analysis of self-compassion-based psychotherapy revealed significant improvements in anxiety and depression. Self-compassion is also a *transtheoretical* mechanism of change because it correlates with improvements in different kinds of therapy, such as psychodynamic psychotherapy, cognitive-behavioral therapy (CBT), acceptance and commitment therapy (ACT), and mindfulness-based cognitive therapy.

How does self-compassion work in therapy? Research indicates that learning self-compassion in therapy increases compassionate responding to personal distress (e.g., self-kindness, common humanity, and mindfulness) and decreases uncompassionate responding (e.g., self-judgment, isolation, and rumination). Uncompassionate mental processes appear to cause or worsen psychological disorders; for example, if we are anxious or depressed, we tend to blame ourselves for how we feel, feel alone in our suffering, and tend to think repetitively about the causes and consequences of our problems. Therefore, the lessened tendency to respond uncompassionately to distress may be considered a putative mechanism of change in self-compassion-based therapy.

Shame reduction is another putative mechanism of change. Shame is closely related to self-criticism and is implicated in a wide range of psychological disorders. Clinical studies consistently show that as self-compassion levels increase in therapy, shame decreases. Therefore, learning self-compassion in therapy can help to alleviate shame associated with anxiety and depression.

Research indicates that the mechanism of change most consistently associated with self-compassion is emotion regulation. *Emotion regulation* is the ability to recognize our emotional states and to modulate their intensity and duration. How does self-compassion regulate emotion? Psychologically, insecure attachment is closely associated with emotion *dysregulation*, and self-compassion appears to mediate the relationship between insecure attachment and emotional distress by providing a sense of emotional security and safety. Physiologically, heart rate variability is considered a marker for emotion regulation (through activation of the vagus nerve), and self-compassion is linked to higher variability.

Finally, self-compassionate individuals seem to regulate emotion neurologically by activating their brain's ventromedial prefrontal cortex (decision-making) and deactivating their amygdala (threat). This is familiar brain circuitry for down-regulating stress and negative emotions.

Who Should Receive Self-Compassion Therapy?

Self-Compassion for Parents of Children in Distress

It can be a challenge for parents when their children are experiencing anxiety and depression. Self-compassion can help. Research shows that parents' ability to be compassionate with themselves is even more predictive of parental well-being than the severity of their child's symptoms. Ideally, parents are also in a position to modulate their children's emotions. For example, when parents are able to regulate their own emotions, they provide reassurance and a sense of stability that helps children cope with their own difficult emotions. Therefore, one way that parents can help children struggling with anxiety or depression is to cultivate compassion for themselves.

Conclusion

Self-compassion appears to be a key factor in emotional health and well-being and an underlying process of change in therapy. It can be learned in therapy via the therapist's presence, the therapy relationship, and home practices. A unique aspect of self-compassion in therapy is the focus on explicitly cultivating an attitude of warmth and kindness toward oneself. This approach might be especially useful for anxious or depressed people who experience shame, self-criticism, rumination, or loneliness. Clinical research on this model is increasing rapidly and shows considerable promise as a way to help individuals cope with the difficulties of life.

Recommended Reading

Gilbert P: The Compassionate Mind. London, Constable, 2009

Neff K, Germer C: The Mindful Self-Compassion Workbook. New York, Guilford Press, 2018

Part VI

Special Populations and Special Topics

71

Children

Rebecca Hamblin, Ph.D.
Karen Dineen Wagner, M.D., Ph.D.

Introduction

All children experience fears, worries, sadness, and mood swings from time to time, but for some, these ups and downs go beyond brief states of distress and begin to interfere with family life, school, friends, and other activities. Nearly one-third of children will develop an anxiety disorder by the age of 18, while nearly one in five will experience a depressive disorder, making these problems extremely common. Common mood and anxiety disorders in children include

- *Major depressive disorder:* a persistent sadness, hopelessness, or loss of interest in activities
- *Persistent depressive disorder:* a persistent sad/low mood lasting at least 1 year and usually with fewer symptoms than major depressive disorder
- *Separation anxiety disorder:* a fear of separation from caregivers
- *Specific phobia:* a fear of specific situations/things such as animals, thunderstorms, injections
- *Social anxiety disorder:* extreme shyness or reluctance to engage with others socially
- *Panic disorder:* a sudden, intense fear or panic that occurs seemingly out of nowhere and happens repeatedly

- *Selective mutism:* an inability to speak in certain situations
- *Generalized anxiety disorder:* a persistent worry or feelings of dread related to a number of situations, such as the future, relationships, or health

Other closely related problems include *posttraumatic stress disorder (PTSD)* and *obsessive-compulsive disorder (OCD).* Fortunately, anxiety and depression do not need to become lifelong problems, and excellent treatment options are available.

What Do Anxiety and Mood Problems Look Like in Children?

Anxiety and mood problems in children often appear differently from those of adults. Whereas adults often are familiar with identifying and describing feelings of depression or anxiety, young children lack the vocabulary and experience to label their emotions. Consequently, they may have trouble communicating their emotions in a productive manner that allows parents to readily assist. Common behavioral presentations of fear and sadness in children include opposition or noncompliance when faced with a situation that causes distress, irritability, tantrums, avoidance, crying, reassurance seeking, oversensitivity to criticism and setbacks, and withdrawal. In other words, fearfulness in children may not be displayed as trembling and avoidance but may present as behaviors more commonly associated with anger and defiance. Similarly, sadness may appear as irritability and outbursts rather than lethargy and tearfulness. Learning how your child responds to different emotions can help you to label those emotions for your child.

Causes of Anxiety and Mood Problems in Children

There is no single cause of anxiety and mood problems in children. Contrary to common belief, a child does not have to experience a traumatic event to develop depression or anxiety. Common causes can include stressors at home or school, genetic and temperamental factors, and ongoing patterns of behavioral avoidance. Many parents struggle with a sense of guilt or disbelief when their child is struggling because they strive to minimize stress and model healthy habits for their children. It is important to know that blaming yourself or your child is unwarranted. Anxiety and depression are no one's fault, but parents have the power to help their children recover.

Distinguishing Age-Typical Fears and Sadness From a More Serious Problem

It is often difficult to distinguish typical development and the ups and downs of childhood from more serious problems. Some childhood fears are expected for a particular age group, such as fear of separation from caregivers, fear of death or dying, shyness or fear of strangers, and transient fears of thunderstorms. Similarly, it is appropriate for children to feel sadness and frustration as a healthy part of life. At what point should caregivers become concerned? First, pay attention to the *duration* of the fear or mood disruption. Does it resolve itself in a reasonable amount of time with caregiver support, or does it persist? Second, examine the *impact*. To what degree do the emotions and behaviors affect relationships and activities? Children should be able to engage with immediate and extended family, attend school willingly, have friends, participate in activities outside of school, sleep and eat well, and show increasing independence. If the problem persistently interferes in one or more of these areas, it is time to seek expert advice. It is always reasonable to seek the help or advice of a health professional if something does not feel right or you simply want some input on your concerns.

Tips For Parents: Dealing With Day-to-Day Fear, Anxiety, Sadness, and Mood Turbulence

If a mood disturbance or anxiety is transient or is not severe enough to warrant clinical concern, parents can help guide their children to identify and effectively respond to difficult emotions and feared situations. One of the most important things to remember is that this is a time to *validate* what your child is feeling. Never criticize or shame a child for their emotions, even when the behavior is not appropriate. Instead, discuss the behavior in light of their feelings and try to help them put a name to their experience, for example, saying, "When you're feeling sad, a helpful thing to do is to try to name what's making you feel sad so we can work on it." Make it an ongoing family endeavor to be aware of how each person responds to stressful events and situations, and model for your child how you would like them to act or respond. Encourage exploration of new places and situations, try new things together as a family, encourage appropriate risk taking, discuss mistakes as a fact of life, and emphasize behavior over outcomes!

Clinical-Level Interventions

When anxiety or depression become impairing to a child's daily functioning, it is time to seek professional advice and treatment. Effective treatments for children are very similar to those for adults and include psychotherapy, medication, or a combination of both. Cognitive-behavioral therapy (CBT) has been shown to be effective to treat anxiety and depression in children. This therapy helps the child to recognize negative or unhelpful thoughts and behaviors that affect their emotions. A core component of CBT for anxiety disorders is called *exposure therapy* (or *exposure and response prevention*), which focuses on progressively and systematically desensitizing the child to the fear or worry by gradually and compassionately having them face the situation they fear. By facing their fears in this way, children learn that their feared outcome is unlikely or that they possess the skills to handle the situation. Research shows this approach is well-tolerated and often results in improvements beyond the immediate treatment target, and these gains tend to be long-lasting. Studies also show that parental involvement in exposure therapy is ideal and leads to better treatment outcomes. Look for a therapist who can describe exposure therapy in detail, is compassionate and patient, and involves parents heavily in treatment.

A core component of treatment for childhood depression is *behavioral activation*. This therapy involves gradually increasing the child's engagement in activities from which they have withdrawn, as well as actively problem-solving any current stressors. Again, most current research indicates that family involvement leads to superior outcomes, and it is important to seek a therapist who includes the parents in treatment. Sometimes treatments for young children focus on training the caregivers to deliver the therapy at home; it is always important and appropriate to inquire about the evidence and effectiveness of a particular therapy for your child. See https://adaa.org/finding-help/treatment/choosing-therapist or https://iocdf.org/find-help for tips on finding a psychotherapist and for listings of psychotherapists in your area.

As with psychotherapy, medication options for depression and anxiety are very similar to one another. The most common class of medications used to treat these conditions in youth is the selective serotonin reuptake inhibitors (SSRIs). Fluoxetine is the only SSRI currently approved by the U.S. Food and Drug Administration (FDA) for treating depression in children (age 8 years and older); however, prescription of other SSRIs is common, and medication choice is based on the clinical history of the child and the most up-to date research. Duloxetine is the only medicine FDA-approved for anxiety disorder in children age 7 years and older, but as with depression, several SSRIs have shown to be effective. Because anxiety and depression commonly co-occur, with one another and with other conditions, your child's doctor may recommend an SSRI that they think is best for the child's presentation. SSRIs work by increasing certain neurotransmitters in the brain and often take 4–6 weeks to reach their full effect. Common side effects include gastrointestinal symptoms, headaches, irritability, agitation, and sleep disturbance. The doctor may consider other classes of antidepressants if SSRIs have not been effective. It is important that the doctor listens closely to your concerns and to those of your child and discusses treatment options and the reasons for their recommendations.

Conclusion

Mood and anxiety problems are relatively common among youth and can appear differently than in adults. There is usually no single identifiable cause, but several treatment options and resources are available for children and caregivers. First-line interventions include medications called SSRIs and CBT. It can be difficult for caregivers to distinguish age-related fears and mood fluctuations from more serious disorders. Concerned caregivers may wish to start by consulting with their child's pediatrician or a child psychologist or psychiatrist. Please see the "Recommended Readings" that follow.

Recommended Reading

Lebowitz ER: Breaking Free of Child Anxiety and OCD: A Scientifically Proven Program for Parents. New York, Oxford University Press, 2021

Rapee R, Wignall A, Spence S, et al: Helping Your Anxious Child: A Step-By-Step Guide for Parents, 2nd Edition. Oakland, CA, New Harbinger, 2008

72

Suicide and Self-Harm in Youth

Jennifer L. Hughes, Ph.D., M.P.H.
Joan R. Asarnow, Ph.D., ABPP

Introduction

Sometimes children and adolescents experience periods of time during which they feel highly stressed, down, sad, or hopeless. These experiences, if they last for a few weeks and impact the child's ability to take part in family, social, and school activities, may indicate an anxiety or depressive disorder. Sometimes, when youth are very upset, they may have thoughts about hurting themselves on purpose or about killing themselves. These kinds of thoughts can sometimes lead to youth harming themselves.

According to the Centers for Disease Control and Prevention (CDC), suicide deaths among U.S. youth have increased in recent years. In 2020, suicide was the third leading cause of death among adolescents ages 15–19 and the second leading cause of death among young adolescents ages 10–14. Suicide attempts in youth are concerning not only because these may cause severe or long-lasting injury but also because youth may have to visit the emergency department or hospital, resulting in time away from family, friends, and school. A history of suicide attempts also puts a child at greater risk for future suicidal behavior. We know that more youth were seen in the emergency department for suicide attempts in late 2020 than during that same period in 2019. In a 2019 national survey of high school students, the Youth Risk Behavior Surveillance System, 18.8% of youth reported having seriously considered suicide, 15.7% had made a plan about how they would attempt suicide, and 8.9% reported having attempted suicide in the past 12 months.

Why Is My Child Experiencing Suicidal Feelings?

It can be hard for parents and family members to understand why their child might be considering suicide. Although there is no single cause, suicide and suicide attempts tend to occur when stressors and health conditions converge and lead youths to feel hopeless and desperate to stop their emotional pain. The most reliable predictors of future suicidal behavior are prior suicidal thoughts, suicide attempts, and other forms of self-harm (e.g., cutting an arm or leg with no intent to die); however, a number of factors may increase the risk for suicide and suicide attempts, including significant mental health disorders, such as depression or addiction; exposure to suicidal behavior in others; family history of suicidal behavior and other behavioral health problems, such as mood disorders and substance misuse; recent psychiatric hospitalization; high social needs, poverty, or community violence; risk-exposure history that includes racism experienced by minoritized youth; child maltreatment and abuse; participating in bullying, which can include being the victim of bullying as well as being a perpetrator; and heavy use or overuse of the internet and social media. Factors that are *protective* against suicide and suicidal behavior in children and adolescents include family cohesion; good access to care; faith and spiritual beliefs; intrapersonal factors, such as cognitive flexibility and emotion regulation skills; and strong interpersonal relationships. In addition to the risky aspects of internet/social media, there are positive aspects such as connection, reduced isolation, and community.

What to Do If Your Child Expresses a Wish to Harm Themselves

If a youth mentions wanting to harm themselves, **always take it seriously**. This includes any comments about dying, self-harming, or attempts to end their life. A first step can be to contact the child's pediatrician or primary care provider. The youth and/or parent can also call or text 9-8-8, the national suicide prevention lifeline, for guidance on the next steps for keeping the youth safe. Other important warning signs include talking about or making plans for suicide, making statements that indicate feelings of hopelessness about the future, appearing in high distress or emotional pain, behavior changes such as withdrawing from social activities or hobbies, changes in sleep, or expressing increased irritability or anger (www.youthsuicidewarningsigns.org). Once a child or adolescent has decided to attempt suicide, they may also appear suddenly calmer; therefore, any change in a youth who has been struggling can be an indication of heightened risk and should signal a need for additional support and protection. If in doubt, parents or family members should do their best to make sure the child is not left alone and is with someone who can protect them.

When a youth is having suicidal thoughts or urges, parents or family members can do several things to help keep them safe. First, it is vital to listen closely to the youth's thoughts and feelings, with the goal of helping them feel understood and supported. It is also important to communicate hope and determination that help can be found. It is important for parents to remember that they do not need to handle this alone, and they may need to reach out to other family members, health or mental health care providers, or responsible individuals who can help them support and protect their child during times of risk. Parents can contact the child's health care provider, such as a pediatric primary care provider or family physician, for assistance in finding proper care for their child; the provider may recommend visiting the local emergency department or refer the child to a mental health provider for suicide-specific care. However, a strong relationship with and the availability of a primary care provider offers another protective support. Youths often list their primary care clinician as a trusted adult and may feel more comfortable discussing problems with someone who has helped them feel better in the past. Most primary care providers have experience with and knowledge about mental health concerns and can be a strong resource for parents to ensure their child has a trusted adult to go to if they feel troubled or unsafe.

When a child presents with suicide risk, primary care providers will generally refer them to a mental health specialist. The care that is recommended will depend on many factors, including an assessment of the severity, intensity, and duration of the child's suicidal thoughts and urges and their ability to stay safe, as well as the parent's or caregiver's ability to keep the child safe. When a youth has expressed suicidal thoughts or has tried to hurt or kill themselves, providers will often develop a safety plan with that youth. A *safety plan* helps the child stay safe by identifying a list of coping strategies and sources of support they can use before or during a self-harm or suicidal crisis. It typically includes coping strategies for managing distress and intense emotions safely, personal warning signs of suicidal crisis, people or places that can provide a distraction and protection, trusted adults the youth can contact for help, and ways to keep the home environment safe. The safety plan is developed in collaboration with the child or adolescent so that it is specific to their coping strategies and their supports, such as parents, extended family, teachers, coaches, family friends, or health care or mental health care providers. It is important for the youth to have copies of the safety plan in places that are easy to access, such as their bedroom, their cell phone, or their binder or locker at school.

Parents and family members can support youth who are struggling with suicidal thoughts, urges, and behaviors by checking in with them, asking directly how they are feeling and whether they are experiencing thoughts or urges. Parents can also seek the help of other family members, such as grandparents or aunts and uncles, to provide additional support for the youth, particularly in situations in which frequent check-ins with the parents might cause the child more distress. Sometimes youth are unable to explain the reasons they have for self-harm. During these check-ins, the parent or other caregiver should let the youth know that they are there to listen, with the goal of supporting them and helping them use their safety plan or solve problems, as needed. It can also be helpful for parents to make time to learn about self-injury and suicidal urges or behaviors.

Another important action parents and family members can take to support children in suicidal crisis is by addressing home safety factors, which means securing potentially dangerous items in the home so that they are not easily available to the youth during suicidal crisis. This can prevent the youth from easily acting on suicidal thoughts or urges, thus protecting them from harming themselves. Potentially dangerous items to consider securing or removing from the home include firearms, ammunition, knives and other sharp objects, ropes, prescription and over-the-counter medications, cleaning products, and drugs and alcohol. Addressing home safety includes considering all areas of the home, such as the garage, basement, tool shed, car, and even the youth's bedroom and backpack. The Lock and Protect website (https://ucla.chsprc.com) is one resource for planning how to make a home safer for children and adolescents who are struggling with self-harm.

Treatment

Interventions are available specifically for children and adolescents who have made a suicide attempt, and these are focused on reducing suicidal ideation and preventing future suicidal behaviors. Common elements of these interventions include a comprehensive assessment to inform treatment, safety planning, family involvement, coping skills training to match the needs identified in that assessment, and the promotion of continuing care. Dialectical behavior therapy (DBT) has been studied in three randomized controlled trials and currently has some of the strongest evidence for reducing repeated self-harm and suicidal ideation among youth ages 12–18. DBT is a manualized, cognitive-behavioral treatment that includes weekly individual therapy for the patient, occasional family sessions for the patient and family, a weekly multifamily skills training group, and phone coaching for the patient and their caregivers. This treatment usually lasts 19–24 weeks. DBT aims to help youth develop more effective emotion regulation, interpersonal, and behavioral skills. Other treatment approaches have also shown promise, particularly those that include outreach to parents to help them support their children.

Conclusion

When your child expresses suicidal thoughts or behaviors, it can be scary and distressing. Remember that you can obtain support for yourself as well as your child. This can include talking to a trusted friend or family member or seeking mental health support from a professional. Doing what you need to do to care for yourself will help you to better care for your child.

Recommended Reading

Asarnow JR, Zullo L, Ernestus SM, et al: "Lock and protect": development of a digital decision aid to support lethal means counseling in parents of suicidal youth. Front Psychiatry 12:736236, 2021 34690841

Substance Abuse and Mental Health Services Administration: Treatment for Suicidal Ideation, Self-Harm, and Suicide Attempts Among Youth. Rockville, MD, Substance Abuse and Mental Health Services Administration, 2020

73

Elderly Patients

Neha Jain, M.D.
David C. Steffens, M.D., M.H.S.

Introduction

Elderly patients are a population that must be considered separately because of the many changes that happen as people age, including physical changes in the body; psychological changes as people come to terms with their achievements, losses, and life events; and, often, spiritual changes as people start to consider the meaning of life and death. Depression and anxiety appear to be more common among people of color, women, those who live alone, and those who have multiple medical problems, including chronic pain and insomnia. Depression and anxiety disorders are common among older adults, although they might present differently and are often overlooked.

Risk of Suicide

Older adults attempt suicide less often than younger adults but typically are more successful at completion. Many older adults who complete suicide are depressed and have recently seen a physician. Sleep issues, anxiety, poor concentration, alcohol use, and pain increase the risk of suicide in older adults.

Risk of Memory Problems

Depression and anxiety appear to increase the risk of developing memory problems and dementia in the future. Some researchers consider depression and anxiety to be early stages of dementia, whereas others consider them to be risk factors. Regardless, this highlights the importance of diagnosing and treating anxiety and depression in elderly patients.

What Do Depression and Anxiety Look Like in Elderly Patients?

Recognizing depression and anxiety in older adults might be more challenging because, unlike younger adults, they may not complain of feeling low or nervous. Instead, they might talk about physical issues such as pain, feeling tired, feeling more forgetful, or not feeling as active as they used to. Older adults might blame their symptoms on "normal aging," medical problems, or medications themselves. They may simply withdraw, not participating in activities or enjoying themselves as much as they used to but still insisting everything is "fine." They may also try to put on a "brave face" when they are with friends and family, hiding the symptoms they experience when by themselves.

Grief and Other Issues

Anxiety and *depression* are broad terms, and often these conditions may coexist with others such as prolonged grief, posttraumatic stress disorder (PTSD), or alcohol use. Psychiatric assessment by a qualified physician might help distinguish clinical depression from grief and worry from an anxiety disorder. Severe anxiety and depression may be associated with psychosis, losing touch with reality, weight loss and infirmity, or a reduced ability to live independently.

Screening and Assessment Tools

Many tools are available for screening and assessment of depression and anxiety, ranging from quick two-question self-report screeners to comprehensive evaluations by a neuropsychologist lasting several hours. The Patient Health Questionnaire–2 (PHQ-2) and Generalized Anxiety Disorder–2 (GAD-2) are shown in Tables 73–1 and 73–2.

Approach to Assessment

Assessment often starts with the older adults' primary care physician or geriatrician, who performs a clinical assessment for depression or anxiety disorders that

Table 73–1. Patient Health Questionnaire–2 (PHQ-2)

Over the last 2 weeks, how often have you been bothered by the following problems:	Not at all	Several days	More than half the days	Nearly every day
Little interest or pleasure in doing things	0	1	2	3
Feeling down, depressed, or hopeless	0	1	2	3

Note. The PHQ-2 score ranges from 0–6. Scores of 3 and above are considered positive on the screen and need further assessment.

Table 73–2. Generalized Anxiety Disorder–2 (GAD-2)

Over the last 2 weeks, how often have you been bothered by the following problems:	Not at all	Several days	More than half the days	Nearly every day
Feeling nervous, anxious, or on edge	0	1	2	3
Not being able to stop or control worrying	0	1	2	3

Note. A score of 3 on the GAD-2 is considered the cutoff.

Resources and information are also available online at the Anxiety and Depression Association of America (ADAA) website (https://adaa.org) and the AARP website (www.aarp.org).

may include more detailed questions about mood, anxiety, day-to-day functioning, and memory. In addition, the physician may order blood work to assess for medical problems that might affect mood and anxiety, such as thyroid issues and anemia. They may then decide either to offer treatment or to send the patient for further assessment with a psychiatrist who specializes in the treatment of older adults. They or the psychiatrist will then discuss the probable diagnosis and various treatment approaches and decide the treatment plan with the patient.

Treatment

A combination of psychotherapy and medication is the best treatment approach for moderate-to-severe anxiety and depression symptoms. Milder symptoms may be managed with psychotherapy alone. Many kinds of psychotherapy have been used for older adults:

- *Behavioral therapy* focuses on building skills that lead to more positive experiences.
- *Problem solving therapy* focuses on specific problems that may be related to anxiety or depression symptoms and on improving the patient's ability to resolve them.

- *Cognitive-behavioral therapy* focuses on the triad of thoughts, feelings, and behaviors and how changing one of these can help the patient change the other two.
- *Interpersonal psychotherapy* focuses on four areas: unresolved grief, role transitions, interpersonal role disputes, and interpersonal deficits.
- *Brief dynamic therapy* focuses on psychodynamic principles of exploring the unconscious and bringing it to awareness, but with a focused, time-limited approach.
- *Reminiscence therapy* and *life review therapy* are also effective in some older populations.
- *Supportive therapy* uses the therapeutic relationship between patient and therapist to improve the patient's ability to cope with life stressors.

There are also specific therapies, such as cognitive-behavioral therapy (CBT) for insomnia. Based on patient preference and availability, psychotherapy may be used one-on-one or in group sessions.

Medications

Medication selection is often based on multiple factors, the most important of which are history of response to a particular antidepressant and the patient's individual constellation of symptoms. Most antidepressant and antianxiety medications are slow acting and may take 8–12 weeks to show full effect. In addition, a slower, more careful titration is often needed in elderly patients to reduce side effects. Common antidepressants and anxiolytics used in older adults are listed in Table 73–3.

Selective Serotonin Reuptake Inhibitors

The selective serotonin reuptake inhibitors (SSRIs) are the most common class of medications used for treatment of both depression and anxiety in older adults. They are safe, effective, and easily available. Common side effects include nausea, stomach disturbance, low sodium levels (leading to dizziness/confusion), and an increased risk of bleeding. Some SSRIs can also affect the heart rhythm. Sometimes, people who do not tolerate one SSRI may do better with another medication from the same class.

Serotonin-Norepinephrine Reuptake Inhibitors

Serotonin-norepinephrine reuptake inhibitors (SNRIs) are often the second-line agent used for patients who may not tolerate SSRIs. Some SNRIs are useful for those with chronic pain. SNRIs can cause an increase in blood pressure and anxiety and are somewhat less tolerated overall compared with the SSRIs.

Table 73–3. Antidepressant and anxiolytic medications commonly prescribed for elderly patients

Class	Generic name	Brand name	Dosage range, *mg*
Selective serotonin reuptake inhibitors	Citalopram	Celexa	10–20
	Escitalopram	Lexapro	5–20
	Sertraline	Zoloft	25–200
Serotonin-norepinephrine reuptake inhibitors	Desvenlafaxine	Pristiq	25–50
	Duloxetine	Cymbalta	20–60
	Levomilnacipran	Fetzima	10–40
	Venlafaxine	Effexor	37.5–225
Atypical antidepressants	Bupropion	Wellbutrin	75–300
	Mirtazapine	Remeron	7.5–45
Serotonin modulators	Trazodone	Desyrel	25–100
	Vilazodone	Viibryd	10–40
	Vortioxetine	Trintellix	5–10
Benzodiazepines	Clonazepam	Klonopin	0.25–2
	Lorazepam	Ativan	0.25–2

Atypical Antidepressants/Serotonin Modulators

Atypical antidepressants include bupropion, mirtazapine, and trazodone. These medications have unique mechanisms of action and are sometimes combined with SSRIs and SNRIs for added efficacy or to target particular symptoms such as insomnia or lack of energy.

Add-On Medications

Occasionally, medications such as antipsychotics or hormonal supplements may be used as add-on agents for treatment of depression or anxiety that does not respond to first- or second-line approaches. These are usually prescribed by experts in psychopharmacology.

Sedatives/Anxiolytics

Traditional sedative/anxiolytic medications, such as clonazepam, are sometimes used for anxiety and insomnia in elderly patients. These agents have a higher risk profile, leading to an increased risk of falls, sedation, and cognitive impairment.

In general, the best approach is to minimize the use of such medications and to use them in as low a dosage and for as short a time as possible. Still, given the length of time required for other medications to achieve their full effect, anxiolytics often serve as helpful adjuncts, especially in the beginning of treatment.

Tricyclic Antidepressants/Monoamine Oxidase Inhibitors

Similarly, tricyclic antidepressants (TCAs) and monoamine oxidase inhibitors (MAOIs) are best avoided in older adults given the higher risk of side effects with these medications, but they may occasionally be prescribed by an expert psychopharmacologist if needed.

Interventional Treatments

Invasive treatments are sometimes indicated for severe depression, which may be associated with psychosis, weight loss, and infirmity.

Electroconvulsive Therapy

Electroconvulsive therapy (ECT) remains the gold standard for treatment of severe depression in elderly patients. ECT procedures are performed in the medical setting under anesthesia. Compared with medications, ECT is often well tolerated in older adults and can be dramatically effective.

Other Interventional Treatments

Other interventional treatments include brain stimulation therapies such as transcranial magnetic stimulation (TMS) and intranasal/intravenous ketamine, although trials of the latter in geriatric depression have had mixed results. Although these treatments are newer and less well studied in older adults, evidence is accumulating for their possible efficacy in the treatment of depression.

Conclusion

Mood and anxiety disorders in older adults are common and often underdiagnosed. It is important to screen for the presence of mood and anxiety problems and to treat them when necessary, while maintaining focus on the elderly person's quality of life.

Recommended Reading

Anxiety and Depression Association of America: Understanding Disorders: What Are Anxiety and Depression? Silver Spring, MD, Anxiety and Depression Association of America, 2023. Available at: https://adaa.org/understanding-anxiety.

Espinoza R, Kaufman AH: Diagnosis and treatment of late-life depression. Psychiatric Times, October 30, 2014. Available at: https://www.psychiatrictimes.com/view/diagnosis-and-treatment-late-life-depression.

74

Group Therapy to Treat Depression and Anxiety

The Best Treatment Approach

Cheri L. Marmarosh, Ph.D.

Introduction

Why is group therapy one of the best treatment approaches for depression and anxiety? That is an important question many people ask when I refer them to group therapy. Most people who struggle with depression and anxiety feel alone and isolated with their symptoms. They have serious concerns that get in the way of their social relationships, limit their ability to focus on their work and professional goals, and inhibit their overall functioning. Often, people with depression and anxiety worry that others will judge them or that they will be burdened by the stigma of being "depressed" or "crazy." On top of their current symptoms, they can feel the shame that comes from our families, culture, and society. When people join a therapy group, however, they immediately meet others who are struggling with similar issues. Unlike friend groups, they can be more honest and open with the therapy group about their feelings or struggles. Unlike individual therapy, they can hear others share perspectives, learn how depression and anxiety interfere with others' relationships, and feel connected to a group. Researchers studying the benefit of group therapy have found it to be as effective as individual therapy for both depression and different anxiety disorders. This chapter will help you decide if group therapy is a treatment approach you may want to pursue. In the following discussion, I review the basics of how group therapy facilitates change, examine the benefit of combined group and individual therapy, and provide ways to find a group if you decide that is a treatment you would like to try.

Group Therapy: Facilitating Change

Many theories exist as to how group therapy facilitates changes for patients with depression or anxiety. Many group therapy texts and courses review these therapeutic factors, which include universality, cohesion, hope, feedback, and existential growth. Positive psychologists have included additional aspects of group therapy that are important, such as gratitude, forgiveness, and revising negative relationship patterns. My focus here is on the similar therapeutic aspects that all group therapies have in common and the therapy factors most relevant to depression and anxiety.

Universality

It is not unusual for people to feel alone when they are struggling with depression and anxiety. Group treatment offers members an opportunity to feel less isolated. In a therapy group I led in a college counseling center, the first thing members did when they met for the first time was talk about their treatment, medications, and how grateful they were to be able to talk about their mental health. Many of them revealed feeling surprised that others struggled with the same issues and thought that it was an unexpected benefit of the group. *Universality*, the sense of not being alone with one's suffering, not only helps adults but can also benefit children and adolescents. Younger people often feel ashamed or isolated with their struggles. Group therapy is the only treatment that brings people together to address their personal struggles and problems.

Cohesion-Group Attachment

In addition to reducing isolation, group therapy provides members with another identity that can bolster them during times of distress—a *group identity*. Similar to how a sports team or club can boost self-esteem, the group therapy identity fosters a sense of cohesion, and members often feel they belong to something bigger than themselves. The group therapy identity can also help members cope with stress when they are away from the group. Many members think of the group when they encounter upsetting situations, experience panic attacks or anxiety, or feel suicidal. The group provides a resource that can bolster against self-harming thoughts and function as a secure base for members. I recall one member who described how a racist remark had triggered a spiral of depressive thoughts. The member was able to think about the therapy group to cope, recalling supportive interactions in the group that reminded him that not all people are racist or devaluing and that he was worthy. Researchers have determined that members who develop strong relationships within the group subsequently develop healthier relationships outside the group a year after therapy ended.

Feedback and Social Learning

Although group therapy can be supportive, it sometimes also can be challenging as members learn how their symptoms impact others. It is not uncommon for people with depression and anxiety to struggle with interpersonal issues that contribute to their condition or are a byproduct of it. For example, many people with depression are unhappy because of being rejected, hurt, or mistreated in a prior or current relationship. Group therapy can help members understand how past experiences have led to their negative view of themselves or others.

Not only do people sometimes develop depression and anxiety after an interpersonal difficulty, but their depression and anxiety can impact other relationships. Many people who are depressed are not aware of how their negativity or withdrawal impacts others. They may not see that they are not as empathic or compassionate to others when they are consumed with anxious or depressive thoughts. A group offers opportunities for members to hear different perspectives. For example, one member became self-critical when another member said something hurtful in the group session. The leader helped the member, along with others who shared this issue, explore how instead of expressing anger when someone said something hurtful, the member blamed themself and avoided conflict and anger. Over time, the group members were able to see how internalizing responsibility for other people's behaviors contributed to their own depression and how avoiding confrontations maintained their low self-worth. Individual therapy cannot offer members different experiences that mimic real life outside of the group. The social interactions in group therapy help us hear, firsthand, how people are engaging in the real world. Gaining insight into how we respond in relationships helps us make changes that can lessen depression and anxiety.

Existential Growth: Meaning in Life

Group therapy also confronts members with existential challenges, such as members' responsibility to make changes in their own lives and be responsible for their actions. In group therapy, members are held accountable for their comments to others, their attendance, their ability to take in feedback from others, and their speaking up and taking risks. As one leader said, "In group therapy, you get what you put into it." Members can start to explore their narrative, who they are, and who they want to be. Their ability to try new behaviors and take control of how they respond in relationships can foster self-esteem and well-being. Members also can gain a sense of purpose when they are able to help someone else who is struggling and can provide resources, information, and guidance to members who need their help. In group therapy, members are not always *receiving* support as in individual therapy; they also *give* support and compassion to others. The act of helping others can reduce depression and anxiety.

Gratitude

Unlike individual therapy, group therapy also allows participants to see others who are experiencing greater losses, more severe symptoms, and different challenges. Members can gain a sense of gratitude by seeing what others are overcoming. In addition, members can start to feel a sense of appreciation for what they do have, even while they are coping with something difficult, such as depression and anxiety. Group therapy also provides the experience of receiving support from multiple people. Many members are touched by the care and genuine curiosity others are willing to give them. In individual therapy, one person—the therapist—gives the person their time and support; in group therapy, members can receive positive feedback, empathy, and positive regard from multiple people.

Forgiveness

In group therapy, it is not uncommon for members to express conflict and navigate ruptures in relationships. The group helps members learn to forgive others and tolerate their own imperfections and mistakes. For example, it is not uncommon for group members to challenge other members and group leaders who say something offensive or discriminating. During the group process, members can learn to be assertive with their feelings and how to forgive people who apologize for hurting them. Forgiving others and oneself can lead to more trust in relationships, less isolation, and less depression and anxiety.

Addressing Maladaptive Relationship Patterns

Similar to individual therapy, effective group therapy facilitates the revision of internal models/schemas of the self and others. Instead of feeling worthless and worried that others will reject or abandon them, members may start to feel they are valuable and to trust that others care. In group, members interact with one another, and this allows relationship patterns to emerge, along with the scripts we have developed to predict what other people will do. Members with depression may learn that they expect negative feedback and criticism and that they push away positive feedback and mistrust it. People with anxiety may learn that they worry so much about the future that they miss out on positive interactions in the present. Group therapy may help members identify interpersonal patterns that maintain their depression and anxiety, and they learn to try new ways of relating that can revise their beliefs about themselves and others.

Combined Treatments: What Is Right for You?

When people are struggling with depression and anxiety, they need support. Sometimes people may want individual and group therapy combined because they are coping with some issues that make them feel vulnerable or in need of more time and attention, such as trauma, acute suicidal ideation, or acute grief. Sometimes people in a group who are coping with depression and anxiety also benefit from taking medications that can alleviate symptoms. It is not uncommon for members to work with group therapists, individual counselors, and psychiatrists to facilitate a well-rounded treatment. Group therapy can enhance any individual therapy for people struggling with anxiety and depression. It can also stand alone as a treatment and has been demonstrated to have equivalent outcomes to individual therapy.

Finding a Group

Finding a group therapist to work with requires a small amount of work. If you have access to health insurance, then you can identify who in your network is conducting groups. Once you identify possible therapists, you can review their credentials and prioritize those who are certified group psychotherapists (CGPs). CGPs are certified by the American Group Psychotherapy Association (AGPA) because they have had the specialized training and supervision to lead groups.

If you do not have health insurance (or even if you do), you can find a group by looking for local community mental health clinics in your area. Sometimes local universities have mental health clinics that treat people in the community. Many of these clinics offer therapy groups that have lower costs and are possibly available online. You can also search for local groups by looking at the CGP listing on the AGPA website. If you are looking for a group for someone in college, most university counseling centers offer group psychotherapy in their clinics.

Conclusion

As you can see, group therapy is an effective and efficient approach to treatment of depression and anxiety. It can be used in combination with individual therapy or stand alone and can help many different needs and patient populations. There are groups for people of different ages, identities, backgrounds, and diagnoses. Unlike individualized treatments, group therapy also provides connection and support and decreases loneliness. Because it addresses more than just patient symptoms, it is the best treatment for people seeking mental health care.

Recommended Reading

Kaklauskas FJ, Greene LR: Core Principles of Group Psychotherapy: An Integrated Theory, Research, and Practice Training Manual (AGPA Group Therapy Training and Practice Series; Block M, Stephens A, series eds). Oxfordshire, UK, Routledge, 2019

Yalom ID, Leszcz M: The Theory and Practice of Group Psychotherapy, 6th Edition. New York, Basic Books, 2020

75

Prevention of Anxiety and Depression in Youth

V. Robin Weersing, Ph.D.
Michelle Rozenman, Ph.D.

Introduction

Scared and Sad Feelings Are a Normal Part of Growing Up

Feeling scared, worried, nervous, anxious, sad, and irritable is common during childhood and adolescence. However, for some youth, these feelings become frequent, intense, or long-lasting and get in the way of their life or the lives of family members. In this chapter, we provide information on when problems with anxiety and depression may first arise and how scientifically supported strategies can be used to address these symptoms. We discuss how parents can support prevention of anxiety and depression and offer guidance on when to see a professional.

When Do Anxiety and Depression Become a Problem?

For most youth, symptoms of anxiety develop earlier than those of depression. Children may have trouble separating from parents, be shy around new people, and struggle with novelty and uncertainty in general. For some, these "normal" fleeting experiences of anxiety may stick around and begin to impact the lives of the child and their family. Depression, irritability, and loss of interest or pleasure in activities more commonly arise later in development, usually during the teenage years. Everyone experiences low mood sometimes, but depressive symptoms that linger and interfere with daily functioning are concerning.

Can We Prevent Anxiety and Depression? How?

Good evidence indicates that we can prevent the development of anxiety and depression in youth who are already *at risk*—those who already have some symptoms of anxiety or depression. We can also prevent anxiety and depression in youth with a family history of these problems.

Data are mixed on whether we can prevent anxiety and depression with "universal" prevention programs. These programs try to prevent mental health problems by offering a class or program to all youth (typically at school), regardless of their symptom level or risk status. Although universal prevention programs do no harm, they do take resources and time and may not be helpful for people who are not at risk. To make the most effective use of family and health resources, experts recommend early and regular mental health monitoring of youth to effectively identify those who may benefit most from prevention and early intervention programs.

Various strategies may help prevent the development of anxiety and depression. These can be grouped into strategies that help youth *learn* about anxiety and depression, *relax* as a way to manage upset feelings and cope with stress, *think* differently about stressors and life problems, and *act* in new ways that improve mood and reconnect them with people and activities. Although all of these may be helpful, the "act" strategies have been shown to make the most difference in the lives of children and adolescents.

Learn

Psychoeducation, or Learning About the Connection Between Thoughts, Feelings, and Behaviors

How we think, feel, and act are all connected. For example, feeling worried, nervous, scared, or sad can lead us to think negative thoughts and avoid or withdraw from things we want and have to do. However, the opposite is also true: if we push ourselves to do the things we want and have to do—even when those things are hard—we end up feeling better and thinking more positively about ourselves and our ability to manage hard situations. Teaching youth and families these connections can help them start to think about how their own thoughts, feelings, and behaviors are linked so that they can keep an eye on thoughts and feelings that might lead to avoidance or withdrawal.

Identifying Emotions

Sometimes it can be hard to know what we and others feel. Practice with identifying and labeling our feelings in various situations—including when we feel anxious or sad—can directly connect how we feel with what is happening around us and how we act in response.

Relax

Deep breathing, tensing and relaxing muscle groups systematically (called *progressive muscle relaxation*), thinking about a peaceful place, and doing self-care activities can help us respond in the moment when we feel scared, nervous, worried, or stressed.

Think

Cognitive Restructuring and Coping Thoughts

Challenging unhelpful threat-focused or negative thoughts with more neutral ones (*cognitive restructuring*) and coming up with coping statements (e.g., "I've done this before, I can do it again") can help us develop a more neutral mindset about difficult situations and a more positive attitude about our ability to cope.

Problem Solving

With problem-solving, youth learn to take a step-by-step approach to identify exactly why a problem is a problem, brainstorm solutions, examine the pros and cons of each potential solution, and actively try out solutions to see if they can solve the problem.

Mindfulness

Mindfulness involves deliberately paying attention to one's thoughts and feelings without trying to change them. It also involves redirecting our attention to what is happening around us (i.e., the things we have to do or want to do) instead of what is happening inside our mind or body. A growing body of data suggests that mindfulness helps us get unstuck from upsetting thoughts and feelings and, with practice over time, can improve stress and mood.

Act

Behavioral Activation, or Scheduling Fun/Pleasant Activities

When we feel scared or sad, it might become difficult to have fun or to be productive. Deliberately scheduling activities that are fun (e.g., playing at the park, baking, family game night), that we have to do (e.g., completing assignments), or that build mastery (e.g., practicing an instrument or sport) can help improve mood and can also help us actively approach instead of avoid or withdraw.

Exposure, or Graded Approach

When we feel anxious, we often avoid things that we want or have to do. By approaching or "exposing" ourselves to the things we are avoiding in a slow, step-by-step way, we get better at tolerating negative thoughts and feelings. For example, a child who is scared of the dark might practice being in a room with less and less light and eventually practice sleeping without the overhead or closet lights on so that they get used to it over time.

Social and Communication Skills

Many children and adolescents who struggle with feelings of anxiety and depression also lack skills and confidence in communication and social interaction. In addition to the other "act" exercises we have described, youth may also benefit from direct instruction on effective communication. To summarize, the "act" strategies involve five key components:

- Encourage your child to do the things that they want and have to do
- Even when they feel worried, nervous, scared, sad, or stressed
- In a step-by-step way
- With many opportunities to practice
- With warm caregiver support for trying even when things feel hard

How Can Caregivers Help?

Many of these prevention strategies focus on the individual child or adolescent themselves. However, caregivers can play an important role in prevention. Caregivers can purposefully implement rewards for desirable behaviors (e.g., going to school even though the child feels nervous) and consequences (e.g., reduced screen time for refusal to do assigned chores). They can also work with a mental health professional to learn how to be an at-home coach for the strategies their child may be trying to implement. It is important for caregivers to also take care of themselves. Treating parental anxiety and depression can help prevent these symptoms in the child. If caregivers notice that their own mental health impacts their parenting or that their child is starting to exhibit the same symptoms they do (e.g., child begins to fear something because the caregiver does), this might be a sign for caregivers to find professional support for themselves.

Experts also recommend yearly visits with the child's pediatrician. Physical health problems can contribute to anxiety and depression, and wellness visits are a great time for a mental health checkup with your child's doctor. For school-age children, caregivers can communicate with teachers about what they are noticing at home and what the teacher notices at school to keep track of any avoidance, withdrawal, or other concerning behaviors.

When to Consult With a Professional

Sometimes it can be hard to tell when it is the right time to consult with a professional, such as a primary care doctor or mental health provider. Additional support might be helpful if your child or adolescent exhibits any of the following:

- Avoidance of important life activities, such as going to school, getting up in the morning, or leaving the house
- Withdrawal or loss of interest in things they used to enjoy, such as spending time with friends or engaging in favorite activities (e.g., sports, art)
- Significant struggles with symptoms to the point that it significantly impacts the lives of family members (e.g., parent misses work)
- Suicidal thoughts/behaviors or self-injurious behavior (e.g., cutting, burning)

Conclusion

Feeling scared and sad is a normal part of growing up. If these feelings are starting to get in the way of a youth's daily life activities or cause a lot of upset, they may indicate a problem. For youth who are already experiencing some symptoms of anxiety and/or depression, various treatment strategies can be utilized. These strategies can be grouped into those that help youth learn about these feelings and how they might get in the way, help them learn to relax in order to manage upset feelings and cope with stress, help them think differently about stressors, and help them act in new ways that improve their mood and reconnect them with the things they want and have to do. Caregivers can help by rewarding desirable behaviors, working with a professional, taking their child to yearly wellness visits with their pediatrician, and, if relevant, getting treatment for their own anxiety and/or depression.

Recommended Reading

Beardslee WR: Out of the Darkened Room: When a Parent Is Depressed: Protecting the Children and Strengthening the Family. Boston, MA, Little, Brown and Company, 2009

Rapee R, Wignall A, Spence S, et al: Helping Your Anxious Child: A Step-by-Step Guide for Parents, 3rd Edition. Oakland, CA, New Harbinger, 2022

76

Premenstrual and Perimenopausal Disorders

Korrina A. Duffy, Ph.D.
Christina Metcalf, Ph.D.
C. Neill Epperson, M.D.

Introduction

Between puberty and menopause, hormonal changes make females more susceptible to depression and anxiety than males. Fluctuating hormones over the menstrual cycle and during the transition to menopause create unique mental health concerns for this population. Our aim in this chapter is to provide patients and their families with information about the prevalence, symptoms, diagnosis, and treatment of premenstrual syndrome (PMS), premenstrual dysphoric disorder (PMDD), and depression and cognitive complaints occurring during the menopause transition.

Premenstrual Syndrome and Premenstrual Dysphoric Disorder

Prevalence

PMS and PMDD are common. In fact, up to 10% of females experience PMS and up to 5% develop PMDD. Approximately 80% of females experience mild premenstrual symptoms in the week or two before their period starts, but their symptoms are mild and tolerable enough that they do not meet diagnostic criteria for PMS and PMDD.

Symptoms

PMS and PMDD are characterized by physical and emotional symptoms. Common symptoms include bloating, headache, breast tenderness, weight gain, irritability, anxiety, anger, depressed mood, mood swings, tiredness, and difficulty sleeping. Although PMS and PMDD are similar, PMDD is more severe. Females with PMDD typically experience a greater number or greater severity of emotional symptoms than those with PMS. As a result, females with PMDD are at a substantially higher risk of suicidal ideation, plans, and attempts.

Diagnosis

For a patient to be diagnosed with PMS or PMDD, their symptoms must occur in the week or two before period onset, improve within a few days of period onset, and become minimal or absent for the rest of their menstrual cycle. Symptoms that occur during this time must impair the person's functioning at work, at home, or in relationships in a manner noticeably different from the rest of the cycle. To be diagnosed with PMDD, patients should be evaluated by a physician and must have at least 5 of 11 specific symptoms, one of which must be an emotional symptom (Table 76–1). PMS is used to describe females who experience physical or emotional symptoms that interfere with their ability to function in their daily life but ultimately do not meet the criteria for PMDD because they do not experience enough symptoms, only experience physical symptoms, or are not adequately impaired by their symptoms. To establish a diagnosis of either PMS or PMDD, the patient needs to monitor their symptoms daily across at least two menstrual cycles using a standard questionnaire, such as the Carolina Premenstrual Assessment Scoring System (CPASS) or the Daily Record of Severity of Problems (DRSP), which can be downloaded for free (see https://tinyurl.com/6ec2zh3d). This monitoring requires an investment of time and effort but is nec-

Table 76–1. Symptoms of premenstrual dysphoric disorder (PMDD)

In most menstrual cycles over the previous year, symptoms must be present in the week before your period starts, improve within a few days of your period starting, and become minimal or absent in the week after your period ends. To diagnose PMDD, clinicians look for at least five of the following symptoms:

1. At least one of the following emotional symptoms must be present and noticeable:
   a. Shifts in emotions that are rapid and pronounced (e.g., mood swings, feeling suddenly sad or tearful, or increased sensitivity to rejection)
   b. Irritability, anger, or increased conflicts with others
   c. Depressed mood, feelings of hopelessness, or self-critical thoughts
   d. Anxiety, tension, and/or feelings of being keyed up or on edge
2. At least one of the following additional symptoms must be present:
   a. Decreased interest in usual activities (e.g., work, school, friends, hobbies)
   b. Difficulty concentrating
   c. Sluggishness, tiredness, easily exhausted, or noticeable lack of energy
   d. Noticeable change in appetite, overeating, or specific food cravings
   e. Sleeping too much or difficulty falling or staying asleep
   f. Feeling overwhelmed or out of control
   g. Physical symptoms, such as breast tenderness or swelling, joint or muscle pain, feeling bloated, or weight gain.

The symptoms must be distressing or interfere with work, school, usual social activities, and/or relationships with others (e.g., avoidance of social activities or decreased productivity at work, school, or home). The symptoms cannot be a worsening of another mental health disorder, such as major depressive disorder or panic disorder, or be attributed to a substance (e.g., medication or drug of abuse) or another medical condition (e.g., hyperthyroidism).

Note. For exact diagnostic criteria, see American Psychiatric Association: *Diagnostic and Statistical Manual of Mental Disorders*, 5th Edition, Text Revision. Washington, DC, American Psychiatric Association, 2022, p. 197.

essary to ensure that symptoms are limited to the week or two before and the initial days after menstruation onset. Some females experience what is referred to as a premenstrual worsening of depression or anxiety, and treatment for these problems can differ from treatment options available to patients with clear evidence of PMS or PMDD.

Treatment

Patients with PMS and PMDD present with a wide range of physical and emotional symptoms that make treating these conditions complex. Because certain treatment options work better for some symptoms than others, more than one treatment may be needed to alleviate all symptoms. Medications, such as certain antidepressants and hormonal contraceptives, may be prescribed to treat severe symptoms.

Antidepressants can be effective in treating mood and anxiety symptoms. Serotonin reuptake inhibitors are the gold standard (i.e., the best antidepressant treatment option with the strongest evidence) for treating PMDD and severe PMS. These medications change serotonin functioning in the brain, which affects mood, anxiety, sleep, and pain. They can be administered throughout the entire menstrual cycle (i.e., continuous dosing) or limited to the 2 weeks before menstruation (i.e., intermittent dosing). When dosed continuously, antidepressants have been shown to be more effective in alleviating certain symptoms than when dosed intermittently. However, intermittent dosing may cause fewer side effects.

Combined oral contraceptives (i.e., those containing both estrogens and progestins) can be effective in treating overall premenstrual symptoms. One type called YAZ has received U.S. Food and Drug Administration (FDA) approval for the treatment of PMDD, which means it was determined to be safe and effective for this condition. The typical regimen of YAZ is 24 days on (with active pills) and 4 days off (with inactive pills). Although YAZ and other combined oral contraceptives are particularly helpful in improving physical symptoms, such as bloating, headache, breast tenderness, and weight gain, these medications are not effective in treating depressive symptoms. Patients also should be aware that the use of combined oral contraceptives such as YAZ can increase their risk for blood clots.

Another treatment option is psychotherapy. An approach known as cognitive-behavioral therapy (CBT) has the best evidence for reducing PMS and PMDD symptoms. CBT works by helping patients learn how their thoughts, emotions, and behaviors impact one another and how to change unhelpful patterns. Patients learn concrete skills over the course of 8–12 sessions that they can then apply on their own.

Lifestyle changes may also improve the symptoms of PMS and PMDD. For example, managing stress and engaging in relaxation techniques, such as deep breathing exercises and meditation, may be helpful. Regular exercise has been revealed to improve emotional and physical premenstrual symptoms. Dietary changes, such as cutting back on salty and sugary foods, are also recommended. Eating a diet that is rich in complex carbohydrates (e.g., whole grains and beans) during the week or two before period onset may be impactful, perhaps due to the ability of these foods to increase serotonin in the brain. Keeping blood sugar levels even by eating smaller, more frequent meals may also help manage some symptoms.

Table 76–2. Stages of reproductive aging

Stage	Menstrual cycle criteria
Premenopause	Relatively regular menstrual cycles
Menopause transition	
Early	Change in length of consecutive menstrual cycles is 7+ days (time between start of one period and start of next period is 7+ days longer or shorter than typical)
Late	No period for 60+ days
Postmenopause	
Early	Begins 12 months after last menstrual period
Late	Begins 6 years after last menstrual period

Perimenopause

Mood and Cognitive Concerns During the Transition to Menopause

Menopause marks the end of the reproductive years for females. A female is in postmenopause when it has been more than 1 year since her last period. However, biological changes leading up to menopause begin years before (see Table 76–2 for the stages of reproductive aging). Because of the fluctuating and decreasing hormones, the menopause transition is marked by a range of symptoms including depression, anxiety, difficulties with attention and memory, hot flashes, and night sweats, as well as changes in weight, energy, skin, hair, and sexual function.

Depression symptoms are common as females transition to menopause, especially among those who have been depressed previously. Females who have been depressed previously are 13 times more likely to experience significant depression symptoms during the menopause transition and 8 times more likely to experience depression in the postmenopause phase than their peri- and postmenopausal counterparts who have never had depression. However, even those females who have not had depression in the past are 2–4 times more likely to experience a depressed mood throughout the menopause transition than before. Generally, depression risk decreases once a female enters postmenopause, especially for those who were never depressed before perimenopause. Although depression symptoms during the transition to menopause are not necessarily different from those in other life stages (Table 76–3), they can be complicated by or overlap with other common symptoms that occur during the menopause

Table 76–3. Symptoms of depression

1. Depressed mood (observed by self or others)
2. Loss of interest in most activities (observed by self or others)
3. Significant and unintentional weight change (gaining or losing at least 5% of body weight in a month)
4. Sleeping too much or difficulty falling or staying asleep
5. Moving much more quickly or slowly than usual to a degree noticeable by others
6. Sluggishness, tiredness, easily exhausted, or noticeable lack of energy
7. Profound sense of worthlessness or unwarranted guilt
8. Difficulty thinking, concentrating, or making decisions
9. Thoughts about death, desires to be dead, plans or attempts to kill oneself

Note. For exact diagnostic criteria of major depressive disorder, see American Psychiatric Association: *Diagnostic and Statistical Manual of Mental Disorders*, 5th Edition, Text Revision. Washington, DC, American Psychiatric Association, 2022, pp. 183–184.

transition. For instance, hot flashes may make it difficult to sleep well at night, which may exacerbate symptoms of depression, such as feeling down or irritable.

Cognitive difficulties are another common problem experienced during the menopause transition and include difficulties with memory, finding words, concentrating, accessing information, and working quickly. Such cognitive difficulties can be a result of aging, but the transition to menopause also contributes. Fortunately, research shows that cognitive function often improves once females enter postmenopause. Sleep disruption—which is frequent in the years leading up to the final period and linked with symptoms such as hot flashes—negatively affects cognitive function. Importantly, the risk of cognitive issues is highest for females who undergo an early natural menopause or surgical menopause before the ages of 40–45 years.

Although mood problems and thinking difficulties are common throughout the menopause transition, these symptoms can be treated to reduce their impact on day-to-day functioning. It is important to discuss your symptoms with your physician or nurse practitioner so that they can identify the best treatment options. To prepare for this conversation with your medical provider, consider tracking your symptoms with information such as how many days per week you experience them, their severity (i.e., mild, moderate, severe), and how they impact your life. Then, share this information with your provider at your appointment so they can create a treatment plan to address problematic symptoms. The next section provides an overview of typical treatment options.

Addressing Bothersome Mood and Cognitive Problems

Front-line treatments for depression during the menopause transition include evidence-based psychotherapies (e.g., CBT, interpersonal psychotherapy) and FDA-approved antidepressant medications (e.g., selective serotonin reuptake inhibitors [SSRIs]).

Cognitive difficulties during the menopause transition will typically resolve themselves without treatment. In some cases, however, medications may help. Available options may include agents classified as serotonin-norepinephrine reuptake inhibitors (SNRIs) and stimulants.

Estrogen hormone replacement therapy (HRT) is the gold standard option for treating vasomotor symptoms such as hot flashes and night sweats. Importantly, females need to take HRT that includes natural progesterone or progestin in addition to estrogen ("combined HRT") to protect the uterus because taking estrogen without progesterone/progestin increases the risk for uterine cancer. Although combined HRT is not currently FDA-approved to treat depression symptoms, promising evidence suggests that it can reduce depressive symptom severity when administered during the menopause transition (but not postmenopause) for depression that emerges during that time. The highest-quality research evidence indicates that, for most females, combined HRT provides benefits that outweigh potential risks; however, some experience negative mood effects when taking progesterone or progestin.

Other wellness strategies, such as getting adequate exercise, maintaining a balanced diet, avoiding alcohol and smoking, and prioritizing sleep, support healthy brain functioning and mood. Mentally stimulating activities—but not games marketed as enhancing cognition—have been found to relieve cognitive decline associated with aging.

For more information about symptoms common to the menopause transition, including depression and cognitive problems, as well as evidence-based treatment options, the North American Menopause Society has freely available research-based information and resources (www.menopause.org).

Conclusion

PMS, PMDD, depression, and other concerns during the menopause transition are common yet need not be simply endured. Females experiencing such problems should talk with their medical provider. Treatments to alleviate or minimize symptoms are readily available.

Recommended Reading

International Association for Premenstrual Disorders: What Is PMDD? Boston, MA, International Association for Premenstrual Disorders, 2019. Available at: https://iapmd.org/about-pmdd.

The North American Menopause Society: Mental Health at Menopause. Pepper Pike, OH, The North American Menopause Society, 2023. Available at: https://www.menopause.org/for-women/menopauseflashes/mental-health-at-menopause.

77

Comorbid Mood, Anxiety, and Substance Use Disorders

Kathleen T. Brady, M.D., Ph.D.

Introduction

Information from various sources, including scientific studies and clinical reports, suggests that mood and anxiety disorders, mood and anxiety symptoms, and substance use disorders (SUDs) commonly co-occur. The interaction between these disorders and symptoms is complex. Mood and anxiety disorders may be a risk factor for the development of SUDs. They also may modify the presentation and outcome of treatment for individuals with SUDs, and SUDs may modify the presentation, course of illness, and treatment outcomes for individuals with mood and anxiety disorders. Mood and anxiety symptoms also emerge during the course of intoxication and withdrawal from substances of abuse. In this chapter, I review the area of co-occurring mood and anxiety disorders and SUDs, addressing the prevalence and diagnostic and treatment issues.

Prevalence

Epidemiological studies conducted in the United States over the past 30 years have consistently found that mood and anxiety disorders and SUDs co-occur more commonly than would be expected by chance alone. The National Epidemiological Survey on Alcohol and Related Conditions (NESARC) is the most recent and largest survey study focused on psychiatric disorders and SUDs in the United States to date, including more than 43,000 adults. The study was designed to distinguish between independent (i.e., not due to withdrawal or intoxication) and substance-induced mood and anxiety disorders. More than 17% (17.7%) of respondents with an SUD in the past 12 months also met criteria for an anxiety disorder. Approximately 15% of those with any anxiety disorder in the past 12 months had at least one co-occurring SUD. More than 20% of participants with any SUD over the past 12 months met criteria for a mood disorder, and more than 19% of those with any mood disorder in the past 12 months had an SUD. Associations between SUDs and specific anxiety and mood disorders were virtually all significantly positive ($P<0.05$). Females are more likely than males to have multiple comorbidities (i.e., three or more co-occurring psychiatric diagnoses in addition to SUDs). The findings of the NESARC were largely consistent with two earlier, large-scale epidemiological studies, the Epidemiologic Catchment Area (ECA) and the National Comorbidity Survey (NCS). In general, these studies found that individuals with anxiety disorders were twice as likely to have an SUD than those without anxiety disorders (odds ratio [OR] ~2.0), with panic disorder being the specific anxiety disorder most likely to be associated with SUD (OR ~3.0). Individuals with mood disorders in general are three times as likely to have a lifetime SUD (OR ~3.0), with bipolar disorder being the specific mood disorder most likely to be associated with SUD (OR ~4.0).

Relationship Between Mood and Anxiety and Substance Use Disorders

Several possible explanations exist for the common co-occurrence of mood and anxiety disorders with SUDs. The *causal hypothesis* suggests that having a mood or anxiety disorder can lead to the development of an SUD, or vice versa. There may be an indirect causal relationship with an intermediary causal agent. Alternatively, factors may exist that are common to both the substance use and mental health conditions, increasing the likelihood that they will co-occur.

The *self-medication hypothesis* posits a direct causal relationship, such that substances are used in an attempt to medicate the symptoms of an underlying mood or anxiety symptom. In some cases, the mood and anxiety symptoms may worsen after the substance use has ceased because the symptoms of withdrawal from many substances include anxiety and mood alterations. Alternatively, substance intoxication and withdrawal can induce a variety of symptoms, including depression, generalized anxiety, and manic symptoms. In most cases, the mood or anxiety symptoms subside and eventually disappear with abstinence, which helps distinguish substance-induced symptoms from true comorbidity. An indirect causal relationship exists if one condition impacts an intermediary factor that, in turn, increases the likelihood of developing the other condition. For example, research has shown that early-onset substance use reduces the likelihood of educational success, which may lead to later-life difficulties (e.g., unemployment) that could predispose to the development of other problems, such as depression.

The co-occurrence of two conditions can also be the result of shared biological, psychological, social, or environmental risk factors. For example, both substance and mental health conditions have been associated with lower socioeconomic status, childhood sexual and/or physical abuse, conduct disorder in childhood, and antisocial personality disorder. It is also possible that a genetic vulnerability to one disorder may increase the risk of developing another.

A growing body of evidence implicates common neurobiological pathways and abnormalities involved in SUDs and mood and anxiety disorders. Using a neurobiological framework, two hypotheses can be postulated to explain comorbidity: 1) SUDs and mood and anxiety disorders may be different symptomatic expressions of similar preexisting neurobiological abnormalities; or 2) repeated substance use, through neuroadaptation, can lead to biological changes that share common elements with the abnormalities seen in mood and anxiety disorders.

Course of Illness

There is a growing awareness that people with co-occurring SUDs and mood or anxiety disorders have a more severe clinical course and worse outcomes than those with uncomplicated mood or anxiety or SUDs. Alcohol and drug use are associated with mood destabilization in individuals with mood disorders. For example, one study comparing participants with co-occurring bipolar disorder and SUD with others who have uncomplicated bipolar disorder found that substance users had an earlier age at onset for mood disorder, more frequent hospitalizations, and more comorbid psychiatric disorders. For anxiety disorders, the situation is similar. Intoxication with stimulants is associated with anxiety and can lead to panic attacks. Withdrawal from opioids, alcohol, benzodiazepines, and other substances is also associated with anxiety symptoms. Once developed, evidence suggests that symptoms of mood or anxiety disorders and SUDs sustain one another, forming a positive feedback loop that can heighten the severity and duration and worsen the treatment response for all disorders. The relationship between SUDs, mood and anxiety disorders, and suicidality has long been recognized. A number of studies have demonstrated that a co-occurring SUD increases the risk for suicide in individuals with either a mood or anxiety disorder. The disinhibition and despair often associated with intoxication likely may lead to an increase in impulsive and self-destructive acts. In conclusion, it appears that SUDs have an adverse impact on the course and prognosis of mood and anxiety disorders, leading to more frequent hospitalizations and treatment-resistant symptoms.

Treatment

Optimal treatment of co-occurring mood or anxiety disorders and SUDs involves the integration of services and effective treatments from both the psychiatric and substance use fields and involves both medications and psychotherapy.

Psychotherapeutic Treatments

Cognitive-behavioral therapies (CBTs) are among the most effective treatments for mood and anxiety disorders and SUDs. Common elements in CBT, regardless of the disorder targeted, include relaxation, coping skills, behavioral activation, problem solving, and sleep hygiene, all of which can help patients who have these disorders. Over the past 20 years, CBT treatments for specific co-occurring conditions have been developed by blending elements from successful treatments for each condition into one treatment manual.

Alcoholics Anonymous and Narcotics Anonymous groups are found in all communities, and active participation can be a major factor in a person's recovery. Individuals with co-occurring mood or anxiety disorders and SUDs should choose 12-step recovery groups in which they are not likely to receive mixed or negative messages about the use of psychotropic medications under the directions of a physician.

The use of nonpharmacological treatments is important for several reasons. First, the ability to self-regulate subjective states and the confidence that can result from successful mastery through behavioral therapy can be extremely helpful to individuals in recovery. Second, learning strategies to self-regulate mood and anxiety symptoms may help patients break out of the mindset of using external agents to combat intolerable subjective states and help them acquire alternative coping strategies.

Pharmacological Treatment

Rapid and continuing progress has been made in the development of pharmacological agents to treat both SUDs and mood and anxiety disorders. Unfortunately, little research has been done on the efficacy and safety of such agents in the treatment of the comorbid condition. In the absence of specific information about pharmacotherapeutic treatment of a co-occurring condition, the best approach is to use a medication with demonstrated efficacy in the mood or anxiety disorder being treated, with special considerations related to the SUD in mind.

These considerations include paying particular attention to potential toxic interactions with drugs and alcohol, should relapse occur, and assessing the abuse potential of the agent being used. Whenever possible, using one medication that has efficacy in the treatment of both disorders is ideal. Growth has occurred in the development of pharmacotherapeutic agents for the treatment of alcohol, nicotine, and opiate dependence; however, little exploration has been done into the use of agents targeting SUDs in individuals with co-occurring psychiatric disorders. Much more systematic investigation in this area is needed.

Conclusion

There is growing interest in the co-occurrence of mood and substance use disorders. Co-occurrence of these disorders is common and has an impact on the prognosis and course of both disorders. The diagnostic issues at the interface of drug or alcohol use disorders and affective illnesses are particularly difficult because of the substantial symptom overlap between substance intoxication and withdrawal and the symptoms of affective disorders.

Over the past few years, advances have been made in the treatment of co-occurring disorders. Further investigation of specifically tailored treatments for patients with co-occurring substance use and other mood disorders is under way. Many advances have been made in the pharmacotherapy of mood disorders in recent years, and this progress will impact individuals with co-occurring disorders because newer agents with less toxicity, fewer side effects, and fewer interactions with substances of abuse will be evaluated in the treatment of the comorbid condition. Specific considerations when choosing a pharmacological agent for use in patients with SUDs include safety, toxicity, and abuse liability.

Although few studies specifically target pharmacotherapy for co-occurring disorders, those that have been conducted indicate that similar pharmacotherapeutic agents work for patients with mood disorders with or without SUDs. In conclusion, although the co-occurrence of SUDs and mood disorders is an important area in which recent developments provide cause for considerable optimism, much work remains to be done.

Recommended Reading

Grant BF, Stinson FS, Dawson DA, et al: Prevalence and co-occurrence of substance use disorders and independent mood and anxiety disorders: results from the National Epidemiologic Survey on Alcohol and Related Conditions. Arch Gen Psychiatry 61:807–816, 2004

Sofuoglu M, Rosenheck R, & Petrakis I: Pharmacological treatment of comorbid PTSD and substance use disorder: recent progress. Addict Behav 39(2):428–433, 2014

78

Comorbid Autism Spectrum Disorder and Anxiety/Depression

Susan W. White, Ph.D.
Jong-Woo Suh, B.A., M.A.
Nicole R. Friedman, B.S., M.A.

Prevalence of Comorbidity

Autism spectrum disorder (ASD) is characterized by difficulties associated with social interaction and communication across diverse contexts and atypical patterns of activities and behaviors, such as repetitive behaviors or narrow focus of interest. When researchers first started tracking the number of autistic people in 2000, ASD was considered to be a relatively rare condition. However, with the steady increase in the estimated prevalence of ASD, it is now considered a more common condition than we once believed. Some researchers argue that the increase in the number of autistic people is due primarily to increased awareness of the disorder, while others argue that other factors have contributed to the increase of ASD in the population. In general, ASD is more common among males than females. In addition, it can be found across all ethnic, cultural, and socioeconomic groups. However, ASD is more likely to be recognized earlier in development among White people and families from a higher socioeconomic status, which is likely attributable to differential access and disparities in the receipt of diagnostic services.

Comorbidity is the presence of one or more conditions in a person. Many autistic people have psychiatric comorbidities. For example, it is estimated that upward of one in two autistic individuals also have at least one other co-occurring mental health disorder. Depression and anxiety are perhaps the most commonly seen co-occurring diagnoses in this population. Internalizing problems, which include both depression and anxiety, limit functional independence and quality of life. In addition, problems related to depression and anxiety are unlikely to abate on their own without treatment and have been linked with other serious concerns (e.g., suicidality).

Depression and anxiety affect autistic people throughout their life span. Scientific evidence, however, suggests that these disorders may become more problematic with age, perhaps due to developmental changes, such as the increasingly complex social milieu of high school and the loss of services upon exiting high school. Although research has produced inconsistent findings to date, there is some indication that anxiety and mood problems may be more prevalent among autistic people who do not have intellectual impairment.

Why Is Comorbidity So Common?

Autistic individuals may be at an increased risk for co-occurring mood and anxiety problems due to characteristics and difficulties associated with having ASD. For example, autistic individuals experience difficulties associated with social interaction and communication across different contexts. More specifically, they may have challenges with taking the perspective of other people during conversations. This can be frustrating to peers and lead to less interaction. In addition, the autistic person may have difficulty anticipating other people's responses. These sociocognitive impairments sometimes prevent autistic individuals from successfully developing and maintaining social relationships and contribute to increased experiences of social rejection and feelings of loneliness. Ultimately, all of these factors may lead to increased mood and anxiety problems.

Autistic individuals also may be at an increased risk for co-occurring mood and anxiety problems due to challenges related to emotion regulation. *Emotion dysregulation*, or difficulty in effectively managing affective and behavioral reactions during stressful situations, is believed to be a primary risk factor for the development of mood and anxiety problems. Biological, genetic, and neural processes may also play a role in the emergence of comorbidity. Symptoms of mood and anxiety problems may arise during adolescence, in part due to uneven neural development. Specifically, the subcortical limbic regions of the brain, which are functionally involved in emotional experiences, may be more heavily engaged during socioemotional processing than the prefrontal regions in autistic individuals, leading to greater sensitivity to stressors and fewer coping resources.

These risk factors are not universal and may vary from person to person. In other words, there are multiple pathways to, for example, a co-occurring diagnosis of depression. It can sometimes be helpful to consider risk factors because this can help inform treatment.

Identification and Diagnosis

It often is unclear whether concerning behaviors represent problems with anxiety or depression or are attributable to ASD. For example, social withdrawal (e.g., spending more time alone), elaborate rituals (e.g., having a multistep bedtime routine involving a parent), and repetitive reassurance-seeking (e.g., checking to be sure the parent is available) can be indicative of internalizing problems, as well as ASD. Concerned family members should consider whether the behavior or symptom represents a "change from baseline"—in other words, look for new behaviors or worsening symptoms as being possible indicators of secondary mood or anxiety problems. Sometimes autistic individuals can verbalize feelings of depression or anxiety (although these words might not be used); often, however, clinicians and family members must rely on observable behaviors in order to identify these problems, especially among people who are minimally verbal.

Diagnostic overshadowing refers to the attribution of all behaviors or symptoms to one disorder (i.e., the ASD diagnosis), without fully considering the impact of one diagnosis on another or the possibility that another condition may be present. Although there is increasing recognition of psychiatric disorders in autistic individuals, three main factors can complicate the diagnosis and even delay the delivery of appropriate treatment: 1) symptom overlap (e.g., ascribing a behavior to ASD that is actually signaling another condition), 2) variability in presentation of ASD core symptoms (e.g., the appearance of symptom changes over the course of development); and 3) indicators of the second disorder being missed because they are atypical in nature (e.g., unusual phobia). Therefore, autistic individuals who display observable changes from baseline must be properly assessed and evaluated for possible co-occurring conditions. To secure an evaluation, you should discuss your concerns with your medical or primary care provider to obtain resources or a referral for psychological assessment in your local area.

Treatment Considerations

Increased efforts have been made to develop and test interventions targeting co-occurring mental health conditions in ASD. This has been approached in two ways: developing new interventions specific to autistic individuals or adapting existing interventions for mental health conditions in other groups for use in autistic individuals. For example, increasing parent involvement, adding visual supports, using more concrete language, or incorporating interests are common modifications to help make therapy more successful for the autistic person.

Cognitive-behavioral therapy (CBT) is an intervention focused on identifying maladaptive thought patterns and sometimes challenging them or identifying more helpful cognitive interpretations in order to alter patterns of thinking, emotional responses, and behaviors. CBT is considered a first-line treatment for mental health problems (e.g., anxiety, depression), and its effectiveness with nonautistic and autistic people has been strongly supported by research. Several studies have supported the use of CBT, with some modifications, for autistic individuals. Clinicians may choose to focus more heavily on the behavioral aspects of ASD, particularly for individuals with lower verbal skills and those who may have more limited flexibility in thinking. In these cases, behavioral strategies may be more helpful to promote socialization opportunities, improve adaptive behaviors, set life goals, and otherwise support healthy lifestyle choices.

Although research suggests that CBT can reduce anxiety and depression in autistic individuals, medications are also often used. CBT is likely more cost-effective and may show more sustained improvements; however, medications are frequently used to treat co-occurring mental health symptoms in autistic individuals. Many of the medication trials have had inconsistent results in terms of their effectiveness in improving symptoms. This may be due to difficulty separating improvements in co-occurring anxiety and depression from core ASD symptoms or associated behaviors. As with nonautistic individuals, a combined approach to treatment (i.e., medication and CBT) likely is optimal for addressing anxiety and depression.

Conclusion

Many autistic individuals, children through adults, struggle with depression and anxiety. Since the early 2000s, awareness of this comorbidity has increased among health service professionals, and the research base has grown steadily. Although differential, accurate diagnosis can be challenging, psychosocial and pharmaceutical evidence-based options are available for treatment. Parents and other family members or caregivers are important as historians (to document and report patient behaviors and symptoms during assessment) and as advocates (in securing appropriate treatment).

Recommended Reading

Spain D, Musich FM, White SW (eds): Psychological Therapies for Adults With Autism. New York, Oxford University Press, 2022

White SW, Maddox BB, Mazefsky CA (eds): The Oxford Handbook of Autism and Co-Occurring Psychiatric Conditions. New York, Oxford University Press, 2020

79

Laboratory Tests

Eric Chen, M.D.
Cristina Montalvo, M.D., M.B.S.
Paul Summergrad, M.D.

Introduction

Researchers have worked for decades to find a laboratory test that would accurately diagnose people with an anxiety or depressive disorder. Unfortunately, no such test has yet been discovered. However, your doctor can order tests to help them confirm whether your symptoms of anxiety or depression are due to a primary psychiatric condition or to a medical disorder. Many different medical conditions can cause symptoms similar to those experienced by people with an anxiety disorder or a depressive disorder. In those cases, the person would be diagnosed with that medical condition rather than with a mental health issue. In this chapter, we focus on tests that your doctor may order to make sure no undiagnosed medical conditions are causing your symptoms. Your doctor may choose to order only some of these tests or even other tests not listed here.

Thyroid-Stimulating Hormone

The thyroid is an organ located in the neck and controlled by the brain that helps maintain our body *metabolism*—how we handle many different functions.

This includes almost everything our body does, including how fast our heart beats, how our hair grows, and how quickly we digest food. The way that our brain controls our thyroid is through *thyroid-stimulating hormone* (TSH). As the name implies, the more TSH our brain makes, the more our thyroid tells our bodies to run, and the less TSH it makes, the less our thyroid tells our bodies to run. When our thyroid is telling our body to run too slowly, it is called *hypothyroidism*. When our thyroid is telling our body to run too quickly, it is called *hyperthyroidism*.

People with hypothyroidism can seem depressed because they may have low mood, low energy, and no appetite. People with hyperthyroidism can often seem as though they have anxiety because they might feel on edge, sweaty, and have a fast heartbeat. By checking a TSH level, your doctor can make sure your thyroid is telling your body to run at the right speed and that your symptoms of anxiety or depression are not due to a thyroid abnormality. Most standard laboratory tests place the upper end of the "normal" range for TSH to be 5 mIU/L (milli-international units per liter) or 5.5 mIU/L. Any values higher than this range suggest hypothyroidism. However, evidence indicates that any level above 3.5 mIU/L is a risk factor for depression and requires thyroid hormone supplementation.

Complete Blood Count

A *complete blood count* (CBC) looks at the different parts of your blood such as your platelets, white blood cells, and red blood cells. *Platelets* help to stop bleeding, while *white blood cells* help to keep your body safe from infection. Both are important to keep you healthy. Your doctor will be interested in your level of *red blood cells*, which carry oxygen around your body. Not having enough red blood cells is called *anemia*. Anemia can make you feel tired, weak, and short of breath, which can easily be confused with an anxiety or depressive disorder. It has also been linked with depression by the chemical changes it causes in your brain! By checking a CBC, your doctor makes sure you do not have anemia. If you do have anemia, more tests may be needed to figure out which type of anemia you have.

Folate

Folate, which is also known as vitamin B_9, is an important vitamin that we cannot live without. Your body needs folate to make new red blood cells. Red blood cells only survive for about 120 days, and if your body cannot make enough new ones, you will become anemic, resulting in symptoms that could be mistaken for anxiety or depression. We obtain folate through our normal diet, in particular from leafy greens, nuts, beans, seafood, eggs, and meat. Common causes of low folate include heavy alcohol use, not eating enough food, poor absorption by our bodies, medications, and pregnancy. By checking your folate level, your doctor makes sure your body has enough of it to function properly.

Vitamin B_{12}

Vitamin B_{12}, also known as *cobalamin,* is another important vitamin that often works with folate in our bodies. Similar to folate, a low vitamin B_{12} level will cause anemia, causing symptoms that can mimic anxiety and depression. Low B_{12} levels also impact the brain and can cause a drop in your ability to think clearly, which can also be mistaken for depression. The biggest source of vitamin B_{12} for us is red meat, as well as poultry, eggs, and dairy products. People with low B_{12} levels are fairly rare because our bodies can store a lot of it. Occasionally, people consuming a vegetarian diet may have low B_{12} levels. By checking your vitamin B_{12} level, your doctor makes sure your body has enough of it to function properly.

Blood Glucose

Glucose is a type of sugar, and it is the body's main source and the brain's sole source of fuel. Our brain, in particular, uses a lot of energy. Despite being only about 2% of our body weight, it uses 20% of our body's glucose! That is why when the blood glucose level in our blood is low, also known as *hypoglycemia,* our brain has trouble doing its job. Periods of hypoglycemia can easily be mistaken for an anxiety disorder because common symptoms include a fast heartbeat, shaking, sweating, and feeling nervous. In extreme cases, hypoglycemia can cause people to become confused and not know where they are or what they are doing. Very high glucose levels, especially in older persons, may also be associated with confusion, fatigue, and sleepiness. Hypoglycemia is most common in people with diabetes when they take too much insulin and can be less frequently due to other medications or certain types of cancers. Blood glucose levels that fluctuate a lot throughout the day are also associated with lower moods. By checking your blood glucose level, your doctor makes sure it is in the normal range.

Electrocardiogram

Our heart uses electrical signals to make sure that it pumps in sync to get blood to all parts of the body. An *electrocardiogram* (ECG) allows your doctor to look at this electrical activity. An ECG reveals multiple things about your heart, such as the speed and rhythm of your heartbeats because problems with these can lead to symptoms of anxiety and depression. For example, sometimes our heart can be "miswired," causing it to beat much faster than it should for short periods of time. Often, people can become sweaty and breathe quickly during this time as well. These periods can easily be mistaken for the type of anxiety seen in a primary anxiety disorder. In other people, their heartbeat can become irregular and feel as though it is skipping beats, causing the heart to pump blood less effectively than usual. This can cause weakness, fatigue, and a lack of interest in doing things, which may look like depression. By checking an ECG, your doctor makes sure your heart is beating properly.

Liver Function Tests

The liver is the main organ in which our bodies break down toxins and make them safe for our bodies to dispose. When your liver starts malfunctioning, toxins can start building up in your blood. Liver malfunction can be due to a variety of causes such as heavy alcohol use, infections, and medication reactions. These toxins can affect your brain, causing changes in how you think and act, which is known as *hepatic encephalopathy*. People with hepatic encephalopathy may seem confused, with poor memory, concentration, and judgment. They may have difficulty staying alert and have issues with sleep at night. Hepatic encephalopathy can cause people to feel anxious and feel more down than usual. All of these symptoms can easily be confused with an anxiety or depressive disorder.

Liver function tests (LFTs) are a group of tests that can give your doctor an idea of what is wrong with your liver. Your doctor may be able to look at which of the tests are abnormal, and by how much, to get an idea of what may be the cause of the liver problem. This can sometimes lead to other diagnostic tests or procedures to treat the liver condition.

Vitamin D

It has long been known that vitamin D helps the body absorb calcium, a mineral that helps build strong bones. More recently, researchers have discovered many more roles for vitamin D than previously thought. For example, researchers determined that it plays a large role in our immune system, which defends against infections. Some studies have even revealed that people with lower levels of vitamin D are more likely to die from the coronavirus disease 2019 (COVID-19) infection. Vitamin D also plays a role in our mood. Multiple studies have shown that lower levels of this vitamin are associated with depression. However, the evidence is mixed as to whether taking vitamin D supplements can help with depression. Although vitamin D levels are not regularly tested, your doctor may order testing if they suspect you have a deficiency.

Testosterone

Testosterone, commonly called the male sex hormone, is most known for causing the development of male features such as facial hair and a deeper voice. It is also responsible for building muscle, strengthening bones, and sexual function. Testosterone plays a similar role in females, but to a lesser degree. Testosterone plays a key role in the quality of life of males. Low levels of testosterone can lead to low sex drive, erectile dysfunction, and weakness, as well as symptoms of anxiety and depression. Multiple studies have shown that testosterone levels tend to be lower in males who are depressed. However, more research needs to be done to determine whether supplemental testosterone is a good treatment for depression in males, and it is not a treatment for everyone. Testing testosterone levels is not regularly done for evaluation of anxiety or depression; however, if you are having symptoms of low testosterone, your doctor may check your level.

Conclusion

Making the diagnosis of an anxiety disorder or a depressive disorder is important to help you obtain the right treatment. However, it is equally important to ensure that your symptoms are not the result of a specific medical condition because these can easily be confused with a mental health issue. By having these tests done, you and your doctor can ensure the correct diagnosis and treatment.

Recommended Reading

Levenson J (ed): American Psychiatric Association Publishing Textbook of Psychosomatic Medicine and Consultation-Liaison Psychiatry, 3rd Edition. Washington, DC, American Psychiatric Association Publishing, 2019

Summergrad P, Silbersweig DA, Muskin PR, et al (eds): Textbook of Medical Psychiatry. Washington, DC, American Psychiatric Association Publishing, 2020

80

Pharmacogenetic Testing

Joseph F. Goldberg, M.D.

Introduction

Patients and their families are often enchanted by the notion of what their genes can tell about them. A *gene* is a stretch of DNA—the coding molecules in our cells that provide the blueprint for creating proteins, enzymes, and other necessary products in the human body. Psychiatric disorders, generally speaking, are often under some genetic influence, but not in the same way as diseases that are strictly inherited, such as muscular dystrophy or sickle cell anemia. In purely genetic disorders, a mutation in a single gene causes an abnormality that results in a distinct syndrome. By contrast, other kinds of diseases have *some* genetic contribution but are not usually the result of a mutation in a single gene making a big impact. These are called *complex traits*, which means that multiple genes, each exerting some small effect, contribute (along with interactions with the environment) to produce a disease state. Most psychiatric disorders follow complex trait genetics.

Genetics and Medication Effectiveness

What does all of this have to do with the field of pharmacogenetics? It is against this backdrop that we ask to what extent medication response may have a genetic or heritable component. If a patient's sibling with depression got better with a particular antidepressant, does that mean that this patient should take the same agent, based on the belief that medication response predictably runs in families? Nobody really knows for sure, with just a few exceptions. Lithium, which is a cornerstone agent used in the treatment of bipolar disorder, seems to have a fairly high rate of *concordance* (meaning that if it did or did not work for a first-degree relative, it should have a similar effect for you). Scant data also exist regarding the use of some selective serotonin reuptake inhibitor (SSRI) antidepressants for depression. Beyond these examples, whether medication response is heritable remains uncertain.

Separate from the heritability of medication response is the more complicated question of whether there may be certain genes—such as those involved in the processing and breakdown of psychiatric medicines, but sometimes even more obscure genes without such obvious roles in brain functioning—that can influence (and inform) that response. At the present time, we have no sure-fire way to predict from a person's DNA what medicine will or will not work for them. However, sometimes genetic testing can predict which agent may work *poorly* for a given patient or be more likely to cause side effects. This is because genes are known to exert control over the enzymes in our gut and our liver that break down (*metabolize*) certain medicines, including most psychiatric medications. When a gene comes in more than one form, these variants are known as *polymorphisms*. A genetic polymorphism could result in a gene that makes a product (e.g., an enzyme or a protein) that works unusually well or poorly in a particular biochemical pathway.

Consider, for example, the polymorphic genes controlling the enzymes that break down and metabolize medications. For most of the population, these genes work normally, and individuals with such genes are called "extensive metabolizers." However, for a small portion of the population (anywhere from 2%–10% and sometimes higher), often differing across ethnic and racial groups, genes can code for enzymes that metabolize a medication too quickly (called *ultra-rapid metabolizers*) or too slowly or even not at all (called *poor metabolizers*). For someone who is an ultra-rapid metabolizer, a normally dosed agent may have minimal effect because their body breaks it down too quickly. Thus, they may need larger-than-usual dosages, or that medicine may not work at all. In poor metabolizers, the body breaks down a medicine too slowly, leading to one of two results: 1) the agent may build up, causing excessive side effects, or 2) medicines that must be broken down for conversion to their more active form may not have an effect. One example of the latter is the antidepressant venlafaxine, which needs to be broken down in the liver to an active metabolite called desmethylvenlafaxine. If that metabolic step does not occur, or it occurs too slowly, the active metabolite will not be formed in sufficient quantities to have an effect.

Genetics and Medication Safety

Pharmacogenetics can be useful in certain situations to ensure medication safety. For example, a gene called *HLA-B*1502* is involved in producing certain cells in the immune system. In people who descend from Southeast Asia, the presence of *HLA-B*1502* increases their chances of developing a uniquely severe and dangerous rash reaction to carbamazepine. The U.S. Food and Drug Administration (FDA) even requires that people of Southeast Asian ancestry undergo testing to determine whether this gene is present before they can be prescribed carbamazepine. Another example involves people who are genetically poor metabolizers for a liver enzyme called cytochrome P450 2D6 (CYP2D6), which breaks down certain medicines. Some psychiatric medicines can cause heart rhythm problems if levels become too high. If such a medicine was metabolized by someone who is a CYP2D6 poor metabolizer, a serious cardiac arrhythmia could result.

Both of these examples are relatively rare. More broadly, people who are poor metabolizers may just incur more side effects from the medications they cannot efficiently metabolize, or they might have a known variation of a specific gene or set of genes that is associated with higher risk of a particular side effect, such as weight gain, immune system suppression, or sexual dysfunction. Knowing a person's pharmacogenetic profile might help predict the chances of certain side effects occurring with certain medicines, but genetic testing to predict side effects is not 100% foolproof, and some studies have failed to show that pharmacogenetically guided treatment leads to fewer or less burdensome side effects.

Is Pharmacogenetic Testing Effective and Useful?

In 2018, the FDA issued a consumer warning against routine pharmacogenetic testing, stating that "the relationship between DNA variations and the effectiveness of antidepressant medication has never been established" (www.fda.gov/MedicalDevices/Safety/AlertsandNotices/ucm624725.htm). What does this mean for patients who have tried one or more medicines for depression or other psychiatric problems and have not experienced a benefit and now wonder whether pharmacogenetic testing can be useful or should be ordered? The short answer is that, unfortunately, no genetic test will magically answer this question. The best of studies tell us that, in people with major depression, using a pharmacogenetics test may boost the chances of a response to a particular medication only by about 5% or so above and beyond knowledge about nongenetic factors that influence response. However, in some instances, pharmacogenetic testing may still answer a specific question about whether one type of medicine may be better tolerated than another or may provide information regarding genetic variations that might be useful to know when deciding whether a specific agent should be dosed higher or lower than usual.

Many factors besides genetics can influence medication response, such as the severity and duration of symptoms, the presence of multiple psychiatric conditions, the person's level of work and social functioning or support earlier in life, or a history of early life adversity or trauma. Also, from among the approximately 20,500 genes in the human genome, less than 10% code for proteins or other products that have an actual function in the human body (e.g., making a neurotransmitter, metabolizing substances, making molecules that nourish brain cells and keep them healthy). Besides the genes that code for enzymes that break down medications, a handful of so-called candidate genes could be relevant to psychopharmacology, such as those involved in manufacturing brain chemicals (e.g., serotonin) or receptors on nerve cells that become activated by these chemicals. However, very little is now known about which genes actually influence these proteins, chemicals, and receptors or how psychiatric medications actually produce their effects, and, as complex traits, their effects are small. In other words, until we have a better understanding about which genes actually (and not just theoretically) influence medication response, it is premature to rely on pharmacogenetic testing when deciding which agents will be most helpful for a given patient.

What Does a Pharmacogenetic Report Tell You?

A typical commercially produced pharmacogenetics report comes in several sections. One section usually describes variants a person may have in the genes that code for the individual cytochrome P450 enzymes that break down medications or can lead to medication interactions. Another section summarizes the genetic variations that are thought to play a role in how a medication affects the body, such as a gene that codes for the serotonin transporter (*SLC6A4*), which is a target of SSRIs, or a gene that codes for brain-derived neurotrophic factor (*BDNF*), which promotes nerve cell growth and whose expression can be influenced by a number of psychiatric agents. Whether or not variations in these genes truly lead to predictably better or worse effects from a given medication remains an active area of research. Manufacturers of pharmacogenetic products usually weave together several or more specific gene variants (in a process called *combinatorial pharmacogenetics*) that they propose may have unique value in predicting the likelihood of medication response. Reports often include a summary page that identifies medicines to "use as directed" or "use with caution." This is a shorthand way of indicating that patients who are poor metabolizers or are ultra-rapid metabolizers of medications that go through specific enzyme pathways may have an inefficient processing system and may consequently experience either a buildup of side effects or lack of efficacy or may eliminate the agent so quickly that benefits may not be achieved at the usual dosages.

Conclusion

Pharmacogenetics for predicting medication efficacy remains a promising area of scientific study, but technology has not, as of yet, advanced to the point that a laboratory can confidently determine from a cheek swab test of someone's DNA the chances that any particular agent is more or less likely to have a desired effect. Although pharmacogenetics sometimes can be help clinicians know which medicines may be less successful, it does not necessarily point to which will work best.

Recommended Reading

Bertino JSS: Pharmacogenomics: An Introduction and Clinical Perspective. New York, McGraw Hill Professional, 2012

Goldberg JF: Do you order pharmacogenetic testing? Why? J Clin Psychiatry 78(8):1155–1156, 2017 28796939

81

Brain Imaging for Anxiety or Depression

Martin P. Paulus, M.D.

Introduction

In this brief chapter, we describe the different techniques that are being used to take images of the brain, with an emphasis on what these techniques measure. After that, we describe basic insights into brain-based circuits that are important for anxiety and depression. We also briefly review how this information can be used to assess risk for these conditions and the effects of treatment. Finally, we outline what still needs to be done to make imaging more impactful on treatments and outcomes in individuals with anxiety or depression.

What Is Brain Imaging and How Is It Done?

It has long been the hope of mental health professionals that imaging the brain can help to better diagnose, prognose, or treat people with anxiety or depression. The first *computed tomography* (CT) picture of the brain was produced on October 1, 1971, in England, of a female patient with a brain tumor. Since then, brain imaging has seen a remarkable evolution. In 1977, physicists and radiologists obtained the first *magnetic resonance imaging* (MRI) brain scan, and in

1979, the first *positron emission tomography* (PET) brain image was obtained. In 1990, the MRI technique was extended to measure changes in how much oxygen is carried in blood vessels, which is called *functional magnetic resonance imaging* (fMRI), and provided a way to measure the activity of the living brain.

Computed Tomography

CT uses X-rays and clever mathematical techniques to compute how easily those X-rays travel through different tissues in the body. This provides a way to display brain *gray matter*, which are the brain's nerve cells; *white matter*, which are the "cable" connections between different brain areas; *blood vessels*; and other details that could not be seen in a living person up to that point.

Magnetic Resonance Imaging

MRI uses a strong magnet and quickly changing magnetic impulses to assess the magnetic properties of different elements in the body. Clinical MRIs of the brain essentially measure the water content of different tissues. Like CTs, MRIs show gray matter, white matter, blood vessels, and other structures in the living brain, but unlike CTs, no X-rays are involved.

Positron Emission Tomography

PET uses a tiny amount of radioactive substance and sensors that measure radioactivity, along with sophisticated mathematical techniques, to create an image of the brain's metabolic activity. In other words, PET imaging shows how much energy different tissues in the brain consume.

Functional Magnetic Resonance Imaging

Finally, fMRI measures changes in how much oxygen is carried in the blood. Because the brain uses about one-fifth of all the energy consumed by a resting body, and oxygen is essential in generating that energy, the brain has an intricate mechanism for moving blood to where it is needed most. fMRI can show which parts of the brain need the most energy at any given time. Since the discovery of fMRI, researchers have used different ways to examine what the brain is doing; for example, showing pictures to a person being studied activates the part of their brain that processes pictures. This approach has been utilized to identify which parts of the brain are important when people think, feel, and act. Thus, for the first time, researchers could directly link what someone experiences internally with changes in their brain that can be measured objectively.

How Does Brain Imaging Relate to Diagnosing Anxiety and Depression?

Anxiety is an internal state. Therefore, when we measure levels of anxiety, we typically ask, "How anxious do you feel?" or "How worried are you?" as well as "How much has this experience interfered with your life?" and rely on the answers to help us identify who has an anxiety disorder. As in other medical specialties, mental health professionals want measures that can be used in addition to a patient's self-report of anxiety to help us diagnose, prognose, or treat that patient. How far have we come?

Using fMRI and clever probes, researchers have clearly delineated the brain systems important for the experience of anxiety and the differences between individuals who have anxiety disorders and those who do not. Much of this work benefited from previous studies in animals and humans with brain diseases or lesions that changed their behavior. A brain structure called the *amygdala* ("almond shape") and the degree to which it is active has been the most important area of study linked to anxiety. Brain imaging studies have shown that the experience of fear and anxiety is associated with greater activation in the amygdala. Moreover, physical responses such as high heart rate, sweating, or shallow breathing also have been linked to activation in parts of this region. Evidence has shown that individuals with anxiety show a relatively greater response in the amygdala when exposed to fearful stimuli (e.g., a spider, a snake, a threatening-looking person). These findings have helped us understand that a magnified response to fearful stimuli is one way to think about anxiety disorders.

Several other brain structures also have been implicated in these disorders. The *insula* is a structure that is particularly important in processing information coming from inside the body, such as how cold you feel or how fast your heart beats. Similar to what has been observed for the amygdala, people with anxiety show a greater response in the insula, which has been interpreted to mean that they are more sensitive to information from inside the body and may process this information with greater concern. Other important brain areas include the *hippocampus*, which is important for how memories are made and recovered, and the *medial prefrontal cortex*, which is critical for self-related processing. Together, these structures form a circuit that tends to overactivate in anxious individuals.

Can we take an image of these structures to help us diagnose or treat people with anxiety disorders? At this time, the answer is "no" for a number of reasons. First, the differences we can observe between people with and without anxiety are subtle, and there is a great deal of overlap in levels of activation between those who have no issues with anxiety and those who do. Second, the processes that contribute to developing an anxiety disorder are complex. We know that both genetic and environmental factors contribute to changes in how brain structures respond to threatening stimuli. Therefore, all anxiety involves a complex mixture of these processes, which results in a mixture of brain imaging findings. Third, no appropriate studies have been conducted that conclusively show brain imaging can help with diagnosing or treating people with anxiety.

Depression is the most common mental health condition worldwide. Feelings of sadness, a loss of interest in previously pleasurable activities, and other symptoms define this condition. Again, the goal of brain imaging is to find objective evidence for internal feeling states that can be used by mental health providers to better help patients with depression. Depressed individuals may have a difficult time experiencing positive events and, in some cases, may be more profoundly affected by negative events. These observations have been used to develop probes, together with fMRI, to identify the brain structures most consistently affected in people with depression. Among the most important structures is the *anterior cingulate cortex*, part of which has been shown to be less active in depression. Other parts of this structure can also be *more* active, particularly when people experience sadness.

Additional evidence has shown that depression emerges because of changes in the way different brain structures interact with one another. The brain structures that make up this circuit include the amygdala, the hippocampus, and the prefrontal cortex, which is important for making executive decisions. Some studies have determined that the functioning of this circuit improves when people no longer feel depressed. However, in other studies, brain imaging has revealed subtle structural and functional differences in these brain areas even in people without obvious symptoms of depression. The most consistent findings from both structural and functional neuroimaging studies are that the brain imaging findings in depression are diverse, which may be due to the fact that depressed individuals are diverse in terms of their genetic makeup and personal histories.

Current research helps us understand that the inner experience of sadness and loss of interest in activities in depression is mirrored by profound changes in the brain affecting multiple brain structures. On the other hand, what was said about anxiety is also true for depression: the current findings are not sufficiently precise and distinct to be used for diagnosis, prognosis, or treatment.

Conclusion

Where do we go from here? Anxiety and depression are internal experiential states that are associated with measurable structural and functional changes in the brain. Unfortunately, these changes are not like those observed in other medical specialties, such as a blood sugar level that helps diagnose diabetes. Instead, we still need to identify whether common patterns exist among people who experience depression or anxiety but have different biological and psychological constellations that contributed to these conditions. Larger studies are necessary to precisely measure anxiety and depression over time and to obtain brain images that can be related to these experiences. It will take these types of studies to determine whether imaging can be used for diagnosis and treatment in ways similar to how hemoglobin A1C is used for monitoring diabetes, blood pressure for predicting heart attacks or strokes, or liver enzymes for determining whether a treatment will have toxic effects on the body.

Recommended Reading

Janiri D, Moser DA, Doucet GE, et al: Shared neural phenotypes for mood and anxiety disorders: a meta-analysis of 226 task-related functional imaging studies. JAMA Psychiatry 77(2):172–179, 2020

Underwood E: Brain scans could help personalize treatment for people who are depressed or suicidal. Science, August 20, 2019. Available at: https://www.science.org/content/article/brain-scans-could-help-personalize-treatment-people-who-are-depressed-or-suicidal

82

Artificial Intelligence and Treatment

Adrienne Grzenda, M.D., Ph.D.

Introduction

Depression and anxiety can be treated effectively with medication, neuromodulation, or psychotherapy or a combination of these approaches. Finding the correct diagnosis and therapeutic approach for each individual, however, can take a long time. Although the stigma surrounding mental health has lessened, many people are still reluctant to seek assistance. Access to mental health care is also a significant barrier. Not enough experienced mental health providers are available to meet the current demand. Selecting the right medication or intervention is a trial-and-error process that may take weeks or even months to optimize. Finally, the conventional methods of monitoring improvement are often inadequate. These factors can impede initiation of or changes to treatment, delaying relief from suffering.

Artificial Intelligence Approaches to Anxiety and Depression

In response to these issues, clinicians and researchers are experimenting with new and augmented approaches to the diagnosis and treatment of depression and anxiety that use artificial intelligence (AI). *Artificial intelligence* is a general term for computer programs or algorithms that can perform tasks that would typically require human intelligence. AI has been around since the late 1950s, but recent advances in computing speed and power have reignited interest in its applications in medicine. A branch of AI called *machine learning* makes it possible for computers to learn without explicit programming. These machine learning algorithms learn from examples in order to make predictions or take actions based on patterns found in the data. Natural language processing (NLP) is an important subfield of AI that focuses on the interactions between computers and human language, especially how we program computers to comprehend speech or text. For instance, machine learning and NLP help digital assistants such as Apple's Siri and Amazon's Alexa respond to the questions asked by their users.

Health care generates enormous amounts of digital data (Figure 82–1). In fact, 30%–40% of all data in the world generated each year comes from health care. *Big data* is a term used to describe collections of very large amounts of data, often of different types (e.g., text and images). Big data are challenging to aggregate and analyze using conventional techniques. Electronic medical records, insurance claims, public health records, practitioners' notes, laboratory results, imaging, genome sequencing, and device outputs are just a few of the sources of health care big data. Smartphones, smartwatches, and other internet-enabled wearables are also increasingly used to collect information. The ability of machine learning and NLP algorithms to rapidly extract insights from complex data is arguably their most important advantage, especially in medicine, where time and resources are frequently in short supply.

For most tasks, machine learning algorithms use one of two types of "learning." A training dataset is used in the *supervised learning* process (Figure 82–2) that contains descriptive variables about each observation or person, otherwise known as *features* (e.g., age, sex, family history of depression), and the outcomes of interest (e.g., depressed or not depressed). The algorithm uses an iterative experimentation process to identify the relationships between the features and the outcomes. This procedure is repeated until its predictions of the outcomes are as accurate as possible (i.e., fewest wrong predictions). Once trained, the algorithm may be applied to new observations to predict unknown outcomes. *Unsupervised learning* is a type of machine learning in which the algorithm is given access to an unlabeled dataset and then searches for similarities between features in that

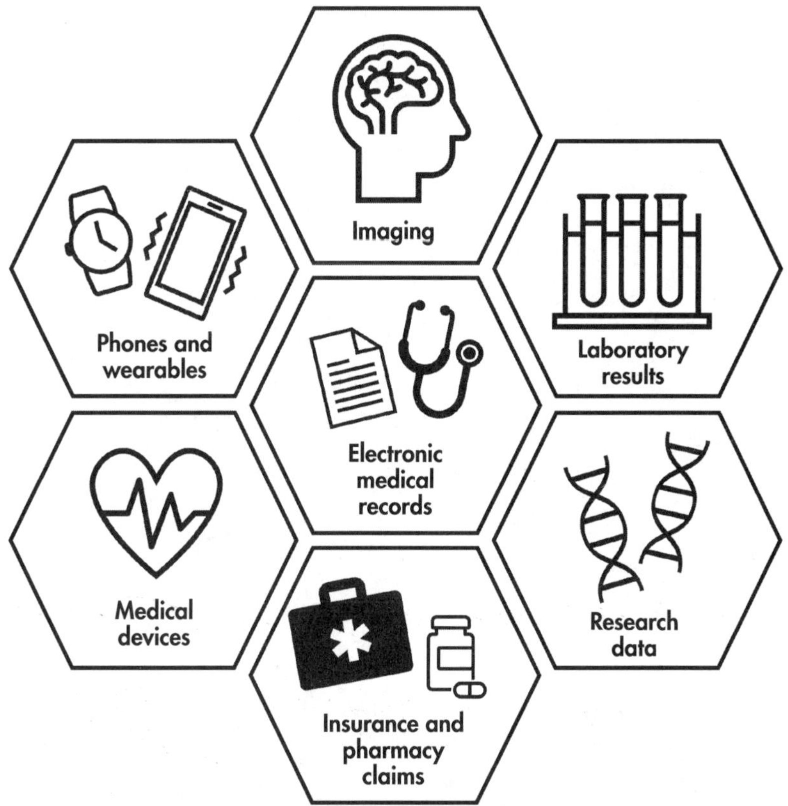

Figure 82–1. Sources of health care big data.

dataset in order to group (or cluster) observations. For instance, an unsupervised algorithm could classify people with anxiety into different subtypes based on their symptoms, sociodemographic information, and prior medications tried. NLP is often used to extract features from clinical notes (e.g., symptoms or medications described in a physician's notes) for input into machine learning models. Complex AI applications, such as OpenAI's ChatGPT, use a combination of supervised and unsupervised learning to accomplish sophisticated tasks.

How Can Artificial Intelligence Help With Mental Health Diagnoses?

AI systems can help address current challenges in the treatment of depression and anxiety in numerous ways, only a few of which are outlined here. Most AI

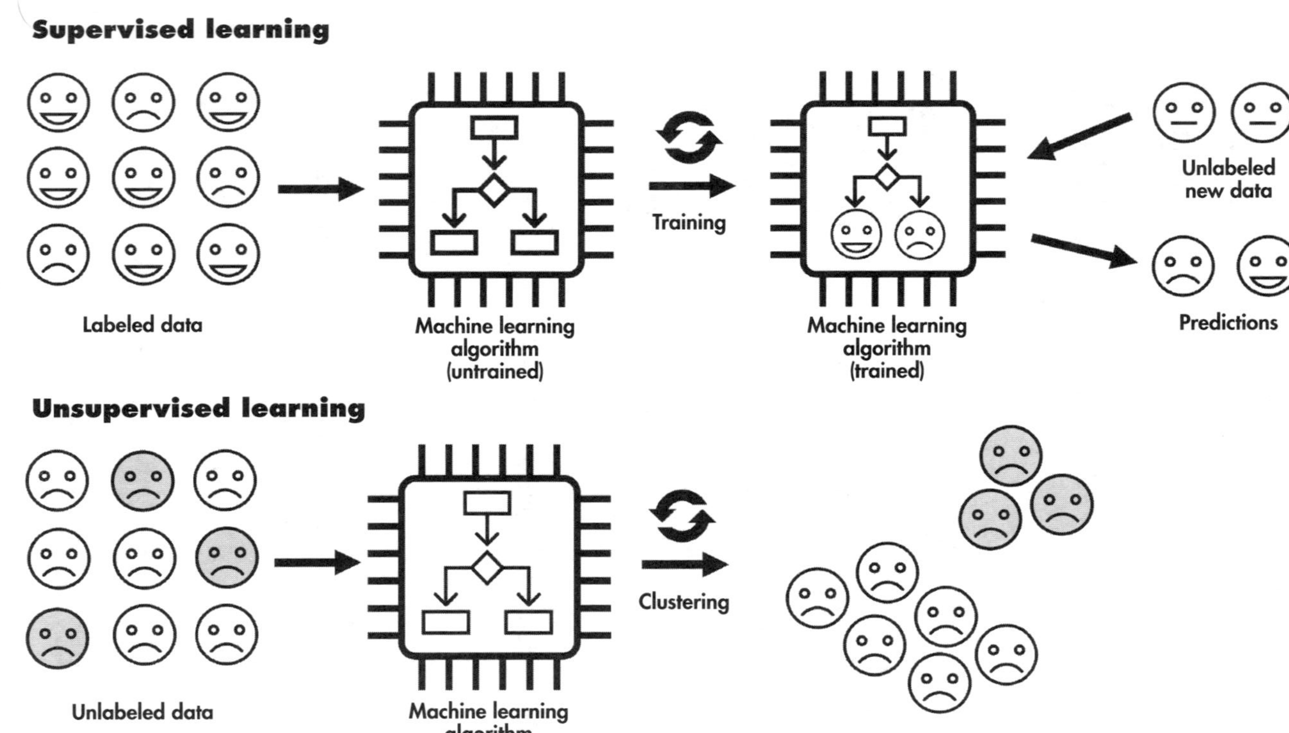

Figure 82–2. Supervised and unsupervised machine learning.

applications in mental health are still in the research phase, but at the rate at which the field is advancing, integration into clinical care is unquestionably on the horizon.

Earlier Diagnosis

Currently, diagnosis hinges on a given patient's self-reported symptoms; expert-determined criteria, such as the *Diagnostic and Statistical Manual of Mental Disorders* (DSM); and the clinician's judgment and observations. Data-driven AI methods can help reduce the amount of subjectivity and variability in the diagnostic process. If a person is experiencing high blood pressure, the diagnosis of hypertension is definitively made based on the result of the blood pressure reading. Objective tests of this nature are currently lacking in psychiatry. Studies have shown success using AI to analyze speech patterns and facial expressions from video-recorded patient visits in order to detect depression or anxiety symptoms and rate their severity. Collecting audio-video data is noninvasive and significantly cheaper than genetic testing or neuroimaging. Eventually, smartphone applications may be able to facilitate instantaneous and anonymous self-screening. AI approaches can also assist in the earlier detection of symptoms by learning informative patterns from high-dimensional data, such as magnetic resonance imaging (MRI) scans and genome-wide gene expression assays. NLP allows researchers to use novel, nonclinical data types, such as social media posts, to detect early illness; for example, people with depression tend to use more negative language in their social media posts.

Personalized Treatment Selection

Two people may describe identical symptoms but may respond differently to the same treatment. Many factors—including brain anatomy and connectivity, genetics, environment, exposures (e.g., life experiences, trauma, substance abuse), and co-occurring medical as well as psychiatric conditions—impact individual variability in treatment response. Unsupervised machine learning can determine whether these factors cluster into distinct biological subtypes that vary in their responsiveness to different treatments. Clinical trials are the current gold standard for determining treatment effectiveness, but trials focus on average treatment effects, usually for one medication or intervention. AI methods, by contrast, can readily integrate data from different treatments to develop individual-level predictions of response. Similar approaches can help predict whether someone may develop intolerable side effects to a medication or calculate the appropriate dosage to maximize benefits while minimizing adverse effects.

Improved Monitoring of Treatment Effectiveness

Typically, monitoring for symptom improvement occurs during follow-up visits, which may happen weeks or months apart. Depression and anxiety can affect a person's memory and recall of recent events and potentially obscure their progress when evaluated in this periodic fashion. The near-universal availability of smartphones makes the continuous collection of mood information from patients feasible. Studies have also shown that people are sometimes more comfortable disclosing sensitive information to an application than to a person. *Chatbots* are AI-driven applications capable of carrying on conversations using text or text-to-speech. They can ask patients questions about mood and medications without making them feel awkward or embarrassed. Rapid translation into preferred languages is also possible, further increasing patient comfort. AI applications can also accumulate background data from smart devices, such as the number of text messages sent, which could signify reduced communication and worsening mood. Researchers are actively investigating how these types of digital markers correlate with mental health symptoms. Collectively, improved monitoring data can provide clinicians and patients with a more comprehensive portrait of progress and facilitate more timely changes to the treatment plan.

Real-Time Interventions

AI-based treatment monitoring is not just about data collection. If worsening mood is detected, a chatbot or application could suggest an immediate course of action (e.g., calling a friend, going for a walk). If emergent symptoms are detected, such as suicidal ideation, the system can alert the provider to follow up immediately with the patient to discuss safety planning or pursue hospitalization. Ecological momentary interventions (EMIs) are treatments provided to patients between sessions in their home environment. EMIs help reinforce concepts and skills taught during therapy. For instance, if person's smartwatch detects a sudden and sustained increase in heart rate, it may suggest high anxiety or a panic attack, triggering a reminder to engage in a breathing exercise. Smart devices also allow dissemination of general alerts, such as reminders to take medications or to attend upcoming appointments.

Improved Delivery of Treatments

The effectiveness of psychotherapy interventions, such as cognitive-behavioral therapy (CBT), depends on how closely the therapy is implemented as intended. AI systems can evaluate how well a provider is adhering to a therapeutic framework and provide immediate feedback, standardizing the quality of delivery.

Combining AI with other technological advances can also augment established treatments; for instance, exposure therapy involves repeatedly exposing someone to the source of their anxiety in a safe environment in order to gradually reduce their discomfort. Recreating the precise objects or content that triggers someone's anxiety can be difficult and costly. Virtual reality (VR) systems can generate immersive, realistic environments using a headset or projection. Treatments that use AI plus VR allow a clinician to tailor the virtual environment to the individual patient. For someone with a fear of flying, exposures might progress from visiting a virtual airport to experiencing a real-time flight simulation.

Discovery of New Treatments

The research and development of new medications is time-consuming and expensive. Researchers start by synthesizing and screening a wide variety of compounds until one achieves the desired effect in cultured cells, then in animal models. The safety, tolerability, and efficacy of the compound are then assessed in humans through clinical trials. This process repeats until the U.S. Food and Drug Administration (FDA) approves the medication for widespread use. The success rate is typically low. AI methods can aid in identifying new medications by generating thousands of theoretical compound structures, then using simulation to predict the likelihood of molecular interactions of interest. The theoretical compounds are then ranked by their simulated scores for desired clinical efficacy or unwanted side effects, eliminating many of the possibilities. As such, a more focused number of compounds would then proceed to synthesis and testing, saving time and money while increasing the chances of success. AI systems can also use large-scale, multidimensional biochemical and molecular data collected from existing FDA-approved medications to predict new uses in the treatment of psychiatric disorders.

Limitations of Artificial Intelligence

AI does have limitations, as well as ethical and privacy concerns, given the sensitivity of the data used. AI systems are sometimes called "black boxes" because it can be challenging to interpret the reasoning behind a system's predictions. It is essential for clinicians to understand the rationale behind recommendations to ensure that systems are behaving in a safe fashion. Regardless of how intricate or nuanced the algorithms that power it may be, an AI system is also only as good as the data on which it has been trained. Data can be flawed, incomplete, and biased. For example, if an AI tool to diagnose anxiety is unable to recognize a set of symptoms because no corresponding features were present in the training data, it might produce false-negative results (e.g., persons with anxiety being predicted as not anxious). These issues are being mitigated by using high-quality training data and close auditing of systems over time.

Conclusion

AI approaches hold enormous potential for addressing chronic issues with the accessibility, delivery, and effectiveness of treatment in depression and anxiety. For patients, AI affords flexibility and choices in how they engage with providers and treatment, as well as increased transparency, which increases patient empowerment. Humans will not be replaced by AI; although AI systems can provide data-driven recommendations for diagnosis and treatment, practitioners are ultimately responsible for evaluating these recommendations in light of their own knowledge, training, and judgment. AI-driven monitoring can provide clinicians with more accurate data about their patients and can automate administrative tasks (e.g., refill tracking, rescheduling visits) to improve the quality of care, increase patient safety, and hasten time to recovery.

Recommended Reading

Fry H: Hello World: How to Be Human in the Age of the Machine. London, Transworld, 2019

Topol E: Deep Medicine: How Artificial Intelligence Can Make Healthcare Human Again. New York, Basic Books, 2019

83

Comorbid Medical Disorders

Alissa Hutto, M.D.
Donald L. Rosenstein, M.D.

Introduction

Psychiatric symptoms frequently co-occur with medical illnesses. Common examples include depression associated with cancer, anxiety in the setting of advanced lung disease, and confusion in patients who become critically ill. In this chapter, we describe psychiatric symptoms and medical illnesses that can exist at the same time, highlight ways to identify the causes of the psychiatric symptoms, and provide recommendations for addressing them.

It is often quite challenging to determine the precise relationship between a mood, anxiety, or cognitive symptom and an underlying medical problem. For instance, anxiety is common among people who have undergone a heart transplantation. It may not be possible to determine whether that anxiety is a psychological reaction to their life-threatening medical experience or a side effect from antirejection medications they are taking.

Co-occurring Medical Conditions

While the relationships between psychiatric symptoms and medical illnesses can be complicated, several medical conditions typically are associated with psychiatric symptoms. Any medical illness that affects the brain can also negatively affect thinking, emotions, and behavior.

Dementia

Dementia can result from conditions that directly damage brain tissue and impair brain function. People who develop dementia may act very differently than their normal selves, even in the early stages of the illness. For example, someone who has frontotemporal dementia might talk less frequently and withdraw from their family and friends, which may be seen by others as a sign of depression. These individuals might also develop unusual behaviors that can be mistaken for mania or a primary psychotic disorder.

Delirium

Whenever a person becomes critically ill, they are at risk for developing delirium, which is a form of acute brain failure. Unlike dementia, which develops gradually and is often progressive, delirium is typically reversible. It usually is caused by underlying medical illness of sudden onset and seen in hospitalized patients but can occur outside of the hospital as well. Delirium affects the brain's ability to focus and to process information, and delirious people may behave strangely while confused. The individual's family or medical team may notice them not eating, not participating in their care, and seeming sad or irritable, and confusion from delirium can also cause great anxiety or cause people to act violently. Delirium can therefore be mistaken for a mood, anxiety, or psychotic disorder. It is essential to identify delirium and treat the underlying medical causes as soon as possible.

Cancer

Cancer can be a particularly devastating disease that affects multiple body systems, including the brain. Even when a person has no primary tumor or metastasis in their brain, cancer puts them at higher risk of depression because of the major functional and financial consequences that are associated with cancer and its treatment. Changes in sleep, appetite, weight, energy, and motivation are common cancer-related symptoms, and these symptoms can affect people's ability to obtain the right care at the right time. Although treating psychiatric symptoms for someone with cancer can be complicated because of the potential for medication interactions, successful treatment is possible and associated with a number of benefits, such as better cancer symptom management and an improved quality of life.

Parkinson's Disease

Parkinson's disease damages the brain cells involved in body movement and emotions, and it can lead to depression and dementia. People with Parkinson's disease move slowly and may not fully express their emotions on their face, which often can make them seem depressed. The movement and cognitive problems of Parkinson's disease can lead to a full, co-occurring major depression in more than 40% of cases. The dopamine-stimulating agents used to treat motor symptoms from Parkinson's disease can also cause anxiety and psychotic symptoms.

Thyroid Disease

Low thyroid hormone levels (*hypothyroidism*) are a common mimic of depression because they are associated with decreased energy and motivation, increased need for sleep, and trouble concentrating. On the other hand, an overactive thyroid (*hyperthyroidism*) can cause a racing heartbeat, nervousness, and insomnia, which together can be mistaken for panic attacks or another anxiety disorder.

Diabetes

Diabetes is a common illness caused by a problem in the way the body makes or uses the hormone insulin. In the early stages of diabetes, fatigue is common and can be mistaken as a sign of a mood disorder. Depending on the type and severity of diabetes, it can be a life-altering diagnosis. Given the loss of control and independence that can come with a chronic illness, people with diabetes are at higher risk for depression. We must be careful giving psychiatric medicines to patients with diabetes because some medications have to be adjusted to avoid diabetes-related kidney damage. Other medicines for depression or bipolar illness (e.g., lithium) can increase diabetes risk. Diabetes and depression can be difficult to manage when they co-occur, but mental health clinicians are able to make treatment plans for depression that take diabetes risk and symptoms into account.

Autoimmune Disease

In autoimmune illnesses, the person's immune system is out of balance and can respond to parts of the body as external or "foreign" threats. Autoimmune disorders can cause mood and anxiety symptoms, especially when the brain and the nervous system are targeted by the immune system. For example, *autoimmune encephalitis* (brain inflammation) is caused by the immune system directly attacking the brain. As a result, any mood, anxiety, perceptual, or cognitive symptom can emerge, making it difficult to diagnose without extensive medical and neurological workup. These psychiatric symptoms often come with other physical symptoms and may be associated with cancer or bacterial infections. *Systemic lupus erythematosus* is an autoimmune disease that can cause encephalitis, although it is associated more commonly with joint, skin, and kidney damage. In *multiple sclerosis* (MS), the immune system attacks nerve fibers in the brain and spinal cord, and depression is common with this disorder. The clinical course of MS can be unpredictable, and both the brain damage itself and the stress of living with MS can affect mood and anxiety.

Autoimmune diseases are often treated with medications that modify the immune system so the body will stop attacking itself. Unfortunately, treatment with immunosuppressants, such as high-dosage steroids, can make someone more susceptible to infections and to psychiatric symptoms as an adverse effect.

Nutritional Deficiencies

Nutritional deficiencies of various vitamins and minerals can result from dietary changes, medication effects, or problems with gastrointestinal absorption, and they can have severe health consequences. For example, low levels of thiamine (vitamin B_1) can have dangerous effects on the central nervous system. Thiamine deficiency can result after gastrointestinal surgery, from excessive alcohol use, or from an inadequate diet. People with low thiamine levels may have trouble concentrating, low motivation, and delirium, which can be mistaken for depression. Similarly, low levels of vitamin D can have harmful effects on mood and energy, which can improve with vitamin D supplementation.

Medication Effects

Many pharmacological treatments for various medical illnesses have psychiatric symptoms as side effects. For example, steroids (e.g., prednisone, dexamethasone) can lead to poor sleep, irritability or elevated mood, and anxiety; stopping steroids suddenly after chronic use can lead to fatigue and low mood. Other immune system medications such as tacrolimus also can cause anxiety or low mood. Several antibiotic and antiviral agents can affect mood and cognition, as can certain antiepileptics and cancer drugs. In addition to causing psychiatric side effects, medications can interact with others that cause weakened effects or even toxicity.

Clues and Cautions

Although numerous illnesses and medications can be associated with psychiatric symptoms, sometimes symptoms of depression and anxiety are quickly assumed to come from a primary psychiatric disorder before a full investigation has been made into other causes. It is true that psychiatric disorders are common, but when providers assume the cause of psychiatric symptoms, this assumption can lead to avoidable suffering due to delays or errors in the diagnosis or treatment of underlying medical illness.

Certain clinical features of the patient's presentation can help providers identify whether psychiatric symptoms are caused by a psychiatric disorder or another medical illness. First, the person's age at symptom onset can be a clue. Major mood and anxiety disorders more commonly develop during childhood or early adulthood. If a patient has mania, major depression, or anxiety disorder for the first time later in life, it may be a sign that a medical illness is at play. Second, the rate of symptom onset can be revealing. Anxiety symptoms and mood symptoms can often take weeks to months to fully develop. If a person develops anxiety or changes in mood within hours or days, it may suggest an acute medical cause. Third, the pattern of symptom severity can also be telling. Once anxiety or mood disorders have developed, the symptoms usually last for weeks to months at a similar level and may slowly improve or worsen. If someone's symptoms have a significantly different pattern, this should encourage evaluation for other medical causes.

What You Can Do

Identifying whether mood or anxiety symptoms are from primary psychiatric disorders or from other medical illness can be difficult, and it is always best to seek a professional opinion. When you or someone you care for is experiencing new-onset mood or anxiety symptoms, it is important to visit a primary care physician, either before or while also obtaining psychiatric care. A basic medical screening would include a physical examination, a set of vital signs, and blood tests, including a complete blood count, a comprehensive metabolic panel, thyroid stimulating hormone, vitamin D and B_{12} levels, and an electrocardiogram (ECG) (see Chapter 79, "Laboratory Tests"). The examination and blood work help rule out some of the important common conditions discussed in this chapter. A baseline ECG and blood work help determine which psychiatry medications are safe.

People often present to their primary care physicians with symptoms that seem obviously related to a psychiatry diagnosis. Clinicians are trained to recognize patterns, and if a pattern fits well, it is tempting to not look for other possibilities. Patients should always feel empowered to voice their concerns and request screening for medical conditions. The primary care evaluation just described is rather low risk and low cost, and missing a medical cause of psychiatric symptoms can be both dangerous and expensive. Ultimately, treatment for mood or anxiety symptoms can be initiated to improve patients' quality of life, even if primary care and psychiatric evaluations have not identified their exact cause.

Conclusion

People who have severe and persistent mental illness, such as schizophrenia or bipolar disorder, are at increased risk for other medical illnesses (e.g., heart disease, cancer, diabetes) that can worsen their psychiatric condition and, as a result, make them less able to follow up with medical care. A careful investigation of the preexisting psychiatric illness and the timing of new or worsening symptoms can make effective treatment possible.

Recommended Reading

Cahalan S: Brain on Fire: My Month of Madness. New York, Simon and Schuster, 2013
Kalanithi P: When Breath Becomes Air. New York, Random House, 2016

84

Virtual Reality

Risa B. Weisberg, Ph.D.
Laina E. Rosebrock, Ph.D.

Introduction

It is likely that you have recently heard a lot of news about virtual reality (VR). You may be surprised to learn that VR has been around for more than 50 years! For much of this time, researchers have been interested in how best to use VR to help people with mental and behavioral health problems, such as anxiety and mood disorders.

Although the use of VR for mental health problems is not new, two main factors have brought renewed interest: 1) recent advances in technology, making the medium both more engaging and more affordable, and 2) a growing gap between the relatively small number of therapists available to provide quality mental health care and the very large number of people seeking help for anxiety and depression. In this chapter, we review VR for mental health and then briefly describe interventions that may be available.

What Exactly Is Virtual Reality?

VR creates three-dimensional, interactive, computer-generated worlds. Typically, this is done via software programs that run on a head-mounted display (or

VR headset) rather than on a flat-screen computer, tablet, or cell phone. These programs replace the sensory input from your actual environment (primarily sight and sound) with input from the software—that is, once you put on a VR headset and launch a program, you can only see what is being presented in the headset, and if you are wearing noise-canceling headphones, you can only hear what the software presents. By replacing your sensory input, VR creates the feeling of being in an entirely different, three-dimensional, life-sized environment.

Many VR headsets are commercially available, and the industry is moving toward making these even smaller and lighter. VR companies are developing ways to replace input from additional senses, such as touch and smell, in order to make virtual worlds feel even more real in the future. VR is currently used in many industries; the most common use is for gaming, and hundreds of games exist on VR platforms, but VR technology also is used to train doctors to complete medical procedures, to help athletes hone their skills and train for games, and to provide distraction and relaxation for patients undergoing painful medical procedures. It is also a powerful tool for individuals seeking to improve their psychological well-being and mental health and a cost-effective way to ensure more people have access to effective psychological interventions.

Virtual Reality in Mental Health Treatment

Anxiety

The earliest use of VR to treat mental health problems was with *virtual reality exposure* (VRE) therapy. As you may have read in earlier chapters of this book, exposure therapy is a very well-researched treatment for anxiety disorders. In *exposure therapy*, patients are asked to enter or engage in situations that they might typically avoid due to anxiety (see, e.g., Chapter 21, "Treatment of Social Anxiety Disorder," and Chapter 25, "Treatment of Specific Phobia"). These exposures most often take place in the real world and thus are called *in vivo exposure*. With repeated exposure to feared situations, anxiety starts to reduce, and people feel more confident in their ability to cope with previously feared scenarios. For example, someone with a spider phobia might be instructed to spend time looking at pictures of spiders, looking at actual spiders, and eventually work their way up to holding a spider. For some fears, however, in vivo exposure can be impractical (e.g., fear of flying), unsafe (e.g., combat trauma), or difficult to control (e.g., social situations with other people).

When it is too difficult to create real-life, in vivo scenarios for exposure therapy, patients and their therapists typically resort to *imaginal exposure*. For example, in treating posttraumatic stress disorder (PTSD), behavior therapists may ask their patients to imagine their traumatic experience repeatedly until it no longer causes distress or until they have learned new ways to view these memories and experiences. Instead of relying on imagination, VR can place the person into a virtual environment that resembles the feared experience or the situation in which the trauma occurred. This can make it easier to conduct the exposure while increasing a patient's sense of presence.

Not only does VRE enable people to face a broad range of feared situations, it is also sometimes seen by patients as preferrable to in vivo exposure. One study reported that 76% of patients would rather participate in VRE than in vivo exposure.

VRE therapy for anxiety disorders has repeatedly been found to be an effective treatment. Numerous research studies have compared it with either a control condition (e.g., a waitlist or placebo therapy) or with traditional, in vivo treatment. VRE for anxiety and related disorders, including specific phobias, social anxiety disorder, panic disorder, and PTSD, has been found to be considerably more effective than control/placebo treatments and just as effective as in-person/in vivo treatments.

Mood Disorders

The use of VR to treat mood disorders is newer and less frequently studied than its use in anxiety disorders. However, studies are beginning to suggest that it may be helpful for these conditions as well. A developing line of research is using VR to deliver *behavioral activation* (BA; discussed in Chapter 57). BA is a form of behavioral therapy that is a front-line treatment for major depression. In BA, patients are encouraged to engage in activities that they previously valued or that led to feelings of accomplishment or enjoyment. Preliminary research suggests that VR-delivered BA, in which patients practice experiencing enjoyable or rewarding scenarios virtually rather than in the real world, may be just as effective for reducing depression symptoms as traditional BA.

Other potential VR interventions for depression, low mood, or sadness are being developed and tested. For example, *cognitive restructuring* (see Chapter 62, "Cognitive-Behavioral Therapy for Social Anxiety") is a technique that teaches patients to question the negative thoughts they may have. Rather than accepting all of their thoughts as facts, patients are taught to examine the evidence for each thought and decide if it is actually true. A patient having the thought, "nothing will ever get better" might be asked to consider what proof they have that this is true. Have things ever improved for them in the past? Do they know other people who have had similar periods of difficulty only to later have their situation improve? This can be very effective, but it is sometimes difficult for patients to hold these internal conversations in their own heads. Researchers and a VR digital therapeutics company (RealizedCare, by which author R. W. is currently employed) are creating and evaluating ways to conduct cognitive therapy via VR, such that patients may speak their thoughts aloud and then, via voice-to-text software, see and interact with them as three-dimensional objects in a virtual world.

Stress Reduction

Mindfulness-based interventions (MBIs) are designed to teach patients to bring their awareness to their present state and to experience the present moment without judgment. A range of MBIs, including mindfulness-based cognitive therapy and mindfulness-based stress reduction, have been found to be effective for reducing stress and depression and demonstrate strong potential for alleviating anxiety. VR is an ideal setting for mindfulness practice. The headset's ability to block out distracting environmental cues can potentially enhance focus and attention. Replacing current sensory experience with immersion in peaceful settings may also assist mindfulness practice. Rather than closing your eyes and imagining sitting on the bank of a river while you meditate, VR can virtually place you on the bank of a peaceful river. Furthermore, audio cues in VR can place a meditation coach or therapist in your ear, right there by the river. A recent systematic review of research on mindfulness in VR found that, overall, VR-based mindfulness practice was associated with a better meditation experience and greater levels of personal mindfulness than was non-VR mindfulness training. Furthermore, more immersive VR-based mindfulness training was more likely to lead to improved mood and reduced stress and anxiety than was less-immersive or non-VR practice.

Where to Find Virtual Reality Interventions

Anyone interested in trying out VR programs to help manage their symptoms currently has two main options: finding a therapist who uses VR to augment treatment (contact companies such as Virtually Better for assistance) or looking for a VR program based on science-supported treatment that can be accessed directly (e.g., oVRcome's programs for exposure therapy) or through the Meta Quest app store or lab (e.g., Tripp or Mindway apps for mindfulness meditation). Some companies are also working with governmental agencies such as the U.S. Food and Drug Administration in the United States and the National Institute for Health and Care Excellence in the United Kingdom to attain approvals that would make VR treatments more widely accessible, either via prescription from any qualified health provider, as an approved over-the-counter device, or within the National Health System in the United Kingdom.

Conclusion

VR is a promising technology that has the potential to automate the provision of effective psychological therapies for anxiety and mood disorders. Research has shown that VR is a highly engaging, effective alternative to traditional methods for treating these disorders. With the demand for treatment far exceeding the number of therapists available, and VR technology becoming increasingly advanced and affordable, we believe that in the near future we will see more development, testing, and use of science-based VR interventions and mental wellness products.

Recommended Reading

Bell I: Virtual reality for mental health: are there any freely available apps that show promise? The Mental Elf, December 8, 2021. Available at: https://www.nationalelfservice.net/treatment/digital-health/virtual-reality-mental-health.

Greengard S: Virtual Reality (The MIT Press Essential Knowledge series). Cambridge, MA, MIT Press, 2019

85

Community Psychiatry

Lianna Karp, M.D.
Luana Marques, Ph.D.

Introduction

In this chapter, we explore tools that can be used to advocate for your care in a community psychiatry setting. We review the systems currently in place, what to expect when seeking care within these systems, and what your rights are as a patient or family member.

Community health centers were created in the 1960s to provide comprehensive care to communities that face extra barriers to health care. These barriers are referred to as *social determinants of health* and include lack of safe housing, transportation limitations, impaired access to education or employment opportunities, language barriers, food insecurity, racism, discrimination, or violence. If these apply to you or your family, you may be eligible to seek mental health care through community psychiatry. Often, the services are only available to people in a specific geographical location—look up the nearest community health center or federally qualified community health center (these receive federal funding for meeting strict guidelines for accessible care) to see if your area is served.

The community psychiatry movement was created to ensure that people with mental health challenges are treated in the least restrictive environment possible, emphasizing the importance of freedom and patient autonomy when seeking care. Instead of the prior model of long-stay psychiatric hospitalizations to provide care, mental health organizations are now attempting to bring treatment to the community so families can stay together and people have fewer major disruptions to their lives when seeking mental health care.

How Do Community Health Centers Work?

Community health centers are "safety net" organizations—meaning that people who do not have insurance, those with public insurance not accepted by other providers, or those who have immigration status affecting their care likely can still obtain care for themselves or their family. One of the defining characteristics of community health is that the care is integrated. Within the same organization, you may be able to access primary care (e.g., pediatric, family medicine), mental health (e.g., therapists, psychiatrists), and substance use treatment providers as well as subspecialty services such as podiatry or dentistry. This allows for coordination across several different specialties, with the goal of making it easy to access quality, team-based care.

Community health centers may be able to meet many other needs beyond basic medical and mental health care, including legal aid, food access, housing resources, employment training, and immigration assistance. A core principle of community psychiatry is a whole-person approach, which acknowledges that environmental factors can significantly impact mental health symptoms. Comprehensive community psychiatric care involves addressing these external factors in addition to routine therapy and medication management.

Mental health care in a community setting is most often provided through a tiered approach in which you likely first will meet with your primary care provider, who performs a mental health screening to determine your specific needs. Then, depending on the severity of your symptoms, you may be referred to additional providers for care. It is important to understand the role of each team member. The following is a noncomprehensive list of providers with whom people may interface when seeking care in the community setting:

- *Individual therapists:* licensed providers who hold a degree or certificate to diagnose and treat mental illness, such as psychologists (Ph.D. or Psy.D.), social workers (L.S.W., L.C.S.W., or L.I.C.S.W.), or mental health counselors (L.M.H.C.)
- *Psychiatrists and psychiatric nurse practitioners:* licensed providers who hold a medical degree as psychiatrists (M.D.) or nurse practitioners (P.N.H.N.P) to diagnose and treat mental illness and who can prescribe psychiatric medications
- *Case managers:* providers who assist in the coordination of care, assessing patients' needs and then connecting them with available resources

- *Behavioral health coaches:* providers who specialize in setting goals to address mental health issues, such as sleep, stress, or relationship challenges, and can assist with prevention of more serious mental health conditions but do not diagnose or treat mental illnesses
- *Recovery coaches:* providers who, like behavioral health coaches, are trained to support goal-setting, in this case for people with substance use challenges
- *Peer specialists:* people who have lived experience (e.g., in recovery from mental illness or substance use disorders) and have been trained to provide peer support, providing unique insight and compassion that comes from shared experiences
- *Community health workers:* trusted members of the community who act as links between clinical care and peer outreach and act as advocates to help care teams understand the cultural context of the community

Care may also extend beyond individual one-to-one provider settings to include support groups (both professionally led as well as peer-led), school-based services, mobile emergency services, and wrap-around teams (which can include providers coming to your home to provide care). Although not exclusive to community psychiatry, several kinds of organizations frequently coordinate with mental health services in the community, such as state and federal agencies that were created to protect vulnerable populations, including those with disabilities or children experiencing abuse.

Preventive Efforts in Community Health Centers

Most community psychiatry efforts focus on crisis stabilization and treatment; however, many preventive efforts aim to foster resilience and provide skills to improve mental well-being, such as programs that train nonprofessionals (e.g., community health workers or peer specialists) to deliver evidence-based therapeutic care. This approach empowers communities to take charge of their own well-being and to harness the power of community members to meet the overwhelming demand for mental health support. Often, these programs are housed within preexisting community organizations such as schools, primary care settings, or faith-based organizations so that there are fewer barriers to access.

Ideal Community Care Structure

When seeking care within community psychiatry, it is important to know your rights. Ideally, care should be culturally sensitive, delivered in your preferred language, and involve shared decision-making between you and your provider.

Most community settings strive to be trauma-informed, meaning that clinical and nonclinical staff are trained to be aware of widespread trauma experienced by the local population. This way, they can recognize the signs and symptoms of trauma, integrate this knowledge into policies and treatment planning, and actively avoid retraumatizing patients by ensuring a culture of safety, trust, and collaboration. Recognition of historical biases and discrimination (based on race, ethnicity, sexual orientation, gender identity, immigration status, and so on) is critical to this approach, as are continued efforts to assess the specific needs of the community and respond accordingly.

Conclusion

Although we have outlined ideal community psychiatry care in this chapter, our description may not always match the reality of the care you receive. Some communities and populations may experience a lack of access to care, including long wait times, inability to access an interpreter in a preferred language, or discrimination within the health care setting. Some organizations may have patient advocacy offices that can help people experiencing these challenges. You can also advocate for yourself or a family member by asking questions, such as "Can we have an in-person interpreter for my mother?" or "Can you please explain your role on my care team?" or "While I am on the waitlist, could I speak to a resource specialist for alternative care options?"

Community psychiatry strives to meet the needs of people who have many barriers to accessing care. You may meet many kinds of care providers from medical doctors to peer specialists, and it is appropriate to ask for assistance getting connected with resources such as legal aid or housing support if needed. Everyone seeking care in this setting deserves affordable, team-based, culturally sensitive, and trauma-informed care.

Recommended Reading

Brister T: Navigating a Mental Health Crisis: A NAMI Resource Guide for Those Experiencing a Mental Health Emergency. Arlington, VA, National Alliance on Mental Illness, 2018. Available at: https://smiadviser.org/wp-content/uploads/2019/04/NAMI01R04.pdf.

Torrey T: Who provides patient and health advocacy? VeryWellHealth, March 15, 2020. Available at: https://www.verywellhealth.com/who-provides-patient-and-health-advocacy-2614914.

86

Suicide

Inna Gonceareno, M.A.
Igor Galynker, M.D., Ph.D.

Introduction

With one death happening every 11 minutes, suicide remains one of the leading causes of death in the United States. On average, every suicide death affects 135 people who knew the decedent, taking an enormous toll on our communities. The most common questions asked when someone dies from suicide are why they took their own life and how we could have prevented it.

What Is Suicide and Why Does It Happen?

Suicide is a complex phenomenon affected by various biological, psychological, and social factors and stressful life events. The Narrative Crisis Model of suicide combines the majority of the factors associated with suicide into a simple three-component model that explains the mental processes leading to suicide. First, some individuals have an increased vulnerability to suicide. Second, after exposure to a stressful life event, they may develop distorted views of their life and of the world around them, called a *suicidal narrative*. Finally, with more stress, they may develop an unbearably painful state of mind called the *suicide crisis syndrome* (SCS), which may ultimately lead to suicide.

Certain long-term risk factors can increase vulnerability to suicide. These include demographic risk factors, such as male sex; middle age; sexual minority status; race and ethnicity, with American Indians/Alaska Natives having the highest suicide rates, followed by White and Hispanic adults; historical risk factors, such as childhood adversity, suicide in the family, history of mental illness, or past suicide attempts; psychological risk factors, including impulsivity, hopelessness, perfectionism, and fearlessness; and sociocultural risk factors, such as acceptability or approval of suicide as a solution to a life problem.

Stressful life events play a key role in triggering the mental processes leading to suicide. The most common stressful life events include work and financial hardship, relationship conflict, serious medical or mental illness, and recent substance misuse. Some stressful life events are uniquely related to suicide in adolescents, such as conflict with parents, ongoing childhood neglect, and bullying. Although some stressors may seem insignificant to outsiders (e.g., receiving a B grade for a college class), their perceived impact on the individual's mental state is more important than the objective circumstances.

The Suicidal Narrative

When stressors accumulate, individuals with an increased vulnerability for suicide increasingly see their lives moving toward "a dead end" at which suicide becomes a viable option. They perceive their life stories as typically following the same pattern of seven stages, described in Table 86–1.

A person's suicidal narrative life story is typically not seen as a "dead end" by others. However, suicidal individuals themselves perceive their life as a narrative with a worthless past; an intolerable, painful present; and no acceptable future. Although all life stories share a common last stage—the perception of having no future—the relative importance of other stages varies. For example, many college student suicides and work-related suicides are driven by unrealistic expectations of success, whereas suicide attempts due to bullying are driven primarily by humiliation, a feeling of loneliness, and the perception of being a burden. Suicidal narrative is a subacute syndrome that may last days or weeks.

Suicide Crisis Syndrome Criteria and Symptoms

The feeling of being trapped in a dead-end life story, which is a coherent thought pattern, brings on an acute suicidal state, SCS, which affects one's mood, ability to think clearly, and physiology, including disruption in sleep and social connections. SCS is a distinct acute psychiatric condition with specific criteria (Ta-

Table 86–1. The suicidal narrative

Stage	Description	Example
Stage 1: Unrealistic life goals	Unrealistically high expectations set by oneself or by others, which are near-impossible to achieve	Making one's first million by age 24, getting straight As, finding a perfect partner, being loved by everyone
Stage 2: Entitlement to happiness	A notion of oneself as special, inflated deservingness only when the unrealistic life goal is achieved	Expecting a happy future and a stellar career that should arrive without much effort
Stage 3: Failure to redirect to more realistic goals	An inability to stop pursuing unrealistic goals when they clearly cannot be achieved and find alternatives	Extended pursuit of a high-risk career path that promises stardom against the odds; an inability to end "doomed" relationships
Stage 4: Humiliating personal or social defeat	A perceived failure from inability to achieve unrealistic goals accompanied by a sense of humiliation, shame, and embarrassment	Being fired from a job, not getting grant funding, being bypassed for promotion, being laughed at on social media, getting a low grade on a test
Stage 5: Perceived burdensomeness	A sense that one's failure to achieve goals makes one a burden to family or loved ones, often to the extent of believing that loved ones would be better off without the individual	Financial dependency on friends or family, moving in with one's elderly parents, being an emotional burden to loved ones
Stage 6: Thwarted belongingness	A feeling of loneliness and disconnection from others due to inability to share the burden of failure	Feeling like an outsider due to unemployment, feeling left behind by friends with more successful careers, getting a divorce, post-migration feeling of alienation
Stage 7: Perception of having no future	An absence of positive thinking and the inability to imagine a viable and acceptable future	An inability to imagine an acceptable future after the life-altering career failure, medical diagnosis, romantic rejection or divorce, incarceration

ble 86–2) that may last days or even hours and signals a high risk for a suicide attempt in the near future.

Critically, suicidal thoughts alone, in the absence of SCS, are not a good indicator that suicide is imminent. The first reason for this seemingly paradoxical phenomenon is that individuals may not have suicidal thoughts or a plan until immediately before their suicide or even not at all. The second reason is that those with suicidal thoughts often hide them and do not seek help from anyone for various reasons, such as fear of involuntary hospitalization, embarrassment, or fear of being labeled "mentally ill."

Because seemingly healthy people without serious psychiatric illness may experience SCS, the diagnosis has been submitted for inclusion in the *Diagnostic and Statistical Manual of Mental Disorders* (DSM) as the first suicide-specific diagnosis.

What Happens If Suicide Crisis Syndrome Is Left Untreated?

The result of untreated SCS, which could be unbearable, is a suicidal act taken in a desperate attempt to end the intolerable emotional pain. Several interventions have demonstrated promise in mitigating suicide risk. The first and foremost goal is to ensure the safety of one's environment, such as by restricting a suicidal person's access to firearms and locking up medications. The next step is to address the acute symptoms of SCS via pharmacological interventions. Currently, only one medication trial is specifically targeting SCS, underscoring the critical need for more such trials to advance treatment options. However, clozapine (atypical antipsychotic), lithium (mood stabilizer), and ketamine (anesthetic) have been shown to alleviate suicidality. Side effects vary depending on the type of medication, and your doctor may adjust the dosage or add another medication to lessen the side effects.

Following prescription of fast-acting pharmacological treatment, safety planning is recommended. During the safety planning session, written individualized steps are created for patients to follow during moments of intense emotional distress and suicidal crisis. Once the acute symptoms have been reduced substantially, psychotherapeutic interventions may be helpful to restructure the distorted life story of the suicidal narrative into a more acceptable life story. The most widely used interventions include the Collaborative Assessment and Management of Suicidality, cognitive-behavioral therapy (CBT) for suicide prevention, and the Attempted Suicide Short Intervention Program.

Given that stressful life events can trigger suicidal behavior, it is important to address a person's reactivity to stressors. Dialectical behavior therapy, mind-

Table 86–2. Suicide crisis syndrome criteria and symptoms

Criterion	Symptom description
A. Frantic hopelessness/ entrapment	Persistent or recurring overwhelming feeling of urgency to escape or avoid an unbearable life situation perceived to be impossible to endure
B. Associated disturbances*	
1. Affective disturbance	Emotional pain; rapid spikes of negative emotions or extreme mood swings; extreme anxiety (a panic-like state) that may be accompanied by unusual bodily sensations, such as nausea, skin crawling; acute anhedonia (i.e., a new or increased inability to experience things as enjoyable)
2. Loss of cognitive control	Intense repetitive thoughts about one's own distress and the life events that caused it; cognitive rigidity (i.e., inability to consider alternative, less negative interpretations); uncontrollable overwhelming negative thoughts, accompanied by head pressure or pain and impairing ability to process information or make a decision; repeated unsuccessful attempts to stop negative or disturbing thoughts
3. Hyperarousal	Agitation (restlessness); hypervigilance (increased sensitivity to the outside world); irritability; insomnia
4. Acute social withdrawal	Reduction of social activity; evasive communication with close others, distancing from family and friends

*Criterion B, associated disturbances, is met if at least one of the described symptoms is present from each of the B1, B2, B3, and B4 criteria.

fulness-based stress reduction, and emotional regulation therapy aim to build skills for tolerating distress and regulating emotions, potentially preventing the relapse of the suicidal narrative or suicidal crisis among at-risk individuals.

Conclusion

Suicide affects all of us. However, our society shies away from talking openly about it, leaving suicidal people to suffer in silence. Understanding the mental processes leading to suicide can help us debunk existing suicide myths, thus reducing the stigma and encouraging people to seek help in their moments of distress. People die from suicide not because they are selfish and want to die but because they want their excruciating emotional pain to end. Knowing the symptoms of the acute suicidal crisis can help us to recognize a person at high risk of suicide and act immediately to save lives.

Recommended Reading

Freedenthal S: Helping the Suicidal Person: Tips and Techniques for Professionals. Oxfordshire, UK, Routledge, 2017

Galynker I: The Suicidal Crisis: A Clinical Guide to the Assessment of Imminent Suicide Risk, 2nd Edition New York, Oxford University Press, 202

87

Inpatient Hospitalization

Carol L. Alter, M.D.
Julie Farrington, M.D.

Introduction

When people experience a health-related problem due to a life-threatening injury or a symptom such as chest pain or require a special procedure such as a surgery, they will often go to the emergency department or be admitted to a general hospital for care. In the setting of a psychiatric emergency, people may also be admitted to a hospital system with specific expertise for treating psychiatric illnesses. People with life-threatening signs or symptoms such as suicidal intent or planning, attempted suicide, or psychiatric symptoms that impair function may need inpatient care within a psychiatric unit. Psychiatric inpatient care has many similarities to any medical inpatient experience, and it has some important differences as well. Symptoms of mental illness can challenge people's experience of themselves such that they have difficulty recognizing the need for care, particularly the need for admission to a hospital to ensure their basic safety. A variety of interventions also are needed to ensure the physical well-being of both the person and those around them, including other patients on the same unit and hospital staff.

This chapter reviews topics related to psychiatric hospitalization, including common reasons for admission; types of admissions, including a need for involuntary treatment; typical procedures on psychiatric units that might differ from general medical care; treatments delivered in psychiatric units; and the role of the family during and after a psychiatric inpatient stay.

Why Would Someone Need Inpatient Hospitalization for Psychiatric Conditions?

All psychiatric conditions present with one or more symptoms such as changes in mood, anxiety or irritability, changes in thought (e.g., slowing, speeding up, or disorganized), and changes in perception (e.g., seeing or hearing things that are not there, believing strongly that people are out to harm you). The presence of any of these symptoms should lead to an evaluation either by the patient's primary care physician or a mental health professional. In most cases, once a diagnosis is made, the symptoms and illnesses can be managed. However, if the symptoms become severe, additional evaluation and treatment may be needed. When a patient is either not functioning or is at risk of harming themselves or others, admission to a hospital may make the most sense.

The most common reason for psychiatric admission is for a patient who has harmed themself, has attempted suicide, or is afraid that they might hurt themself. However, there are many other reasons for admission. If patients have severe symptoms related to mood, anxiety, addiction, impaired thinking, or psychosis that are getting in the way of functioning, then a psychiatric admission may be either helpful or essential to make sure that they are safe. If they have symptoms or behaviors that make it difficult to get out of bed or go to school or work or that are dangerous, such as self-harm, overusing alcohol or drugs, or harming or threatening other people, then it is important for them to be evaluated to determine whether an admission would be helpful.

All hospital emergency departments can evaluate patients with these symptoms. Many communities have mobile crisis teams, or the police or emergency services personnel can help transport patients to an emergency department for evaluation. In that setting, the mental health provider or other physician will assess the symptoms and obtain the person's medical history, conduct a physical examination, and obtain routine laboratory work. They may also order additional tests, such as a computed tomography (CT) scan, magnetic resonance imaging (MRI) scan, or an electroencephalogram (EEG). These types of medical evaluations are done to ensure that the person does not have any active physical health problems that either could account for the symptoms or must be addressed. Patients might present to the emergency department with psychiatric symptoms as well as changes in awareness, chest pain, or a seizure or loss of consciousness. In all cases, it is important to obtain a thorough physical evaluation as well as a psychiatric evaluation.

The mental health team then considers whether an admission would make sense for the patient. This largely is based on whether they have safety concerns and whether the patient could benefit from the services typically offered in an inpatient psychiatric setting. In almost all cases, hospitalization is recommended only if the patient cannot remain safe at home or benefit from outpatient care. Although not all patients who come to the hospital are threatening to self-harm, most have such severe symptoms that they cannot care for themselves.

Can I Decline Inpatient Psychiatric Care?

Even with such severe symptoms, many patients are reluctant to agree to care within a hospital. In cases in which the person does not want help and is committed to harming themselves, does not believe that they need help, or cannot even communicate their desires, they may be hospitalized involuntarily. The requirements for admitting patients involuntarily vary on a state-by-state basis, and federal laws may also apply. In most cases, the physicians can make this assessment, or family members, law enforcement, or others may be involved in this process.

The steps for involuntary admission include checkpoints for preserving individual rights while allowing intervention if certain risks are present. In general, several steps are taken for a patient to be admitted involuntarily:

- An individual determines that the patient requires emergency "detention." Depending on the state, this can include a mental health professional, a family member, a physician, or a law enforcement officer. The patient is either already in a hospital setting or is transported to a hospital securely (by police or ambulance), with a request to the court for emergency detention.
- In most cases, when a request for involuntary admission is made, the hospital has 48–72 hours to conduct a medical evaluation and make a determination about patient safety and the need for involuntary hospitalization. Each state defines the criteria that a patient must meet in order to be involuntarily hospitalized.
- A legal process then occurs, which may include court hearings at 3 days and 14 days postadmission, to determine whether the patient can be released.

Treating a person involuntarily with psychotropic medications is a separate legal process, although this is often done in parallel with involuntary hospitalization.

If a person has been involuntarily committed, they may be changed to voluntary status or released from the hospital if they no longer meet the commitment criteria. This entire process can be very traumatic for both the individual and their loved ones. Forcible custody, physical restraints, and powerful emergency medications are potential aspects of the experience. Being served court papers in the hospital is also stressful. The social worker and court-appointed attorney assigned to the person can be helpful sources of information for family. The goal is health and safety, with a thoughtful balance of individual autonomy and societal responsibilities.

The Substance Abuse and Mental Health Services Administration has a 38-page document with references that provides more in-depth information about the historical evolution and legal ramifications of psychiatric commitment; this document, *Civil Commitment and the Mental Health Care Continuum*, can be accessed at www.samhsa.gov/sites/default/files/civil-commitment-continuum-of-care.pdf.

What Is Inpatient Psychiatric Care Like?

Inpatient psychiatric units have many policies and procedures aimed at keeping patients safe and providing the best opportunity for the care team to determine the best diagnosis and treatment plan for each patient. On most inpatient units, regardless of whether they admit individuals voluntarily or involuntarily, patients will have their personal items checked, and there may be limits as to which items they can keep with them. Clothing items such as belts, scarves, or shoelaces may be prohibited because these present a safety risk. Cellular telephones are usually held at the nursing station or with security (to protect the confidentiality of other patients). Visitors may be limited for the first few days. Most patients will share a room with another patient. They will be provided with meals, and the facility may have limits on outside food being brought into the unit. In most cases, patients are required to remain on the unit, and the usual length of stay is less than a week for acute psychiatric units; if the patient is stable and clinically able, they may be able to have privileges off the unit as they near discharge.

Patients are examined by nursing, social work, psychiatric, and other medical staff. They undergo several intakes and receive a physical examination and, in most cases, laboratory testing. Once the treatment team has evaluated the patient, the team will discuss their findings and recommend treatment. Depending on the types of symptoms and history of illness, this evaluation period may take 1–2 days. In addition to receiving medications, if indicated, patients also participate in various groups, including psychotherapy, occupational or recreational therapy, or mindfulness. Although hospital stays are brief, they do provide an opportunity for patients to gain a better understanding of their illness and to receive interventions aimed at stabilizing their symptoms, improving their safety, and helping identify effective long-term treatment outside the hospital.

Families play an important role in patient care. In most cases, families are contacted by the nursing or social work staff to obtain information about the patient's current symptoms, past history, and social functioning and to prepare for their discharge. Family can include those who are related to the patient or anyone who is close to or provides support for the patient. Because most hospitalizations are brief, planning for care after discharge is a critical component. Family support and involvement is an important factor in that success. A study that examined the role of family support found that family involvement in discharge planning led to improved follow-up after hospitalization, which improves the chances for ongoing improved outcomes.

Family members should expect contact with the staff while the patient is hospitalized. The patient will need to provide permission for the family to speak with the treatment team. If permission is given, the family can reach out to the nursing staff to learn how the patient is doing and to receive information about visiting, treatment, and discharge planning. The family should also speak with the treatment team to learn about the patient's diagnosis and the treatment the patient is receiving.

Ongoing Care Once Released From Inpatient Treatment

Once the patient leaves the hospital, it is essential that they continue treatment. At a minimum, this requires outpatient visits with a psychiatrist who can maintain the treatment started at the hospital and make changes based on patient response over time. Some people may be safe enough for discharge but still need more intensive interventions, such as partial hospitalization or intensive outpatient treatment. Both are offered to patients in the outpatient setting and may last a few weeks or longer and can help patients make a transition to requiring less monitoring and intervention.

Conclusion

Although the vast majority of psychiatric illnesses can and are treated in the outpatient setting, inpatient hospitalization is an important resource for individuals whose symptoms are so severe that they cannot care for themselves or are a risk of harm to themselves or others. Hospitalization can provide a chance to review the current diagnosis and adjust or change treatment, and it provides important support to patients so that they can return to school, work, or family.

Recommended Reading

Dale K: What it's like in a mental hospital. Psycom, July 15, 2021. Available at: https://www.psycom.net/what-a-psychiatric-ward-is-really-like.

Glover S: What to expect during an inpatient stay. NAMI Blog, August 3, 2022. Available at: https://www.nami.org/Blogs/NAMI-Blog/August-2022/What-to-Expect-During-an-Inpatient-Stay.

88

Residential Treatment, Intensive Outpatient, and Partial Hospitalization Programs

Raymond Kotwicki, M.D., M.P.H.

Introduction

Sometimes the "bookends" of psychiatric treatment services available to help patients and their families do not match the level of oversight and interventions needed at the time. Inpatient psychiatric hospitalization in a locked medical/surgical hospital may be too restrictive and even traumatizing for someone who does not require that intensive level of monitoring for safety. Similarly, the traditional model of community-based outpatient care, in which a psychiatrist and a therapist assess and treat patients every 1–3 months, may not provide enough support for patients experiencing a relapse of symptoms. Intermediate levels of care, including psychiatric residential programs, partial hospitalization programs (PHPs), and intensive outpatient programs (IOPs) offer treatment options that may better match the intensity of services patients require in the least restrictive environment that ensures safety. Understanding these alternative levels of care will help patients and families identify when it may be prudent to explore treatment options beyond just hospitalization and outpatient services.

What Are Residential Treatment, Partial Hospitalization, and Intensive Outpatient Programs?

Residential Treatment Programs

Unlike most psychiatric hospitals, psychiatric residential treatment programs are voluntary, unlocked facilities. Patients or their guardians must consent to the treatment provided in such programs and legally have the right to discharge themselves from services unless they are deemed to be in imminent danger of hurting themselves or others in the community. Residential facilities can be either public or privately funded and may or may not include services to help treat substance misuse. Most residential programs have psychiatric physicians, master's-level clinical therapists, psychiatric nurses, and bachelor's-trained support staff to provide consistent coaching and reinforcement for patients. During the daytime, patients typically attend groups that focus on specific psychotherapy modalities and help them develop new skills, insights, and alternative, healthy ways of coping with mental illness and life stress. Because patients enrolled in residential services literally live at the treatment facility, staff support and reinforcement of therapeutic objectives outside of the primary treatment hours are critical for continuity of care and for optimum clinical response. Individual appointments with the patient's psychiatric physician and primary therapist occur one or more times each week between the therapeutic group sessions. The average length of stay in psychiatric residential treatment programs varies significantly, and treatment may last 1–6 months depending on the treatment model, individual patient goals, and progress toward meeting those goals.

In addition to the daytime psychotherapeutic groups and individual psychotherapy sessions, many residential programs also offer adjunctive therapies that augment the treatment experience, such as horticultural therapy, music therapy, drama therapy, and other activities that inspire movement, social interaction, and healthy use of leisure time. These supplemental therapies give patients a break from the demanding work of group psychotherapy and immersive psychiatric treatment while also allowing them to interact with others in "real-world" experiences. For example, if a patient who has social anxiety is participating in a music therapy group in which she has to take a turn singing a solo, this offers her the opportunity to apply the skills she is learning in her cognitive-behavioral therapy (CBT) groups to manage the automatic negative thoughts, catastrophic generalizations, and physical symptoms of panic that define her social anxiety. Repeated opportunities to apply new skills and healthy means of coping with circumstances help patients improve in their applications of those skills. Over time, the anxiety-provoking situations become less threatening, and healthy coping strategies become increasingly accessible. Use of an around-the-clock treatment paradigm in which staff are available to help patients acquire and apply new knowledge and behaviors to optimize results is known as a *therapeutic milieu.*

The therapeutic milieu is the hallmark of every psychiatric residential program, and its consistent application throughout all hours of the day differentiates this level of treatment from every other. In a psychiatric hospital setting, the treatment goal often is to stabilize the symptoms and ensure the safety of patients in the short term. Interventions may include involuntary extension of treatment for severely ill or safety-compromised patients, use of indicated medications before patients possess the capacity to understand their purpose or importance, or even physically restraining a symptomatic patient so they do not become physically aggressive and cause harm to themselves or others. Although necessary at times, these interventions are often paternalistic and frightening. Patients feel out of control—or controlled—and serve a relatively passive role in their recovery and safety planning. Being in such an environment can be extremely helpful to manage acute crises, but most patients and providers would not describe these environments as *therapeutic.*

On the opposite end of the treatment spectrum, outpatient treatment may be extremely helpful while patients and families are in session, but their abrupt return to often unshifting living circumstances, workplace, and social groups often challenges the continuity of their therapeutic work and progress. Their environments and circumstances may be caustic and triggering, and patients may struggle to practice healthy skills and new methods of coping with the difficulties in the real world without additional support. An old adage in psychotherapy suggests that someone can only control and change themselves and not others. Consequently, these unsupportive environments may not provide opportunities for patients to exert the new ways of managing problems that they have learned in outpatient therapy. The outpatient level of care may be highly appropriate for the patient who is relatively skilled and stable in their mental illness, but it may not provide sufficient support and coaching for patients who are just beginning to learn and apply therapeutic strategies.

For this reason, the beauty and effectiveness of residential psychiatric treatment lie in its therapeutic milieu. The core pillars of psychiatric treatment—biological interventions, psychotherapy, skills building, and modulation of feelings and experiences—and the ability to practice them are offered simultaneously. Trained staff are available continuously to assist with patient needs, and all other patients are similarly footed in the residential environment. Crises can either be prevented or managed therapeutically, and patients develop confidence in their independent skills and abilities with repeated practice. Residential psychiatric treatment is analogous to a "study abroad" program in high school or college in which students are immersed in a new, supportive culture to truly integrate a new and foreign language into their way of life. Residential programs immerse patients in their recovery from mental illnesses or substance use disorders.

A focus on holistic health in residential psychiatric treatment programs is paramount. A common misunderstanding is that when people with mental illness are symptomatic and struggling, attention to physical health and lifestyle choices is less important or is impossible. This philosophy is incorrect in many ways and, critically, neglects the sophistication and autonomy of most mentally ill people. Programs that do not prioritize nicotine cessation, healthy eating and active living, sexual health, preventive medical care, and even regular dental care in concert with psychiatric treatment miss the mark. Lifestyle modifications that promote quality of life and prolong living are not simply components of quality holistic health care but also improve the psychiatric outcomes and prognoses of residential patients. No matter the acuity of their symptoms, every psychiatric patient deserves and needs to be educated and expected to integrate holistic health interventions into treatment. Residential programs allow patients to adopt and practice these health behaviors concurrently with their psychiatric treatment. In residential programs, holistic health is literally a patient's full-time job.

One final and critical feature of evidence-based residential psychiatric treatment is the ability of data to help make decisions. Working with the same patients for months in residential care enables clinicians and other scientists to meaningfully measure symptoms, functionality, social relationships, cognition, and other imperative aspects of the patients' lives in order to predict their capabilities and help develop wrap-around services after discharge. *Wrap-around services* are interventions and strategies for successful living that patients require after discharging from the residential therapeutic milieu. For example, if validated psychological tools indicate that a residential patient whose major depression has been treated to remission nonetheless continues to experience poor concentration and slight memory difficulties, that patient may need an independent educational plan to help address these residual executive functioning issues when they return to college. Sobriety plans, vocational assistance, scheduling appointments with a financial counselor or attorney, and even securing community-based medical services may all be components of wrap-around services. Using measurements and analyses to determine the needs of discharging patients helps guide the next steps in residential patients' rehabilitation and can also objectively guide the timing for the next steps in treatment.

Partial Hospitalization Programs

For many patients who are well enough to graduate from residential services, PHPs are the next logical step. PHPs include aspects of individual and group therapies, adjunctive therapies, and rehabilitating in a therapeutic milieu similar to those of residential programs; however, the domiciliary/residential aspect of the treatment day is replaced with a return to life in the "real world." Most PHPs are required to offer 4–5 hours of programming every day to meet insurance reimbursement standards. Once those hours have been met, patients leave the PHP facility to return to their home or other living environment for the rest of the evening or the weekend. PHPs balance intensive daytime psychiatric treatment with independent living for patients who do not require around-the-clock staff coaching and watchful oversight. Another useful aspect of PHP treatment is that issues and problems that arise from life at home can be brought back to treatment the next day for consultation. For instance, if a patient with dysthymia slept well in the residential facility in which they felt safe and protected but experiences significant insomnia in their home bed because they fear being alone in a downtown neighborhood, PHP staff can coach the patient on sleep hygiene strategies and the skills of CBT for insomnia that are specific to their sleeping arrangement at home. PHP allows patients to experiment with applying skills and changing components of their lifestyles in vivo and then re-engage in the therapeutic milieu in order to examine the results. PHPs can take place within residential programs, at hospitals, or even in freestanding office buildings, given that no patients stay in the facility overnight.

Intensive Outpatient Programs

When patients are well enough to return to work, school, or some other regular daytime commitment in addition to continuing psychiatric treatment, they may be ready to engage in an IOP. Many IOPs are connected with PHPs and actually include the same curricula and patients in a "step-down" model in which these patients progress from the PHP to the IOP based on improvements in their symptoms and functionality. The difference between IOPs and PHPs is typically the amount of time patients spend in treatment. Most IOPs require participation in treatment for 3 hours a day for at least 3 days per week. During the balance of their time, they are expected to engage in some other purposeful activity such as returning to work or school or volunteering. The utility of IOP treatment capitalizes on the mix of real-world experience—in this case, during work, school, or other occupational activities—with the therapeutic milieu for consultation and support. Frequently, the social and functional demands of daytime responsibilities exacerbate or contribute to patients' experiences of their mental illnesses or substance misuse. Having the opportunity to engage in resilience-challenging activities while concurrently being in intensive psychiatric treatment can be a powerful mechanism for applying new, healthy ways of managing old problems.

How Do These Three Programs Work Together?

For many patients, the step-wise transition from residential treatment to PHP and then to IOP produces the best results. Tapering the relative amount of time and support from the therapeutic milieu while gradually increasing the responsibilities and pressures of real life enables people to truly recover from their illnesses by learning how to manage setbacks and prevent relapses in the future. Should a patient in PHP or IOP have a relapse in the community, they are always able to increase their level of care to residential treatment if appropriate in order to prevent hospitalization. Most patients engage in this continuum of care for several months to a year so that the therapeutic changes are integrated into their lives, practiced effectively, and permanently ingrained into their behavior in a durable way.

Choosing a Program That Is Right for You

When researching residential, PHP, and IOP programs for yourself or a loved one, there are several important variables to consider. Foremost, ensure that the treatments provided are evidence-based from a medical perspective, utilizing thoroughly researched and reviewed techniques and approaches. Unfortunately, some well-intentioned programs do not use psychotherapies, psychiatric medications, and other rehabilitation interventions that have been proven effective through valid research. Consulting with psychiatric physicians who are familiar with research and evidence-based practices can help families differentiate between programs that are founded on science and those that are not.

Second, try to match the specific diagnoses and needs of a potential residential, PHP, or IOP patient with the targeted treatment offerings of each program. For instance, some residential psychiatric programs specialize in treating patients with obsessive-compulsive disorder (OCD) and therefore have a campus, staff, and policies built specifically to address the needs of these patients. Such a program would not be ideal for someone who is diagnosed with borderline personality disorder and requires very different physical space, staff expertise, and psychotherapeutic interventions. Aligning diagnoses with interventions is essential to optimize treatment results.

A third factor to consider when choosing a residential, PHP, or IOP program is geography. Sometimes, it is clinically essential for individuals to participate in programs near their family, school, or other community-based services so they can reintegrate the therapeutic milieu back into their community of origin. In other cases, such as patients with substance misuse, leaving a community filled with triggers (e.g., friends with whom they misused substances) or other dangers that may cause relapse (e.g., their dealer) may be more therapeutic by providing a fresh start during their rehabilitation. This determination is made on a case-by-case basis, with thoughtful consideration of all the social connections and opportunities provided by various potential treatment locations.

Conclusion

In the psychiatric treatment landscape, residential treatment, PHPs, and IOPs serve as an extremely important piece of the care continuum. These options often prevent inpatient hospitalization for patients with acute symptoms and may offer more intensive treatment for patients whose needs cannot be met by outpatient care. Perhaps the most compelling aspect of these intensive programs is their focus on helping patients cultivate new skills and ways of coping to maximize functionality while simultaneously engaging in symptom-focused treatments. The therapeutic milieu provides opportunities to practice these changes in a relatively controlled environment before reintegrating into the community, and outcome data suggest that this model of rehabilitation is both effective and enduring.

Recommended Reading

Blau GM, Caldwell B, Lieberman R: Residential Interventions for Children, Adolescents, and Families: A Best Practice Guide. Oxfordshire, UK, Routledge, 2014

Houvenagle D: Clinician's Guide to Partial Hospitalization and Intensive Outpatient Practice. Berlin, Springer, 2015

Index

Page numbers printed in **boldface** type refer to tables or figures.